Development and Women's Reproductive Health in Ghana, 1920–1982

This book investigates the history of women's reproductive health in Ghana, arguing that between the 1920s and 1980s, it was largely driven by discourses of development and population control rather than a concern for women's health or rights.

Between the 1920s and 1980s, the choices that Ghanaian women made regarding their reproductive health were defined by development policy and practice. Spanning the colonial and immediate postcolonial periods, this book demonstrates that whilst the substance of development discourse shifted over time, principles of development continued to be used to impact and legitimise reproductive health policy and practices well after independence. The book explores Ghana's pluralist health system, the introduction of maternal and child welfare, the dominance of the Red Cross in Ghana's maternal and child health landscape, nationalist pronatalism and global population activism. In order to understand how global iterations of development and health policy impacted ordinary lives in Ghana, the author uses evidence from multiple 'levels,' including private papers, national archives and records of international and transnational organisations. Providing balanced archival perspectives, the book includes extensive oral history interviews carried out with both rural Ghanaian women and traditional birth attendants, as well as with midwives, doctors and family planning fieldworkers.

This book will have an important impact on a number of historical fields including Ghanaian history, global health history, global histories of population and family planning and histories of development. It will be of interest to researchers and students in the history of public health, development, Africa, Ghana and gender.

Holly Ashford completed her PhD in History at Cambridge University, UK.

Routledge Research in Health and Healing in Africa and the African Diaspora

Health and healing have been critical in African and African-descended communities across the globe. As a result, this series will publish monographs and edited volumes on aspects of health and healing on the African continent and in the African Diaspora.

We welcome proposals on a variety of topics in particular, public health, global health security, health care delivery, innovation in health, epidemics, women and children's health, masculinity and health, mental health, traditional healing, and community initiatives. We seek publications from a range of disciplines and in some cases are interdisciplinary in nature from the social sciences, public and global health, clinical sciences, and the humanities. In addition, we seek research and analyses from area studies that transcends health issues, including African Studies, African American Studies, Caribbean Studies, and Women and Gender Studies and work that is transnational and that in some cases straddles more than one country or region.

Series Editor:
Donna A. Patterson, Delaware State University, USA

Spiritual and Mental Health Crisis in Globalizing Senegal
A History of Transcultural Psychiatry
Alice Bullard

Development and Women's Reproductive Health in Ghana, 1920–1982
Holly Ashford

For more information about this series, please visit: https://www.routledge.com/Routledge-Research-in-Health-and-Healing-in-Africa-and-the-African-Diaspora/book-series/HHAADA

Development and Women's Reproductive Health in Ghana, 1920–1982

Holly Ashford

Routledge
Taylor & Francis Group
LONDON AND NEW YORK

First published 2023
by Routledge
4 Park Square, Milton Park, Abingdon, Oxon OX14 4RN

and by Routledge
605 Third Avenue, New York, NY 10158

Routledge is an imprint of the Taylor & Francis Group, an informa business

British Library Cataloguing-in-Publication Data
A catalogue record for this book is available from the British Library

ISBN: 978-1-032-22784-9 (hbk)
ISBN: 978-1-032-22786-3 (pbk)
ISBN: 978-1-003-27416-2 (ebk)

DOI: 10.4324/9781003274162

Typeset in Times New Roman
by Deanta Global Publishing Services, Chennai, India

Contents

Tables

Figures

Abbreviations

BHS	Basic Health Services
BRC	British Red Cross
CPP	Convention People's Party
DMS	Director of Medical Services
DMSS	Director of Medical and Sanitary Services
DTT	Demographic Transition Theory
ECA	United Nations Economic Commission for Africa
FAO	Food and Agriculture Organization
FGCW	Federation of Gold Coast Women
FGW	Federation of Ghana Women
GAW	Ghana Assembly of Women
GCLMCW	Gold Coast League for Maternal and Child Welfare
GCRC	Gold Coast Branch of the Red Cross
IAW	International Alliance of Women
ILO	International Labour Organization
IO	International Organisation
IPPF	International Planned Parenthood Federation
IUD	Intra-uterine Device
LN	League of Nations
LNHO	League of Nations Health Organization
MCH	Maternal and child health
MH	Ministry of Health
MO	Medical Officer
MP	Member of Parliament
NCGW	National Council of Ghana Women
NFPP	National Family Planning Programme
NGO	Non-governmental organisation
NIEO	New International Economic Order
NLC	National Liberation Council
NRC	National Redemption Council
PHC	Primary Health Care
PMC	Permanent Mandates Commission
PML	Princess Marie Louise Hospital, Accra

PP	Progress Party
PPAG	Planned Parenthood Association Ghana
SCIU	Save the Children International Union
SMC	Supreme Military Council
TBA	Traditional birth attendant
UGCC	United Gold Coast Convention
UNDP	United Nations Development Program
UNFPA	United Nations Fund for Population Activities
UNICEF	United Nations International Children's Emergency Fund
USAID	United States Agency for International Development
USSR	Union of Soviet Socialist Republics
WHO	World Health Organization

Acknowledgements

I have been extremely fortunate to write this book, which would not have been possible without extensive support from those around me. More people have helped me emotionally, intellectually and financially than I have space here to acknowledge. The book is undoubtedly the product of conversations, collaborations and communities I have been a part of over the last few years. I am grateful to Gareth Austin, who lent his constant support and gave invaluable insights. Alison Bashford made a major contribution to this project's beginnings. Simon Szreter and Kate Skinner, who examined my PhD thesis, saw the project's potential and asked perceptive questions.

There are a number of scholars around the world who I am grateful to for engaging with this research at different points and in different places. Particularly Nicole Bourbonnais, Cyrelene Amoah-Boampong, Yuliya Hilevych, David Bannister, Anne Hugon, Alison Downham Moore, Sarah Walters and many others have supported me and taken the time to share their thoughts on my work. I have been fortunate to be surrounded by excellent peers. I am particularly grateful to Keri Lambert, who gave me the courage to start my research in Ghana back in 2015; George Severs, Damilola Adebayo, Noah Oehri and others who provided a vibrant community at Cambridge and beyond.

This study would not have been possible without funding from the Arts and Humanities Research Council. I am also grateful to Cambridge University History Faculty and The Graduate Institute of International and Development Studies, which have also supported me financially in the course of this research.

In Ghana, I owe immense thanks to William Akuetteh Otoo, Moses Andoh, Abiza Isaah and Cerdick Ofori Antoh, who acted as research assistants and translators, allowing me to carry out oral history interviews with 60 Ghanaians. To these 60 people I am also extremely thankful; I hope that I have done justice to their lives, thoughts and opinions in these pages. I am appreciative of all the kindness I experienced throughout my time in Ghana. Archivists across the world went out of their way to help me. There are too many to name here, but I am thankful to them, especially for their patience as I requested seemingly endless documents.

I am especially appreciative of the support given by my family. I know that this would have been impossible without them. Their constant encouragement has kept me going. Kris has been a vigilant editor. He, my parents, Jill and Ben, and my brother James have always been on the end of a phone, saying the right thing, for which I am incredibly thankful.

Introduction

Between the 1920s and 1980s, women's reproductive health choices in Ghana were driven by development policy and practice. As the godfather of family planning in Ghana, Fred Sai, reminds us, choice is a subjective notion.[1] The freedom to choose is dictated by economic, social and cultural circumstances. This is, therefore, a social history at its core. It explores the circumstances in which women made choices about reproductive health. Concepts of development, population and women's reproductive health were intimately intertwined during this 60-year period. I tell the story of desires for population increase, the implementation of maternal and child welfare, the growing medicalisation of pregnancy, nationalist pronatalism, family planning and, throughout, the diversity of healthcare options women could choose and the structural limitations to that choice. Development placed limitations on these choices by cultivating a hegemonic morality that, at different points in this history, promoted biomedicine, population growth or restriction of that growth. At times, 'tradition' was championed in the name of development; at other times, that champion was 'modernity.' As we will see, development was a malleable and shifting concept, firmly intertwined with biological and social reproduction.

In November 1970, the government of Ghana launched the National Family Planning Programme (NFPP) – the first such programme in West Africa. The National Liberation Council (NLC), a military government that ruled Ghana from 1966 to 1969, prioritised the production of a 'Population Policy' in 1969. This Policy determined that women's fertility must be limited in order to allow for economic development. The NFPP was designed to achieve this. Clinic numbers quickly grew, and the Health Ministry received requests from nurses and doctors for contraceptives and information. Midwife Gladys George wrote to the Medical Officer of Health in Koforidua following Christian Home Week: she had held discussions on limiting births, sex, and contraception and reported that 'people were delighted and asked interesting questions.' She proposed to run a clinic in her small town.[2] But from the outset, the Programme did not serve all Ghanaian women. In its early years, most women had not heard of – or were not interested in – the NFPP. Mary Boanno, who lived in a rural village in Central Region, explained: 'we didn't have family planning then … it was recently that we were told we should consider family planning so we can take care of children well

DOI: 10.4324/9781003274162-1

... during that time we were just giving birth.'[3] Even with the establishment of a supposedly national health programme, women's reproductive health choices and ability to choose varied widely. Some were unable to access family planning services, some could but chose not to, and others took advantage of the new clinics, whilst some tried out new pills or contraceptive devices only to discover they did not work for them personally. Women were driven to make certain choices about their reproductive health because of family pressures, public discourse or practical constrictions.

At the launch of the NFPP, J. H. Mensah, the Minister for Finance and Economic Planning, announced to the country that Ghana had taken 'a bold decision to tackle one of the most pressing issues of our time ... the unprecedented growth of the world's population poses one of the greatest threats to mankind.'[4] The NFPP was not first and foremost about women's or children's health needs – the Policy was about development. The Population Policy had been a promise: by limiting fertility, national development would follow. Indeed it was *fertility* that the Policy targeted, which is why there is a third node in the relationship between development and population: health. Specifically, women's reproductive health. Policies that link development to population almost always use women's reproductive health measures as a solution, as I explore in this book.

The creation of the 1969 Population Policy, and subsequent NFPP, was certainly not the first time in Ghana's history that the connection had been made between the development of the country, or colony, its population and women's reproductive health. As this book shows, the need to control population size has been linked to development since at least the 1920s in Ghana. The first ante-natal clinics introduced in Ghana from 1921 were driven by fears that weak population growth would stifle development. Ghanaian women in the 1920s and 1930s embraced maternal and child 'welfare' campaigns as status markers for belonging to a progressive, developed segment of society, in contrast with their less fortunate sisters. Clinics became sites through which identity politics were articulated. The centralised and 'modern' hospitals of the late colonial period welcomed women with gynaecological and obstetric disease but also saw an increase in admissions for 'normal labour.' When Ghana achieved independence in 1957, its first prime minister and later president, Kwame Nkrumah, called upon women to give birth and drive Ghana's development through the provision of a healthy new labour force and citizenry. But the global fixation on development following World War II started a frenzy over the idea of limiting population growth, forcing change in women's reproductive health.[5] Leadership and funding for population activities came primarily from the United States, channelled through international and transnational organisations.[6] By the 1960s, the global movement for limiting population growth was swelling and reaching out into every corner of the earth with funding, so-called experts, contraceptives and a pervasive ideology, which claimed that development relied on limiting population growth.

Women's fertility had been of interest to successive colonial governments, non-governmental organisations (NGOs), ordinary Ghanaian people, African leaders, international organisations (IOs), philanthropists and others for decades.

By addressing a period of 60 years, transitioning from colonial to postcolonial, 'civilizing mission' to development, from imperialism to socialism to neoliberalism, I show the longevity of the relationship between development, population and women's reproductive health in Ghana. This book also explores a period in Ghana's history which has received comparatively little attention: the 1970s.[7] Probably due to deficiencies in Ghana's Public Records and Archives Administration Department (PRAAD), this decade has been understudied by historians. This book ends in 1982 although the story connecting women's reproductive health to development and population does not. The 1980s saw a new era for Ghana in many ways, especially when it comes to health. Structural adjustment caused severe disruption to Ghana's economy and changes in the way healthcare was organised, making it unaffordable to some.[8] Furthermore, the 1980s saw the first cases of HIV/AIDS in Ghana, which fundamentally changed global health approaches to sexual and reproductive health due to 'AIDS exceptionalism.'[9] I explore some of this and reflect on current discourses on demographics in a short afterword.

In order to represent faithfully the choices that women had and those that they made, I juxtapose policy decisions with women's experiences. Top-down development policies had been affecting Ghanaian women's reproductive lives since the 1920s. But these policies dealt almost exclusively with biomedical care and therefore need to be viewed in the context of Africa's remarkably pluralist healthcare system.[10] On a global level, women's fertility came to be seen as something to be 'fixed' so that development could 'happen' for families and nations. It was linked inextricably to production: what food, land, resources were available for the population and how it would impact 'development.' I build on Sarah Walters's concept of 'moral demography' by arguing, as she does, that we need to understand demography according to a wider range of factors impacting women's lives. Importantly, this includes 'perceptions of "modernity."'[11] We will see throughout this book that demographic records as well as hegemonic influences on decisions women ought to make over their fertility were tied in with aspirations for modernity.

In what follows, I address in more depth each of the nodes of the triangular relationship I explore: reproduction, development and population. This book will uncover how women's choices over their reproductive health have been constrained or legitimised by varying development discourses, drawing on new archival research, oral histories and a crosscutting approach to existing literature.

Reproduction and Health in Ghana

Dr Tlaleng Mofokeng framed the right to sexual and reproductive health as both a freedom and an entitlement: the freedom to have control over one's health and the entitlement to equitable provision of health protection.[12] In many ways, I am interested in exploring both sides of this equation. I will unpack the evolution of healthcare in Ghana from a time when government health systems were reserved for European men, showing that access to healthcare was never equitable and rarely seen as a right. Instead, health provision in the context of reproduction has been a woman's responsibility – family members, birth attendants, so-called traditional healers – whilst state-led systems have only provided certain versions of healthcare for certain members of the community. It is the question of 'freedom' that interests me more, though. Since at least the 1920s, development agendas have reached into the intimate lives of Africans and have affected family, reproduction and health. The compulsion for development, which only grew stronger throughout the twentieth century, legitimised certain forms of reproduction and certain methods of healthcare that accompanied it. Women's choices and the control they had over their own bodies were impacted by this.

Women's reproductive lives incorporate events across the life cycle including but not limited to puberty, menstruation, pregnancy, childbirth, infertility, menopause. However, source material refers overwhelmingly to health interventions that focus on pregnancy and childbirth, which reflects the concerns of those that feature in these pages. For this reason, 'reproductive health' in this book refers mainly to discussions of fertility, pregnancy, childbirth and childrearing.

Scholarly interest in reproduction in Ghana centres around the importance of high fertility for Ghanaian families. Socially, economically and culturally, the importance of reproduction and the 'skills associated with motherhood and marriage' have historically been prioritised for women both in Ghanaian communities and by the country's successive governments.[13] High fertility has been 'a major preoccupation' in Akan society since the precolonial period.[14] Procreation was the principal objective of marriage, and most Ghanaians married. In 1960, 91% of women and 65% of men above age 15 had been married at some point. Those in towns were much more likely to marry later or not at all.[15] Procreation was not limited to marriage though, with extramarital sex widely practised and somewhat tolerated. Many interviewees noted a change in morals, whereby older generations would not tolerate pre-marital sex.[16] However, the Akan were matrilineal, so the children of daughters were generally welcomed regardless of the circumstances.[17] Perhaps more significant than sanctions put on pre-marital sex were those surrounding sex and pregnancy, which were seen as unacceptable before girls' initiation rites, linked to puberty.[18] On the other hand, as Jean Allman has shown, rights and responsibilities within the conjugal family – rather than the matrilineal *abusua* – grew in Ashanti due to the expansion of cocoa and cash, missionaries' impact on conceptions of marriage and family, and the impact of schooling on the family economy.[19]

The 1920s was the first time when African women's reproductive lives were 'medicalised' in different ways across the continent. The medicalisation of motherhood is a process through which women become 'patients' and reproductive events are defined as medical conditions and treated as such. The medicalisation of reproduction arguably reduces a 'complex cultural and social phenomenon' to a mere procedure or a bodily experience.[20] Indeed, the introduction of biomedicine into some African settings isolated people from social aspects of healthcare.[21] Social networks have been incredibly important to women's reproductive lives as families have provided herbal, religious and social remedies to reproductive ills.[22]

But it became clear through interviewing Ghanaian women that most encountered biomedicine as part of a pluralistic attitude to healthcare. Biomedicine melded with social expectations, for example, as fatherhood became a more responsible role during the colonial period,[23] men insisted that women attend antenatal clinics or bore responsibility for hospital fees.

As scholarship turned to the body as a site of 'intervention or inscription' in the 1990s,[24] a range of historians began to frame colonial history through interventions made on women's bodies. These interventions were often in response to demographic concerns in colonial Africa.[25] One of the most influential insights in this field came through Nancy Hunt's exploration of the medicalisation of birth in the Belgian Congo. Hunt crucially observed that social and biological reproduction were connected. She showed that social and cultural conventions of puberty in the Congo were essential to biological puberty and parenthood. These ties were broken through medicalisation, or through reforming reproduction as colonial officials attempted to do. In order to understand reproductive health, as historians we must cast our net wider to consider both the social and physiological aspects of it.[26] Whilst most historians of reproductive healthcare in Africa point to desires for population increase as a factor motivating intervention, few triangulate this with development, and none demonstrate the consistency of this relationship throughout the twentieth century, as I do.

Colonial rule saw an expansion of medical services in the Gold Coast.[27] At first, hospitals and dispensaries overwhelmingly treated male patients. Women came under the oversight of medical care, specifically because of their reproductive roles. They instantly began to shape these services, insisting on cures for their children rather than preventative care, which has historically dominated medical services for women.[28] Anne Hugon has produced a detailed account of reforms in motherhood in the colonial Gold Coast. She recounts how the establishment of a series of medical institutions, alongside the professionalisation of midwifery, set the tone for state provision of reproductive health from the late 1920s.[29] But the colonial state was not alone in seeking to reform reproductive habits. 'Women's Work' campaigns, usually led by women missionaries, sought to modify family life and marriage alongside religious belief. Jean Allman has shown that in response to lessons on mothercraft in Ashanti, women quietly resisted this invasion of their private lives.[30] I build on these important insights into women's healthcare, contextualising them through their relationship with development and population; I also expand on them by moving beyond colonial rule.

Whilst parenthood was a path to social adulthood for men,[31] motherhood was a crucial role for women in Ghana throughout the period covered in this book.[32] A study carried out in the 1980s found that Ghanaian women 'felt complete' through motherhood. Others, and this was frequently corroborated by my own interviewees, relied on children to look after them in old age.[33] Whilst we can certainly point to continuities in the desire for children, women's choices have also been historically specific. Motivations for childbearing and its execution have undergone dramatic changes. As will be explored in Chapter 4 especially, once Ghana became an independent nation, reproduction was tied up with citizenship and with nationalism. But even as a new kind of citizenry was being built under Nkrumahism, women's lives remained governed by expectations of marriage and motherhood.[34] Like in Kenya, where Lynn Thomas writes that 'few participants in twentieth century Kenyan politics were ever able to neatly separate issues of land, labor, and political control, from those of gender, sexuality and reproduction,' reproduction has remained a central concern in Ghanaian politics.[35]

Visions of Development

Development has many coinciding intents in this study: economic growth; gendered social reconfiguration; anti-(neo)colonial resistance; modernisation. These development aspirations are all imagined through different modes of social and biological reproduction. Throughout the period, women's reproductive health was bound up with demographic questions, in which development planners took particular interest. Alison Bashford reminds us that population is not only a question of sex; reproduction is – perhaps more significantly – an economic issue.[36] In practice, this means that these aspects were not separated in the minds of many development planners. Even whilst organisations and individuals disagreed over what was best for women's reproductive health, they all agreed that reproduction was crucial to their vision of development. Reproductive health initiatives were shaped by the changing development concerns of communities, the colonial and postcolonial governments in Accra, and non-governmental (NGOs) and international organisations (IOs). At different times in the twentieth century, development practice in Ghana has targeted women's reproductive lives; it has hidden women's needs, subsuming reproductive health within larger development goals.

Development changed the choices that women had regarding their healthcare. Principles of development were used in the twentieth century to legitimise certain reproductive health practices and to demonise others. Arturo Escobar showed that 'development' was not an ahistorical process of social or economic change, but a historically situated event, that depended on a representation of the 'other' as underdeveloped. Development, from the 1950s to 1970s, he argues, was ubiquitous, the world was 'colonized by development discourse.'[37] Discourses of development were used to construct a global second-class, the underdeveloped, who had fallen victim to their state. Escobar was among scholars in the 1990s who, rather than discussing the merits of individual development projects, framed development as a discourse. This is a helpful way of understanding it as a phenomenon and as a legitimising tool. '[D]iscourse,' he reminds us, 'produces permissible modes of being and thinking while disqualifying and even making others impossible.'[38] Whilst I apply this reading of development, I also push back against a rigid division of those wielding power through this discourse and those victimised by it. As we will see, many Africans, particularly but not solely political leaders, appropriated development as a powerful discourse for their own means. For example, in the 1930s Africans in the Gold Coast used the language of development to back the colonial government into a corner over maternal and child welfare services. Development also became a powerful driver in Ghana's decolonisation and postcolonial history as governments used it to secure legitimacy for nation-building.[39]

It is an important goal of this book to understand how development works and impacts lives. This builds on James Ferguson's study of development projects in Lesotho, which has become crucial in terms of understanding how development functions. Ferguson showed that through development, state power could expand and be strengthened through 'services' and 'local governing machinery.'[40] This power was given an apolitical and bureaucratic veneer because of its links to 'development,' something that was accepted as simultaneously positive and apolitical. Development discourse, he argued, had the power to prescribe action. Ferguson unpacked this action and the consequences of this legitimising power by exploring what development 'does' rather than what it says it does.[41] In other words, he explored the actual results of development projects which were, at times, wildly different from the original goal. Similarly, Escobar argues that the practice of development *actually* produced 'massive underdevelopment and impoverishment, untold exploitation and oppression.'[42]

Dependency theorists of the 1970s argued that post-war development echoed imperialism by condemning ex-colonial territories to 'periphery' status and exploiting their economic resources.[43] Indeed, women reflecting on the results of development in Africa have long pointed out that many projects have actually had negative impacts on women, especially on their economic independence.[44] Through development initiatives, a problematic binary was established, which valued women's labour as reproductive and men's as productive. Where reproductive work could previously be spread across the entire life cycle by sharing it among women, new employment constraints and the propensity for migration to urban centres changed this.[45] We know that interventions in reproductive health often have results that were not envisaged by their authors.[46] I therefore emulate Ferguson's approach in this book, searching for development projects' actual outcomes.

Development is carried out by actors to encourage growth or progress. In other words, it is something which is *done*. Yet it also has an aspirational dimension; it is an ideal, something to strive for. In this book I show that development has been malleable. It has been utilised as a concept by different actors, in different times and places. Examining development through the lens of reproduction and reproductive health means that we have no choice but to see development as a social and moral category as well as a means of economic growth. Indeed, Ghanaian historian Adu Boahen suggested that development without attention to human welfare, development cannot be defined as such; it must be more than just economic growth.[47] But economic growth itself attained a positive moral status as it became universally sought after in the twentieth century.

Development came to be articulated morally. In the Ghanaian context, Kate Skinner has shown that taking part in development projects was often a way for people to display good character and awareness of 'better ways of living.'[48] In the sphere of reproduction and sexuality, this was particularly important because of the strong moral codes already applied here. Vivienne Adams and Stacey Leigh Pigg have explored the relationship between sexuality and development, finding that the latter often aims to construct 'social and behavioural change' legitimised through science which was internationalised through colonialism.[49] In other words, the internationalisation of technical work such as development planning and western science does legitimising work in the social sphere. Adams and Pigg importantly show how development does *moralising* work, an aspect of development which is often underemphasised and which I explore throughout this book.

Like Ferguson, Frederick Cooper highlighted the bureaucratic nature of development in the period following World War II. Development was used as a last-ditch attempt by French and British colonial powers to hang on to their possessions in Africa.[50] Furthermore, the first global institutions for development were established,[51] and the world was divided into the developed and the underdeveloped, beginning with the Truman Doctrine and escalated by the United Nations.[52] In the post-war world, capitalist nations saw social progress and economic growth as essential to safeguard democracies globally.[53] Modernisation theory dominated during this period: the idea that all nations were at a certain stage in the one-way trajectory of progress towards high productivity, consumption and state welfare.[54] The fact that this theory has been widely criticised does not take away from its power during the twentieth century. The terminology that emerged during this period of development fever: 'Third World' or 'developing world' has mainly been replaced; scholars and international agencies are now more likely to refer to 'low-income countries' or to the 'global south.'[55] However, the sentiment behind these words arguably mirrors earlier terms.

I have referred a few times so far to women's freedom to choose within their reproductive lives. This builds on Amartya Sen's concept of 'development as "freedom,"' which invites us to acknowledge different kinds of development, taking into account shared norms and values. It sees development as the removal of 'unfreedoms,' of which economic poverty is only one.[56] However, although Sen frames development as 'freedom,' some of his ideas are prescriptive. He champions empowering and educating women as the key to reducing fertility and decreasing infant mortality.[57] But this formula presents women's freedom as advantageous because it benefits society at large, especially by stemming population growth. Furthermore, as Chandra Mohanty has lamented, this conception of development continues to foreground women's *fertility* as a concern rather than their rights or needs as individuals.[58]

Population Questions

According to the Ghana Statistical Service, the country's population in September 2021 was 30.8 million people.[59] This represents a growth rate of 2.1% since 2010, the slowest growth period since independence. Ghanaians' household sizes have also dropped dramatically since 2000 from 5.1 people per household to 3.6.[60] This suggests that Ghanaians are having less children and are less likely to live in extended families than at any other point in history. Demographic changes in Africa cannot be ignored: the population of the continent grew six-fold in the twentieth century, making it the fastest growing on earth.[61] Africa maintains this status in the 2020s.[62] However, as Akosua Adomako Ampofo has stressed, there has been and remains a dominant discourse on population in Africa: lowering fertility is linked to prosperity. But the viewpoints of those on the continent, especially women, have been underrepresented in scholarship. Too much demographic discourse frames women's reproductive health needs according to this dominant discourse and the need to solve the 'population problem.'[63] In this book I show that, far from being a contemporary phenomenon, this discourse is deeply rooted in Ghana's history and, in many ways, has colonial origins.

Historians of Africa continue to disagree over the continent's demographic history. The difficulties lie in the lack of documentary evidence, which is exacerbated further back in time we look. Throughout the period covered in this book, census records in Ghana were extremely unreliable, especially in earlier decades – they were even more so in other areas of Africa.[64] Historians of demography in Africa have found creative ways to deal with this, particularly looking to collect data at the local community level.[65] These studies, though, have focused on how to find an 'accurate' demographic history of Africa; this book is instead interested in why data about the population was collected and what was done with the demographic 'knowledge' of various actors.

In the early twentieth century, Africa's – including Ghana's – population density was low in comparison to almost everywhere else in the world.[66] In fact in the 1950s the colonial office cited this as a primary reason not to promote birth control in West Africa, as will be explored in Chapter 4. Within Ghana, there were varying levels of population density (Table 0.1). The Western Region[67] was particularly sparsely populated and consistently characterised as underdeveloped.[68] In comparison, population density in Eastern Region and Ashanti have consistently been higher. The importance of cocoa to these regions from the beginning of the twentieth century made them wealthy and caused a shift in labour patterns.[69] Cash-crops, particularly cocoa, were farmed principally by the farm owner

Table 0.1 Population Density by Region, 1960

Region	*Population (thousands)*	*Population %*	*Population Density (persons/square km)*
Accra	492	7.3	192
Western	626	9.3	25
Central	751	11.2	35
Eastern	1,094	16.3	54
Volta	777	11.5	37
Ashanti	1,109	16.5	44
Brong-Ahafo	588	8.7	15
Northern	532	7.9	8
Upper	757	11.3	28

Source: Robert Szereszewski, 'Regional Aspects of the Economy,' in *A Study of Contemporary Ghana*, ed. W. Birmingham, I. Neustadt, and E. Omaboe, vol. 1 The Economy of Ghana (London: George Allen & Unwin Ltd, 1967), 90. I have adapted the figures to apply to square kilometres rather than miles in the original source.

himself (most were male), with the help of spouses and children. A gendered division of labour endured throughout the twentieth century whereby women were responsible for reproduction and domestic work and typically worked in the informal trade economy as well. Meanwhile, men dominated extra-subsistence trade and the wage economy.[70] This incentivised both migration to and reproduction in these regions. Despite increasing investment in education and employment of wage labour, children's labour remained important in rural economic activities.[71]

From a rural versus urban population point of view, the latter grew dramatically in the twentieth century (Table 0.2).[72] Although fertility in urban areas was likely to be lower,[73] migration and better medical services facilitated growth. Towns and cities were a rapidly growing site of industry, trade and an expanding urban, educated elite.[74] There were significant concerns over migration at certain points in Ghana's history. In the late colonial era officials began to worry about overcrowding and lack of recourses in cities. Migration from beyond the nation's borders also caused issues, particularly during postcolonial economic recessions, which saw the rights of the non-autochthonous population threatened.[75] As this book shows though, the principal explanation for population growth has been fertility. For this reason, demographic and development questions have brought women's reproductive health sharply into focus.

Tabless 0.3 and 0.4 provide an overview of census data between 1921 and 1984. Whilst historians generally agree that colonial censuses are significant

Table 0.2 Urban Population, 1921–1960

	1921	*1931*	*1948*	*1960*
Accra	41,100	60,700	133,200	388,231
Kumasi	38,000	35,800	77,700	220,922
Sekondi-Takoradi	9,500	22,400	43,700	120,793
Cape Coast	14,900	17,700	23,000	56,730
Tamale	3,900	12,900	16,100	57,946

Source: Dennis Austin, *Politics in Ghana, 1946–1960* (Oxford: Oxford University Press, 1964), 4.

Table 0.3 Population in Census Years 1921–1948

Population Census Years 1921–1948 (thousands)			
	1921	*1931*	*1948*
Total Gold Coast	2,528	3,227	4,610
Gold Coast Colony	1,140	1,901	2,483
Ashanti	455	647	916
Northern Territories	707	992	1,206
Togoland	210	329	429

Source: The numbers in this table are taken from the revised estimates of the population of the Gold Coast in table 8 of the following article: Frankema and Jerven, 'Writing History Backwards or Sideways.' I have adjusted the regional figures in line with the adjustment made by the authors to the overall population.

Table 0.4 Population in Census Years 1960–1984

Population Census Years 1960–1984			
	1960	*1970*	*1984*
Total	6,726,820	8,559,313	12,296,081
Greater Accra	491,820	851,614	1,431,099
Northern	1,288,920	727,618	1,164,583
Eastern	1,094,200	1,261,661	1,680,890
Western	1,377,550	770,087	1,157,807
Ashanti	1,109,130	1,481,698	2,090,100
Brong-Ahafo	587,920	766,509	1,206,608
Volta	777,280	947,268	1,211,907
Central	n/a	890,135	1,142,335
Upper East	n/a	542,858	772,744
Upper West	n/a	319,865	438,008

Source: Awusabo-Asare, 'Population and Housing Census National Analytical Report,' 72; *1960 Population Census of Ghana. Advance Report of Volumes III and IV*, Accra, 1962.

undercounts,[76] the 1960 census has been viewed as a slight overcount, given the new incentive of possible allocation of public goods according to population.[77]

There was significant population growth from the 1920s onwards as Africa recovered from demographic decline linked to the process of colonisation.[78] By 1984 the population of Ghana was nearly five times that in 1921. The causes of this growth have been debated. Some, like David Patterson, argue that fertility remained stable throughout this period, whilst the positive effects of colonial medicine caused population growth through lowering mortality rates.[79] Given the lack of widely available antibiotics until at least the 1950s, and the slow growth of systematic maternal and child health (MCH) programmes, a significant drop in infant and maternal mortality rates from the 1920s seems unlikely. John Caldwell pointed to the reduction in famine, modern transport systems and the concentration of people in towns to explain population growth.[80] E. V. T. Engmann highlights a correlation between areas of high development and population growth, pointing particularly to industrial and administrative centres as well as cocoa-growing areas.[81] Indeed, some scholars consider that fertility rates *did* increase due to higher demand for labour and the interruption of indigenous fertility control methods such as breastfeeding and postpartum abstinence.[82]

Despite the apparent population growth, interwar colonial officials in Ghana aspired to still greater growth; partly this was to increase the availability of labour and partly as a key indicator of development. Scholarship has drawn attention to similar aspirations across British, French, Belgian and Portuguese African colonies.[83] Indeed, like Samuël Coghe's study of early-colonial Angola, the case of Ghana shows us that fears of de- or underpopulation were far more prevalent than neo-Malthusian concerns among interwar colonial officials.[84] Indeed, despite growth, population *density* remained comparatively low, meaning that competition for land was not a factor driving down birth rates.[85] Other factors though, such as the increase in monogamous relationships and changes in women's labour patterns, may well have had this effect as the colonial state grew stronger from the 1920s onwards.[86]

In the latter half of the twentieth century, population control became almost as ubiquitous as development itself. It became a global phenomenon, with international and US-based philanthropic organisations targeting African countries from the 1960s onwards, with varying results.[87] Concern over population growth was based on Demographic Transition Theory (DTT) which became prescriptive, driving policy almost as soon as it was written in the 1940s. Broadly speaking, DTT posits that industrialisation and the consequent improvement in living standards will cause population growth as mortality rates decline. A decline in fertility rates will follow as a result of various effects of modernisation: individualism, education, urbanisation and consumer aspirations. Importantly, this theory has been applied universally, and in a context of normalised economic planning. As population policymakers became impatient waiting for modernisation to result in a drop in fertility in so-called 'underdeveloped nations,' DTT was turned on its head. Now, policymakers argued, high fertility needed to be curbed in order to *allow* modernisation and economic development.[88] Family planning programmes were frequently designed and delivered on the basis that rapid population growth would prevent economic development. Yet, surprisingly few studies root the inequities inherent in global population activism in local African histories, which I will address.

One of the most important points to emerge from recent scholarship on birth control is its transnational nature.[89] From the 1950s onwards, certain organisations, such as International Planned Parenthood Federation (IPPF) and Population Council, attained a global reach. Meanwhile, individuals working in population activism or family planning fieldworkers shared ideas and devices across borders, sometimes aided by these organisations and sometimes of their own volition.[90] When we look at family planning and population control on a global level, it becomes obvious that reproduction has been stratified.[91] Scholars have highlighted tensions over eugenic aspects of population control programmes across the globe, frequently along racial lines.[92] Population control efforts concentrated on developing countries and, in particular, racialised bodies. This is a crucial dynamic to keep in mind when exploring the extent to which women had a choice over their reproductive health. Mahmood Mamdani's 1972 single-village study in India argued that population control was a 'weapon of the political conservative,' because it acted as a substitute for social and economic change.[93] Mahmood argued that overpopulation discourses were not to do with the quantity of people, but their 'quality.'[94] The observation is striking, emphasising the biases in overpopulation discourse which are explored especially in Chapter 5 of this book. I also connect these population discourses to a longer history in which 'underdeveloped' populations were controlled.

Reproductive justice campaigners frame a person's 'safe and dignified fertility management, childbirth, and parenting' as a human right.[95] This is a far cry from population growth limitation policies that were not concerned with individual rights but with global economic growth. On the other hand, we must remember that family planning was welcomed by certain individuals, families, health practitioners and nations. Nicole Bourbonnais rightly argues for a more nuanced view. Family planning was embraced by some, and opposed by others for religious, racial and political reasons.[96] Paying attention to women's agency in reproduction highlights the fact that the envisaged effects of family planning might not play out in reality,[97] African women have used contraceptives as a way to guarantee the survival of more healthy children rather than to limit births.[98]

When discussing health programmes linked to population control, historical actors refer to 'family planning,' 'population control,' 'contraception' and 'birth control' at times interchangeably. However, these terms have different implications. 'Family planning' refers to limiting and spacing children within a family, whereas 'population control' refers to macro-level control of demographic changes. 'Family planning' is frequently used as a euphemism for the latter. Meanwhile, 'contraception' refers to technologies, not necessarily used in the context of the 'family,' nor to control births. 'Birth control,' on the other hand, implies that its primary purpose is – usually – to avoid pregnancies and births but does not necessarily refer to contraception. I use historical terms relevant to their context.

Sources and Methodology

Underpinning the arguments made in this book is a wide range of evidence, including documentary and oral evidence across multiple 'levels.' When writing this book, I was interested in the interaction between development discourses at international and national levels and the impact they had on ordinary women's reproductive lives. In order to illustrate the disparities between these levels I collated evidence from international organisations, national archives, personal papers, oral histories, newspapers and so on. By doing so, I show that Ghanaian actors belong to a global history of reproductive health. They belong to networks that transcend national borders and are impacted by ideologies that do the same.

There has been much debate over how to integrate the 'global' and the 'local.' Some historians of family planning have done this successfully, such as Bourbonnais' study of birth control in the Caribbean, which shows how transnational activism was translated into the local implementation of family planning.[99] Due firstly to imperialism, and then internationalism and globalisation, the question of healthcare in Ghana has always been impacted by ideology, innovation and ideas beyond its borders. I am inspired by Alison Bashford's assertion that childbirth was the ultimate 'glocal' event because it remains 'culturally specific' despite being

> massively medicalised … as a key element of and for new kinds of primary care, by colonial, postcolonial, communist, socialist, liberal states alike, and through all kinds of international organisations and transnational health foundations.[100]

A study of women's reproductive health provision in Ghana would not be complete without attention to the global movement and this book transcends a national framework.

I put emphasis on southern Ghana, whose regions have a certain amount of cultural and linguistic homogeneity. Except for the Ga, the area is inhabited by Akans, matrilineal groups whose languages are mutually intelligible. The principal reason for restricting the focus geographically is to allow certain generalisations based on cultural and social similarities. The second reason is the different developmental trajectories experienced by regions in the north of the country. This, as David Bannister has shown, meant that health institutions there had a distinct history.[101] Particular attention is paid to Western and Central regions (as they were before 2018), since oral histories were carried out in villages there. It is worth noting, however, that many of the women I interviewed had led mobile lives, often experiencing pregnancy and childbirth in different circumstances. Jean Allman and Victoria Tashjian's observation that 'the boundaries between urban, suburban, and rural were extremely fluid in life histories,' certainly resonates.[102]

The process of interviewing Ghanaians – mainly Ghanaian women – was illuminating. Documentary evidence that depicted the long arm of development stretching into women's villages, families and bodies was undermined by the testimony of women who rarely experienced it, carried with them immense and intergenerational knowledge of herbal remedies for reproductive health issues and who appeared oblivious to government messaging telling them to have more or less children dependent on its current development ideology. As Anne Stoler notes, the sense and order that colonial archives tried to bring to their subjects' experiences was undermined by the messiness of people's lives.[103] I saw at once the variety of recourses that women had for their healthcare and the simultaneous tragic results of not having access to certain medical aid.

What Ghanaian motherhood looked like has varied enormously according to a range of factors such as ethnicity, mothers' employment, whether mothers were single or married, whether those marriages were monogamous or polygynous, religion, education, social status.[104] Even whilst appreciating the structural determinants of women's health choices, oral histories are testimony to the fact that women's experiences were by no means homogenous.

I interviewed women between the ages of around 55 and 95 although it is difficult to know exactly as the majority of women did not have an accurate record of their age. This meant that I could gather some testimony about the entire period this book covers as women referred back to their mothers' or grandmothers' experiences. I deliberately chose to interview a majority of women living in rural areas (Figure 0.1). These were the women most underrepresented in archives, and I was determined that their voices be heard. Listening to women's testimony certainly complicated the seemingly objective story that archives offered. They reminded me of the need to read archival sources 'against the grain,' especially in an ex-colonial, African context, where the power relations between those constructing archives and the histories of those within them remained so unequal. Interviews were carried out in the southern area of the

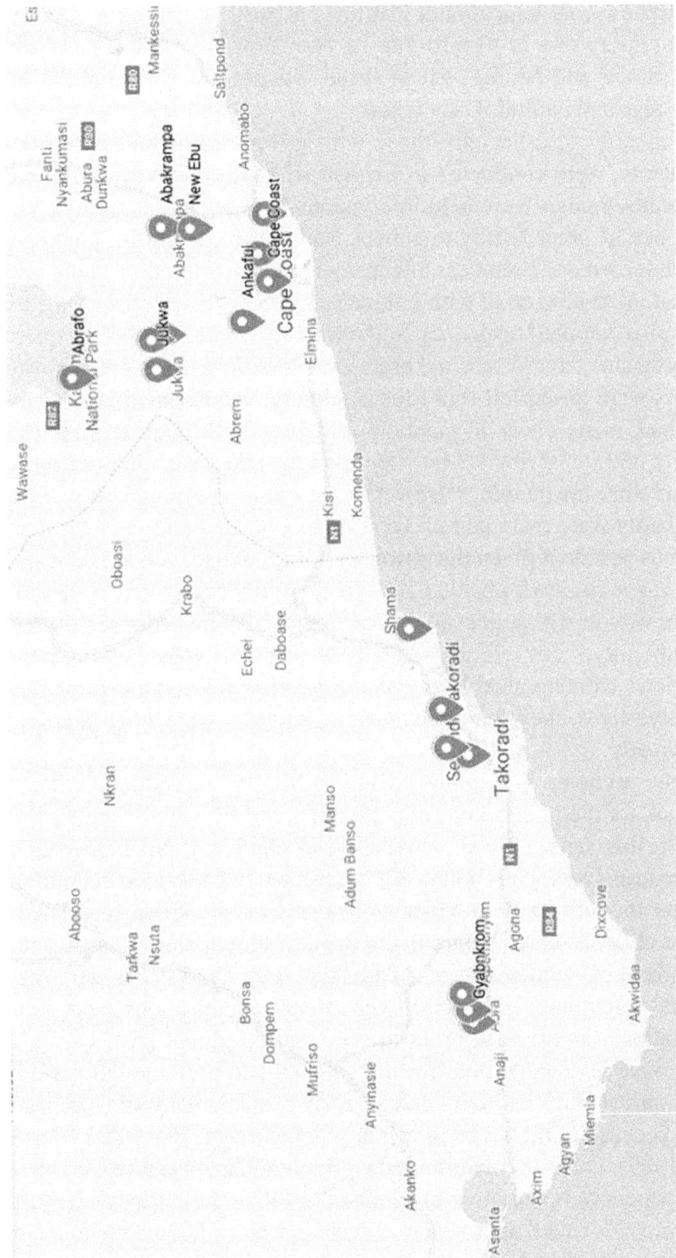

Figure 0.1 Interview Locations, October 2017–July 2019.

Western Region, in the villages: Adjumako, Mpatase, Abra and Gyabenkrom. Most of the women I spoke to in these villages worked as farmers, either on rubber plantations or farming foodstuffs. I also carried out interviews in Aboadze, where the vast majority of people worked in fishing. The second group of interviews was carried out in Central Region. This area of the country is characterised by its urbanity, its educational institutes as well as fishing and farming.[105] I carried out interviews in Abrafo, Jukwa, New Ebu, Ankaful, Barabadze, Koforidua, Abakrampa and Moree. All of these villages are within about 25 kilometres of the regional capital, Cape Coast.

Some of the interviews, especially those with government-trained (retired) midwives and doctors, were conducted in English with only the participant and myself present. Many though were held in compounds or outside houses in villages in the presence of other family members. Some of those family members had opinions of their own and doubtless affected what women felt they could talk about. The fact that interviews dealt with intimate and deeply emotional moments of women's pasts also coloured responses. Some women avoided answering questions about sex, pregnancy avoidance and pregnancy loss. In some cases, the way in which questions were posed left room for ambiguity. When asked how many children women had, many chose to mention only those still living at first. The work of translators and transcribers who supported me when carrying out these interviews was therefore invaluable.[106] However, they also presented issues. Two of the three translators were men, and all were more educated and younger than interviewees. This is pertinent given the power dynamics of age, gender, race and education at play, as is my own position as a young, childless, white, well-educated woman. The way in which questions were posed by translators sometimes caused further ambiguity – not referring directly to women's vaginas, for example. Whilst interviews were invaluable as a source to show women's experiences of their reproductive lives, they, like documentary sources, were imperfect and had to be read critically.

Delving into the archives to explore Ghanaian history, reproduction stares back. Once you look for them, questions of population, fertility, family and health are everywhere. In this sense, Stoler's invitation to explore what is unwritten in the archive because '"everyone knew it"' is crucial.[107] Unwritten 'common sense' assumptions about the way in which Ghanaian women experienced fertility, pregnancy and childbirth are prolific in the documentary material I accessed. I, like other historians of women and of Africa, therefore had to consider what lay behind authors' intentions. I accessed international organisations' and philanthropic organisations' archives in order to see Ghana's global past. Ghana's national archives were invaluable both for the colonial and postcolonial period. However, much archival material from Ghana's early postcolonial years has been destroyed mainly because of the series of military governments that ruled Ghana in the 1970s and 1980s. Other archives including international organisations, private papers, newspapers were therefore invaluable for filling these gaps as well as for achieving my multi-levelled approach to evidence, which allowed me to meld local, national, international and transnational stories.

Organisation

The organisation of this book is informed by the varying, malleable and contradictory ideologies of development that have defined Ghana's twentieth-century history. Chapters 1 and 2 investigate a period in the 1920s and 1930s when population concerns led to the first implementation of systematic biomedical health services for women and children. This absolutely has to be understood in the context of a transnational push for maternal and child welfare that was linked to a rise in women's international organisation, developmental humanitarianism and imperial oversight. As such, Chapter 1 explores how colonial officials, African leaders and the League of Nations were all invested in concerns over women's fertility. The convergence of this concern is articulated through exploring what it meant to count the population in 1920s colonial Africa and what it meant to encourage high fertility. It argues that demographics were already intimately intertwined with development for a variety of actors.

Chapter 2 shows that when nascent maternal and child welfare services were threatened by global economic depression, African leaders evoked paternalist and humanitarian language to fight for their survival. Developmental humanitarianism during this period had decidedly social and moral overtones. Ghanaian women, as subjects of humanitarian discourse, were shoehorned into the role of victim, which shaped the provision of healthcare. Humanitarian discourse also constructed hierarchies of African women: those 'progressive' women who were involved in maternal and child welfare and those 'backward' women who needed to be helped by their more enlightened sisters. The interaction of development with women's reproductive health therefore fixed women's position in elite civil society, especially in Ghana's towns.

Chapters 3 and 4 begin to cross the divide of colonial and postcolonial Ghana. A diarchic government involved both British colonial authorities and elected African leaders from 1951 to 1957. Women's reproductive health was therefore caught up in a desire for modernisation, which was both characteristic of late colonial policy and Ghanaian nationalism. In Chapter 3 it becomes clear that the 1950s saw women accessing hospitals and clinics in larger numbers than ever before. But there was a clash between large-scale modernisation and a push for 'community development' that retains the moral overtones of the 1920s and 1930s maternal and child welfare campaigns. In 1957, Ghana achieved independence, and Kwame Nkrumah's Convention People's Party (CPP) took control. Their visions for national development and the perceived need for population increase are explored in Chapter 4.

Chapter 5 does the important work of analysing the Population Policy (1969) and National Family Planning Programme (NFPP) (1970). Not only was the Population Policy part of economic development planning, the NFPP also sought social and moral development through its discourse about precisely who it served and why. This development programme did the work of categorising women and men through their readiness to engage with 'modern' technologies and ideas associated with family planning. Once more, we see the stratification of women in society into those who engaged with biomedical services and those who did not.

Although the NFPP targeted urban areas overwhelmingly, other healthcare initiatives were desperately needed in rural areas. The 1970s saw a severe economic decline, a factor that led to the establishment of Primary Health Care (PHC) as the government's health policy. PHC was part of wider calls for community-driven development in the 1970s, especially relevant in Ghana, where, just as NFPP was getting off the ground in 1972, a second military coup put Colonel Acheampong and the National Redemption Council (NRC) in charge of the country. The NRC was determined to achieve self-sufficiency and officially rejected foreign interference and neocolonial control. Despite this, global debates in MCH – especially the uses of 'traditional' birth attendants – loomed large in Ghana. I emphasise that PHC saw MCH and family planning become a core component of localised healthcare, where women's caring roles were leant upon.

Notes

1 MacFarlane, Deborah, Interview with Dr Fred Sai for *Smith College Population and Reproductive Health Oral History Project*, 11 March, 2004, 76.
2 PRAAD, Koforidua, ERG 5/1/41: Letter from Gladys George, Midwifery Superintendent, to Medical Officer of Health, Koforidua, March 1969.
3 Interview with Mary Boanno and Martha Abena, Abrafo, Central Region, 23rd July, 2019.
4 PRAAD, Koforidua, 5/1/41: 'Address by the Hon J H Mensah Minister of Finance and Economic Planning of the Occasion of the Formal Launching of Ghana's National Family Planning Programme – 22nd May, 1970,' 1.
5 John Sharpless, 'Population Science, Private Foundations, and Development Aid: The Transformation of Demographic Knowledge in the United State, 1945–1965,' in *International Development and the Social Sciences: Essays on the History and Politics of Knowledge*, ed. Randall Packard and Frederick Cooper (Berkeley: University of California Press, 1998), 176–202; Matthew Connelly, *Fatal Misconception* (Cambridge, MA: Harvard University Press, 2009); Emily Callaci, '"Injectable Development" Depo-Provera and Creation of the Global South,' *Radical History Review* 2018, no. 131 (1 May 2018): 82–104; Simon Szreter, 'The Idea of Demographic Transition and the Study of Fertility Change: A Critical Intellectual History,' *Population and Development Review* 19, no. 4 (December 1993): 659.
6 Emily Klancher Merchant, *Building the Population Bomb* (Oxford: Oxford University Press, 2021), 27.
7 This was discussed in a panel at Ghana Studies Association conference, July 2022, convened by Elisa Prosperetti and Clare Nicholas. Jennifer A. Hart, *Ghana on the Go: African Mobility in the Age of Motor Transportation* (Bloomington and Indianapolis: Indiana University Press, 2016); Bianca Murillo, *Market Encounters: Consumer Cultures in Twentieth-Century Ghana, New African Histories* (Athens: Ohio University Press, 2017); Alice Wiemers, *Village Work: Development and Rural Statecraft in Twentieth-Century Ghana* (Athens: Ohio University Press, 2021).
8 Kodjo Senah, 'In Sickness and in Health: Globalization and Health Care Delivery in Ghana,' *Research Review* 17, no. 1 (2001): 87.
9 Vinh-Kim Nguyen, *The Republic of Therapy: Triage and Sovereignty in West Africa's Time of AIDS*, 1st edition (Durham, NC: Duke University Press, 2010), 13. See also John Iliffe, *The African AIDS Epidemic: A History* (Oxford: James Currey, 2006).
10 Steven Feierman and John M. Janzen, 'Introduction,' in *The Social Basis of Health and Healing in Africa*, ed. Steven Feierman and John M. Janzen, 30 (Berkeley: University of California Press, 2009), 1–23.

11 Sarah Walters, 'African Population History: Contributions of Moral Demography,' *The Journal of African History* 62, no. 2 (July 2021): 184.
12 Ebenezer Durojaye, Gladys Mirugi-Mukundi, and C. G. Ngwena, eds., *Advancing Sexual and Reproductive Health and Rights in Africa: Constraints and Opportunities* (New York, NY: Routledge, 2021), x.
13 Felix Odei Akuffo, 'Teenage Pregnancies and School Drop-Outs. The Relevance of Family Life Education and Vocational Training to Girls' Employment Opportunities,' in *Sex Roles, Population and Development in West Africa: Policy Related Studies on Work and Demographic Issues*, ed. Christine Oppong (Portsmouth, NH: Heinemann, 1987), 157.
14 Gareth Austin, *Labour, Land and Capital in Ghana: From Slavery to Free Labour in Asante, 1807–1956* (New York: University of Rochester Press, 2009), 56.
15 P. A. Tetteh, 'Marriage, Family and Household,' in *A Study of Contemporary Ghana*, ed. W. Birmingham, I. Neustadt, and E. Omaboe, Vol. 2 (London: George Allen & Unwin Ltd., 1967), 201–2.
16 Interviewees often had children outside of marriage. See also: T. E. Kyei, *Marriage and Divorce among the Asante: A Study Undertaken in the Course of the Ashanti Social Survey (1945)* (Cambridge: African Studies Centre, 1992), 11, 47.
17 Tetteh, 'Marriage, Family and Household,' 204.
18 Wolf Bleek, 'Family and Family Planning in Soutehrn Ghana,' in *Sex Roles, Population and Development in West Africa: Policy-Related Studies on Work and Demographic Issues*, ed. Christine Oppong (Portsmouth, NH: Heinemann, 1987), 140.
19 Jean Allman, 'Fathering, Mothering and Making Sense of "Ntamoba": Reflections on the Economy of Child-Rearing in Colonial Asante,' *Africa: Journal of the International African Institute* 67, no. 2 (1997): 205.
20 Beth Maina Ahlberg and Asli Kulane, 'Sexual and Reproductive Health and Rights,' in *African Sexualities: A Reader*, ed. Sylvia Tamale (Capetown, CA: Pambazuka Press, 2011), 328.
21 Megan Vaughan, *Curing Their Ills: Colonial Power and African Illness* (Cambridge: Polity, 1991).
22 M. J. Field, *Religion and Medicine of the Ga People* (Oxford: Oxford University Press, 1961); Kofi Appiah-Kubi, *Man Cures, God Heals: Religion and Medical Practice among the Akans of Ghana* (Totowa, NJ: Allanheld, Osmun & Co. Publishers, 1981); Patrick Twumasi, 'Ashanti Traditional Medicine,' *Transition* 41 (1972): 50; Patrick Twumasi, *Medical Systems in Ghana: A Study in Medical Sociology* (Tema: Ghana Publishing Corporation, 1975).
23 For changing attitudes to fatherhood, see Jean Allman, 'Fathering, Mothering,' 296–321.
24 Kathleen Canning, 'The Body as Method? Reflections on the Place of the Body in Gender History,' *Gender & History* 11, no. 3 (1999): 500.
25 Janice Boddy, *Civilizing Women: British Crusades in Colonial Sudan* (Princeton, NJ: Princeton University Press, 2007); Carol Summers, 'Intimate Colonialism: The Imperial Production of Reproduction in Uganda, 1907–1925,' *Signs* 16, no. 4 (1991): 787–807; Lynn M. Thomas, *Politics of the Womb: Women, Reproduction, and the State in Kenya* (Berkeley: University of California Press, 2003).
26 Nancy Rose Hunt, *A Colonial Lexicon: Of Birth Ritual, Medicalization, and Mobility in the Congo* (Durham, NC: Duke University Press, 1999) see chapter 1; see also Nancy Rose Hunt, 'Placing African Women's History and Locating Gender,' *Social History* 14, no. 3 (1989): 362.
27 Stephen Addae, *The History of Western Medicine in Ghana 1880–1960* (Edinburgh: The Pentland Press, 1997).
28 K. David Patterson, *Health in Colonial Ghana: Disease, Medicine, and Socio-Economic Change, 1900–1955* (Waltham, MA: Crossroads Press, 1981), 23–24.
29 Anne Hugon, *Être mère en situation coloniale: Gold Coast, 1910–1950*, Histoire contemporaine 28 (Paris: Éditions de la Sorbonne, 2020); Anne Hugon, 'Korle Bu and the

Midwives Hostel as a Site of Memory for Ghanaian Pupil Midwives, 1930s–1950s,' *Ghana Studies* 7 (2004): 43–58.

30 Jean Allman, 'Making Mothers: Missionaries, Medical Officers and Women's Work in Colonial Asante, 1924–1945,' *History Workshop* 38 (1994): 23–47.

31 Stephan F. Miescher, *Making Men in Ghana* (Indianapolis: Indiana University Press, 2005).

32 Throughout this book I am most interested in biological motherhood, given the focus on reproductive health. It is worth mentioning that there was a high prevalence of fostering children and of communal care of children in Ghana throughout the period covered in this book.

33 Oppong, *Seven Roles of Women*, 78.

34 Jeffrey Ahlman, *Living with Nkrumahism: Nation, State, and Pan-Africanism in Ghana* (Athens: Ohio University Press, 2017). Ahlman explores the gendered nature of Ghanaian citizenry under Nkrumah in chapters 3 and 5 particularly.

35 Thomas, *Politics of the Womb*, 6.

36 Alison Bashford, *Global Population: History, Geopolitics, and Life on Earth* (New York, NY: Columbia University Press, 2014), 3.

37 Arturo Escobar, *Encountering Development: The Making and Unmaking of the Third World* (Princeton, NJ: Princeton University Press, 1995).

38 Ibid., 5.

39 Stephan F. Miescher, '"Nkrumah's Baby": The Akosombo Dam and the Dream of Development in Ghana, 1952–1966,' *Water History* 6, no. 4 (1 December 2014): 341–66.

40 James Ferguson, *The Anti-Politics Machine: Development, Depoliticization and Bureaucratic Power in Lesotho*, New edition (Minneapolis, MN: University of Minnesota Press, 1994), 253.

41 Ferguson, *The Anti-Politics Machine*, 28.

42 Escobar, *Encountering* Development, 4.

43 Walter Rodney, *How Europe Underdeveloped Africa* (Abuja: Panaf Publishing, Inc., 1972); Gilbert Rist, *The History of Development: From Western Origins to Global Faith*, trans. Patrick Camiller (London: Zed Books Ltd, 2008), 113–22.

44 Ester Boserup, *Woman's Role in Economic Development* (London: George Allen & Unwin Ltd, 1970).

45 Christine Oppong, Christine Okali, and Beverley Houghton, 'Woman Power: Retrograde Steps in Ghana,' *African Studies Review* 18, no. 3 (1975): 71–72.

46 Caroline H. Bledsoe and Fatoumatta Banja, *Contingent Lives: Fertility, Time, and Aging in West Africa* (Chicago, IL: University of Chicago Press, 2002).

47 Adu Boahen, 'Human Rights, Democracy and Economic Development in Ghana,' in *Africa in the Twentieth Century: The Adu Boahen Reader*, ed. Adu Boahen and Toyin Falola (Trenton, NJ: Africa World Press, 2004), 462–63.

48 Kate Skinner, '"It Brought Some Kind of Neatness to Mankind": Mass Literacy, Community Development and Democracy in 1950s Asante,' *Africa* 79, no. 4 (November 2009): 492.

49 Vivianne Adams and Stacey Leigh Pigg, 'Introduction: The Moral Object of Sex,' in *Sex in Development: Science, Sexuality and Morality in Global Perspective*, ed. Adams, Vivianne and Pigg, Stacy Leigh (Durham, North Carolina: Duke University Press, 2005), 12.

50 Frederick Cooper, *Decolonization & African Society: The Labor Question in French and British Africa* (Cambridge: Cambridge University Press, 2008); Frederick Cooper, 'Modernizing Bureacrats, Backward Africans, and the Development Concept,' in *International Development and the Social Sciences: Essays on the History and Politics of Knowledge*, ed. Frederick Cooper and Packard, Randall (Berkeley: University of California Press, 1998), 64–92.

51 Amy L. S. Staples, *The Birth of Development: How the World Bank, Food and Agriculture Organization, and World Health Organization Have Changed the World 1945–1965* (Kent, OH: Kent State University Press, 2006).
52 Escobar, *Encountering Development*, 3–4.
53 Rist, *The History of Development*, 94.
54 Ibid., 94–98.
55 For an interesting discussion on the emergence of the term 'global south,' see Arif Dirlik, 'Global South: Predicament and Promise,' *The Global South* 1, no. 1 (2007): 12–17. Dirlik notes that the term has given rise to 'south-south' development initiatives and that the conception of the 'south' remains malleable. However, it is a term that remains embedded in historical antecedents that imply the need to 'catch up' through economic development, something which in the context of neoliberal hegemony gives rise to further inequity.
56 Amartya Sen, *Development as Freedom* (Oxford: Oxford University Press, 2001), 3–9.
57 Ibid., 189–201.
58 Chandra Talpade Mohanty, 'Introduction,' in *Third World Women and the Politics of Feminism*, ed. Chandra Talpade Mohanty, Ann Russo, and Lourdes Torres (Indianapolis: Indiana University Press, 1991), 6.
59 Ghana Statistical Service, *Ghana 2021 Population and Housing Census Volume 1: Preliminary Report*, September 2021, 5.
60 Ibid., 8.
61 Shane Doyle, 'Demography and Disease,' *The Oxford Handbook of Modern African History*, October 1, 2013, 41.
62 Edward Paice, *Youthquake Why African Demography Should Matter to the World* (London: Head of Zeus, 2021), xv.
63 Akosua Adomako Ampofo, 'Whose "Unmet Need"? Dis/Agreement about Childbearing among Ghanaian Couples,' in *Re-Thinking Sexualities in Africa*, ed. Signe Arnfred (Uppsala: Nordic Africa Institute, 2004), 115–16.
64 Ewout Frankema and Morten Jerven, 'Writing History Backwards or Sideways: Towards a Consensus on African Population, 1850–2010,' *The Economic History Review* 67, no. 4 (2014): 907–31.
65 Shane Doyle, *Crisis & Decline in Bunyoro: Population & Environment in Western Uganda 1860–1955*, Eastern African Studies (Oxford: James Currey, 2006); Sarah Walters, 'Counting Souls: Towards an Historical Demography of Africa,' *Demographic Research* 34 (15 January 2016): 63–108; Frankema and Jerven, 'Writing History Backwards or Sideways.'
66 Gareth Austin, 'Resources, Techniques, and Strategies South of the Sahara: Revising the Factor Endowments Perspective on African Economic Development, 1500–2000,' *The Economic History Review* 61, no. 3 (2008): 590.
67 Throughout this book I refer to Ghanaian regions as they were at a particular time. In 2018 the country was restructured and divided into 16 regions.
68 *Colonial Annual Reports, No. 1504, Gold Coast Report for 1929–1930*, Government Printer, Accra 1930, 1.
69 Austin, *Labour, Land and Capital*, 12.
70 Ibid., 305. The exception to this was trade in food. See also Takyiwaa Manuh, ed., 'Ghana: Women in the Public and Informal Sectors under the Economic Recovery Programme,' in *Mortgaging Women's Lives: Feminist Critiques of Structural Adjustment*, ed. Pamela Sparr and Takyiwaa Manuh (London: Palgrave Macmillan, 1994), 61–77.
71 Gareth Austin, *Labour, Land and Capital*, 310–12.
72 According to the 1948 census, Accra had a population density of around 15 times that of the next densest areas in the colony. *Gold Coast Census of Population 1948 Report and Tables*, Accra, 1950, 12.

73 Emmanuel Kwaku Akyeampong, '"Wo Pe Tam Won Pe Ba" ('You Like Cloth but You Don't Want Children') Urbanization, Individualism and Gender Relations in Colonial Ghana,' in *Africa's Urban Past*, ed. David Anderson and Richard Rathbone (Oxford: James Currey, 2000), 222–33; J. C. Caldwell, 'Family Formation and Limitation in Ghana: A Study of the Residents of Economically Superior Urban Areas,' in *Family Planning and Population Programs: A Review of World Developments*, ed. Bernard Berelson (Chicago, IL: University of Chicago Press, 1966), 595–613.
74 Dennis Austin, *Politics in Ghana, 1946–1960* (Oxford: Oxford University Press, 1964), 9.
75 Ousman Kobo, '"We Are Citizens Too": The Politics of Citizenship in Independent Ghana,' *The Journal of Modern African Studies* 48, no. 1 (March 2010): 67–94.
76 Frankema and Jerven, 'Writing History Backwards or Sideways,' 913.
77 Gareth Austin, 'Quantifying Transitions in Ghanaian Demographic and Labour History 1800–2000: A Contribution to Comparative History' (Fourth European Congress on World and Global History, Paris, 2014), 7.
78 Cheikh Mbacké, 'The Persistence of High Fertility in Sub-Saharan Africa: A Comment,' *Population and Development Review* 43, no. 1 (2017): 331; Doyle, *Crisis & Decline in Bunyoro*, 2.
79 Patterson, *Health in Colonial Ghana.*
80 J. C. Caldwell, 'The Social Repercussions of Colonial Rule: Demographic Aspects,' in *UNESCO General History of Africa, Vol. VII, Abridged Edition: Africa Under Colonial Domination 1880–1935*, ed. Unesco International Scientific Committee for the Drafting of a General History of Africa and Adu Boahen (Berkeley, CA: University of California Press, 1990), 204–6.
81 E. V. T. Engmann, *Population of Ghana, 1850–1960* (Accra: Published for the University of Cape Coast by Ghana Universities Press, 1986), 7.
82 Dennis D. Cordell and Joel W. Gregory, *African Population and Capitalism: Historical Perspectives* (Madison: University of Wisconsin Press, 1994).
83 Nancy Rose Hunt, '"Le Bébé En Brousse": European Women, African Birth Spacing, and Colonial Intervention in Breast Feeding in the Belgian Congo,' in *Tensions of Empire: Colonial Cultures in a Bourgeois World*, ed. Frederick Cooper and Ann Laura Stoler (Berkeley: University of California Press, 1997), 287–321; Karl Ittmann, *Problem of Great Importance* (Berkeley: University of California Press, 2013), 21; Samuël Coghe, *Population Politics in the Tropics: Demography, Health and Transimperialism in Colonial Angola* (Cambridge: Cambridge University Press, 2022).
84 Coghe, *Population Politics in the Tropics*, 16.
85 Austin, 'Resources, Techniques, and Strategies South of the Sahara,' 590–91.
86 Cordell, Gregory, and Piché, 'African Historical Demography,' 16.
87 Connelly, *Fatal Misconception*; Bashford, *Global Population*; Callaci, '"Injectable Development" Depo-Provera and Creation of the Global South'; Sharpless, John, 'Population Science, Private Foundations, and Development Aid: The Transformation of Demographic Knowledge in the United State, 1945–1965'; Klancher Merchant, *Building the Population Bomb*; Jennifer Johnson, 'The Origins of Family Planning in Tunisia: Reform, Public Health, and International Aid,' *Bulletin of the History of Medicine* 92, no. 4 (2018): 664–93; Maria Dornemann, 'Seeing Population as a Problem. Influences on the Construction of Population Knowledge on Kenyan Politics (1940s–1980s),' in *A World of Populations: Transnational Perspectives on Demography in the Twentieth Century*, ed. Heinrich Hartmann and Corinna R. Unger (New York, NY: Berghahn Books, 2014), 201–51; Elisha P. Renne, 'Interpreting Population Policy in Nigeria,' in *Reproductive States: Global Perspectives on the Invention and Implementation of Population Policy*, ed. Mie Nakachi and Rickie Solinger (Oxford: Oxford University Press, 2016); Randall Packard, *A History of Global Health: Interventions into the Lives of Other Peoples* (Baltimore, MD: Johns Hopkins University Press, 2016), 181–202.

88 Szreter, 'The Idea of Demographic Transition and the Study of Fertility Change,' 664–66.
89 Connelly, *Fatal Misconception*; Bashford, *Global Population.*
90 Caroline Rusterholz, *Women's Medicine: Sex, Family Planning and British Female Doctors in Transnational Perspective, 1920–70* (Manchester: Manchester University Press, 2020); Nicole C. Bourbonnais, 'Population Control, Family Planning, and Maternal Health Networks in the 1960s/70s: Diary of an International Consultant,' *Bulletin of the History of Medicine* 93, no. 3 (2019): 335–64.
91 Faye Ginsburg and Rayna Rapp, 'Introduction: Conceiving the New World Order,' in *Conceiving the New World Order: The Global Politics of Reproduction*, ed. Faye D. Ginsburg and Rayna Rapp (Berkeley: University of California Press, 1995), 1–18.
92 Nicole Bourbonnais, *Birth Control in the Decolonizing Caribbean: Reproductive Politics and Practice on Four Islands, 1930–1970* (Cambridge: Cambridge University Press, 2016); Susanne Klausen, *Race, Maternity and the Politics of Birth Control in South Africa, 1910–1939* (New York: Palgrave Macmillan, 2004); Laura Briggs, *Reproducing Empire: Race, Sex, Science and U.S. Imperialism in Puerto Rico* (Berkeley: University of California Press, 2003).
93 Mahmood Mamdani, *The Myth of Population Control. Family, Caste and Class in an Indian Village* (New York: Monthly Review Press, 1972), 18–19.
94 Ibid., 14.
95 Loretta Ross and Rickie Solinger, *Reproductive Justice: An Introduction* (Berkeley: University of California Press, 2017).
96 Bourbonnais, *Birth Control in the Decolonizing Caribbean.*
97 Amy Kaler, '"Who Has Told You to Do This Thing?" Toward a Feminist Interpretation of Contraceptive Diffusion in Rhodesia, 1970–1980,' *Signs* 25, no. 3 (2000): 677–708.
98 Bledsoe and Banja, *Contingent Lives.*
99 Nicole Bourbonnais, *Birth Control in the Decolonizing Caribbean*, 2.
100 Alison Bashford, 'Bioscapes: Gendering the Global History of Medicine,' *Bulletin of the History of Medicine* 89, no. 4 (28 December 2015): 693.
101 David Bannister, 'Public Health and Its Contexts in Northern Ghana, 1900–2000' (PhD thesis, School of Oriental and African Studies, 2017).
102 Jean Allman and Victoria B. Tashjian, *I Will Not Eat Stone: A Women's History of Colonial Asante*, Social History of Africa (Portsmouth, NH: Heinemann, 2000), xxix.
103 Ann Laura Stoler, *Along the Archival Grain: Epistemic Anxieties and Colonial Common Sense* (Princeton, NJ: Princeton University Press, 2010), 1.
104 Christine Oppong, *Seven Roles of Women: Impact of Education, Migration and Employment on Ghanaian Mothers* (Geneva: International Labour Office, 1987), 87–91.
105 Engmann, *Population of Ghana, 1850–1960*, 37.
106 Research assistants: William Akuetteh Otoo, Moses Andoh, Abiza Isaah and Cerdick Ofori Antoh.
107 Stoler, *Along the Archival Grain: Epistemic Anxieties and Colonial Common Sense*, 3.

1 Hoping for Growth

Population and Development in Colonial Gold Coast 1920–1939

Matters of fertility, infant mortality and population increase were at the forefront of hopes and fears of colonial officials and African communities in the colonial Gold Coast. The colonial archive tells a relatively straightforward story: problems with fertility and mortality were usually attributed to Africans' ignorance or immorality. Colonisers provided solutions as a result of humanitarian impulse, for its own sake, but mainly for the economic exploitation of the colony. Meanwhile, the impulse to expand individual polities informed African public health practices. Concerns over women's reproductive health were directly linked to a desire for population growth, an aspiration on which the aims of Africans and colonial officials converged. The colonial state began to provide maternal and child welfare services, which were embraced by certain sections of the population but sat among wide-ranging health solutions.

I consider three conceptualisations of development in the interwar period. Firstly, African leaders desired political expansionism and growing populations. Secondly, colonial powers sought to expand the economic productivity of their territories. This meant consolidation of control and a reliable and numerous work force. Thirdly, the beginnings of formal international oversight, especially through the League of Nations, meant that imperialism was pushed into 'trusteeship'. Colonial subjects' welfare was measured through maternal and infant mortality patterns. These notions of development converged around women's reproductive health. This illustrates an antecedent for the mid-century discursive environment in which population and development were intrinsically linked, albeit now with a concern for *overpopulation*, and the value of rooting this concern in a longer history.

Colonisers linked perceived population stagnation to diseases of infancy, lack of biomedical health services, ignorance among African health providers, venereal disease, infertility and malnutrition. Because of this, the framework for healthcare was gendered. In the colonial archive, ignorance was implicitly *female* ignorance. Its antithesis, biomedical healthcare, was located in domestic social development projects. Ultimately, through the lens of reproductive health, the colonial state began to engage women more closely. As the colonial medical service and members of civil society began to implement biomedical services for women and children, certain sections of African society became more integral

DOI: 10.4324/9781003274162-2

to them. However, colonial archives reveal instances of indigenous public health and medicine, usually disregarded by Europeans. African political leaders frequently supported healing practices in their territories because of their benefits to reproductive health and potential for increasing the population. Although this was doubtless playing into what colonisers wanted to hear, we also clearly see concerns over infant mortality and fertility.

Fertility, Fear and 'Fetishes'

In the 1920s and 1930s, biomedicine and women's reproductive lives rarely intersected on the Gold Coast. True, there were exceptions; emergency cases might end up at one of the sparsely placed hospitals or elite women might see a private doctor. But reproductive health was most commonly administered by family or community members. Menstruation was greeted in most societies with instruction to girls about their bodies and motherhood. The Queen Mother often had to be notified and a ceremony with parading, dancing and gifts accompanied girls' first menstruation.[1] Menstruating women were commonly housed separately.[2] During pregnancy, most women took herbs. The different medicines that should be prepared at each stage of pregnancy were widely known.[3] Most women stayed with their mother's kin or *abusua*.[4] When the time came to give birth, women were attended by a family member, a well-known birth attendant referred to as *maame* or a spiritualist who attended births, *okonfuo*.[5] Birth attendants helped deliver babies, washed them and showed women how to breastfeed. They might use herbal remedies, rituals or prayers. Once the baby came, women were usually cared for by their mothers and did not leave the house for seven days.[6] They typically breastfed babies for around two years or until they became pregnant again. One of the most fraught events in women's reproductive lives was instances of infertility.[7] Giving birth was an obligatory part of women's lives. Intervention appears to have been particularly common to aid conception.[8] This might mean visiting a spiritualist, or taking herbal remedies recommended by a priest or herbalist. Akans ensured high fertility through polygyny, community contributions to child-rearing and early marriage. In this sense, they had been practising family planning long before it was 'introduced' in the 1960s.[9]

As these practices suggest, fertility was a concern. Certain names given to children highlight worries. One Akan testified: 'the child of a woman whose children die in infancy may be called Donko ... because it is like a slave who may not stay but will run away.' Another name was 'Sumina' or dung hill, implying that 'the child is like rubbish and may be thrown away.'[10] Some parents, who had lost many of their children, would scar the faces of new babies so that the ancestors would think them ugly and not want to take them back to the spirit world.[11] Although there is some evidence of practices at this time that were designed to limit fertility, the overwhelming sense from the colonial record is that women and men were concerned about what is referred to as 'barrenness,' 'sterility' and 'impotence.' As Allman and Parker highlighted in their study of Tongnaab, the 'importance of childbirth' was paramount in communities and linked specifically to the prominence of shrines.[12]

There were economic reasons for enhanced fears over fertility and infant mortality in this period. Cocoa transformed the Gold Coast economy in the twentieth century. It became a major cash crop by the mid-1920s, contributing to half the world's supply.[13] The value of cocoa exports increased exponentially from 1900 to 1930, becoming the colony's major export.[14] As agricultural output increased, so too did the demand for family labour.[15] Labour for cocoa production was largely provided by the conjugal family, even after the practice of employing wage labour became widespread in the 1920s.[16] An increased proportion of labour was allocated to the production of marketable goods. Pressures on the 'traditional household economy' were 'without precedent' by the 1910s and 1920s.[17] The desirability of having a large family was therefore felt by families: children usually worked on family farms. Efua Ata, who married in the 1930s, stated, 'in the past we wanted many children'; she stressed that there was no reason not to have children since there was no need to buy anything and no school fees: 'the men did all kinds of jobs like going into the bush to get meat.' In fact, she explained, having many children was the desired outcome of marriage. For the husband, 'because the man goes to the farm so he will need the assistance of the children.'[18]

Children were especially valuable to their mother's family, given the Akan matrilineal system. Akosua Maame, giving testimony in 1945, said, 'I am the only sister of my brothers and so they would like the family to increase and they forced me to marry … because they wanted children.'[19] Here the reproductive goal of marriage is emphasised, as is the control that men held over women's reproductive lives. In a similar case, Kofi Bonan's father was concerned that all his nephews were 'idiots' and would not be able to 'take charge of the *abusafo*' after he died. As a solution to this, he married his niece to his son so that their children would inherit this responsibility.[20] In both cases, older men sought to secure reproduction to ensure the family's prosperity. In Kofi Bonan's case, the children that he hoped would result from the marriage of his son and niece would be related to him through the matrilineal *and* patrilineal lines. This perhaps reflects the shift in priorities for men around the 1930s as the responsibility of fathers took over that of uncles.[21]

Looking back at the 1920s, one man opined that children had higher value at that time. He said that then, children were the 'highest blessing' a woman could hope for, and if she had a child, a woman would 'continue to stay with the husband however poor.' In contrast, he said, the 'modern woman' in the 1940s wanted 'high heeled shoes, costly earrings and other ornaments' and would 'try her luck' with a new man to get them. In fact, women's sterility was 'held to be an implicit betrayal of her people, and she feels it as such, her concern being shared by her matrilineage.'[22] When women were blamed for the lack of children, it was more than a nuclear family matter, but a 'betrayal of her *people*.' In other words, an increase in people was linked to the prosperity of the entire lineage and possibly the wider community.

Matters of reproduction and fertility were among the most common reasons to visit religious shrines.[23] In most cases, lack of fertility was considered curable. Margaret Field wrote about the Ga: 'a woman who is afflicted with barrenness goes to all kinds of medicine men.' She describes women visiting medicine-men, carrying out certain rituals and taking herbal baths to conceive.[24] Here the 'blame' for childlessness lies with the woman. The Ashanti Social Survey shows that childlessness was one of the main reasons for divorce. Men interviewed, without exception, assigned the cause of infertility to the woman.[25] However, a significant number of women surveyed testified that they left their husbands because of childlessness. These women then usually sought other partners with whom they could reproduce.[26] Indeed, Kyei states that if men did not do their duty 'in all matters of procreation', divorce likely followed.[27] Akan society did not attribute the cause of infertility solely to women. Indeed, for all of the shrines and medicine-men that claimed to offer cures for 'bareness' and 'sterility' in women, 'impotence' in men was mentioned nearly as often.[28]

However, shrines functioned to control women's sexuality. The *Bompata* shrine in Eastern Province was said to cure reproductive health issues in men and women.

> If a woman is suspected of having allowed a man, other than her husband to have connection with her ... she is taken to the fetish & when she put white clay on the fetish she divulges the name of the man.[29]

Presumably, this public mechanism of calling out adultery was a means of avoiding it in the first place. Childlessness was also connected to morality, and its cure social rather than biomedical. Health issues were 'a means for detecting threats to social unity' in Ghanaian society.[30] Similarly to the example above, in Twifu, in the Central Province, in 1930 'there [wa]s a belief that adultery sometimes causes a woman to have difficulty in giving birth to a child. In such cases she must mention the man's name during her pangs and the child will be born without difficulty.'[31] Ga women also named the child's father during labour.[32] This suggests paternity was important across Akan and Ga societies despite their respective matrilineal and patrilineal systems. More importantly it shows that medicine was not simply a matter of applying physical interventions, or herbal remedies, but took a more holistic outlook. Complying with communal, moral norms, in this case, offers a cure for a physiological problem, which was widely believed to be effective.

'To prevent from Witchcrafting ... and increase people'

The colonial archive reveals a number of conflicts between colonial officials and local leaders regarding so-called 'fetishes.' Many argued that shrines were essential to community well-being. In 1936, Kobina Anan wrote to the District Commissioner of the Central Province regarding *Senya Kopoh*. He argued, 'the above fetish is so good to prevent from Witchcrafting [sic.] and increase people' and asked that the shrine be allowed to remain.[33] Anan's argument to the Commissioner reflects the community's fears as well as the colonial government's inclination to 'increase people.' Many applications refer to the deterrence of sorcerers or witches. The Twi word for witch: *bayi* has an interesting etymology linking it to fears over reproduction and infant mortality. The word *oba* meaning child and *yi* meaning to remove, put together express the idea of a child being taken away.[34]

Indeed women gave birth to many children as insurance against high levels of infant mortality. Tales of high mortality became well known and began to act as proverbial tales against having too few children. One example is the banishment of *Nkroma*. In 1912, a report reached the District Commissioner from the Basel Mission that there was a widespread practice throughout the Wenchi district of an 'ancient Fetish custom,' which involved killing every woman's ninth-born child.[35] A representative of the Omanhene of Wenchi explained that:

> It is said our ancestors came out of a hole in the ground. One *Nkroma* [ninth child] first came out of the ground. He stood aside and saw many people coming from the hole. He saw so many he shouted "Too many are coming" and when they heard it they were alarmed and the majority returned to the ground. It was then determined as he had frightened them back there should never be another *Nkroma* in their country.[36]

The banishment of the *Nkroma* is directly related to the belief that these children prohibited others from coming, and the population increasing. The practice could be read as an idiomatic explanation as to why women had 'too many' children: they did not usually all survive but 'returned to the ground.'

In the early 1920s, District Commissioner of the Western Province, W. Kilby, collected evidence regarding a group of women accused of witchcraft in Jenase. Four of the women accused admitted to having formed a group of witches. Their descriptions of practising witchcraft all emphasised links to reproductive issues and infant mortality. Two women in the group who 'have' witches described them as protecting their children and their reproductive health. Ajua Soh stated, 'I had a witch – every woman in Sefwi has a witch. My witch protects my children.'[37] However, the majority of cases described harm coming to infants or pregnant women connected to paying debts. One of the women, Bua Kuwah, was accused of having sold her daughter's womb to pay off a £4 debt. Another woman, Ya Ejoe, described how she had conceived three times but 'each time Bua Kowah took the child to pay the debt.' Witchcraft, in this case, was clearly understood as a threat to *young* children: 'the oldest I have known killed was about three feet tall,' and to women's pregnancies. Allman and Parker have argued that witchcraft 'provided the standard, mundane explanation' for deaths, especially those of children.[38] In this case, it also explained the importance of surviving children and anxieties over reproduction.

Unsurprisingly then, shrines were consulted to protect against witchcraft. In 1926 in Eastern Province a 'fetish' was discovered that the Police Commissioner assumed to be a copy of *Hwe-me-so*, a witch-finding cult described at length by Tom McCaskie.[39] The Police Commissioner witnessed activities at the shrine during which a pregnant woman was assured that 'all would be well with her and that she had not long to wait.' The mother of two sick children was also assured that 'they would recover.'[40] McCaskie found in his study of anti-witchcraft cults that witch-finding was often 'tailored ... to meet local needs, anxieties and aspirations.'[41] In other words, when 'native doctors' promised to protect against witches who threatened infantile deaths or sterility, this reflected local communities' anxieties as they aspired to produce more living children. The loss of a pregnancy or the death of a child is a tragedy on an individual level and explains recourse to shrines and medicine-men. However, the communal or political leaders' appeals to the colonial government, defending these practices, indicated they acted as social 'cures' for reproductive problems. The desire to reduce infant mortality and increase fertility went beyond individuals.

Let us explore that further: in late 1921, the Commissioner of the Central Province arrested and convicted a group of people for practising *aberewa*, which had caused a 'good deal of unrest in the country' in the past and was currently 'causing a great concern' in Winneba.[42] The history of *aberewa* as an anti-witchcraft cult has been well documented.[43] Those involved with this anti-witchcraft medicine said that they had the support of the Omanhene of Akia Kotoku, and Commissioner decided to hear him out. The Kotokuhene explained that the medicine was needed there because 'infant mortality has been very high: Before ... I had 100 children – then I had another 100 – but all are dead except 50.' The Kotokuhene described how ten people had confessed to witchcraft and murder, for which they had to pay £2 and slaughter a sheep. As well as neutralising the effects of witches, the fetish had another function. '[A] barren woman washed with Fetish gives birth to many children.' Kobina Foli, Odikro of Akrosu, stated that the Omanhene obtained the medicine for the town and 'the barren women are giving forth now.' This example clearly indicates communal fears over reproduction. The medicine was brought with the specific object of combatting infant mortality and infertility. In fact, infant mortality in Central Province was considerably high in the 1920s; findings showed in 1931 that 45.4% of children died before puberty.[44] What is more, recourse to shrines was judged to be effective. When the Commissioner instructed the Omanhene to 'give up' the fetish, he argued that 'before the Fetish came many died, now they don't die.'[45]

In another case, Kobina Anan applied to the District Commissioner to be allowed to continue his 'fetish' that would protect from witches; he specifically mentioned that the result would be to 'increase people.' A similar argument was made when the Native Tribunal Office at Moree wrote to the Central Province Commissioner about a shrine in their town. They stated, 'it is evidently fact that since the installation of the said fetish, the citizens of the town have enjoyed better living in health and consequently increased the population.'[46] Clearly, beyond the fertility of individuals, one of the positive effects of shrines was their ability to increase the population. This was emphasised by those applying for permission to keep them. Population increase was seen positively by the communities concerned *and* as an advantageous argument to make to colonial officials for shrines' preservation.

Similarly, men applying for licences as 'native doctors' in 1920s Central Province frequently cited their ability to cure reproductive ills. In December 1923, Kofi Adam applied for a licence arguing that his 'medicine [was] good for women who don't bleed.'[47] A few months later, Kofi Andzi applied because infants in Moree were 'in danger' of being 'destroy[ed] by night spirits.' Kofi Andzi's application was supported by the Omanhene of Moree, who stated that his methods were especially effective with infants.[48] Elsewhere, an application was made on behalf of two 'native doctors' who 'can give medicine to a woman to conceive.'[49] These frequent applications in the early 1920s coincided with a period of population decline in the colony, caused partly by an influenza outbreak, according to the Census Officer in 1931.[50] This could explain heightened concerns over reproduction and fertility. Indeed, one popular medicine called *gyemi*, translated by the Assistant District Commissioner as 'save me,'[51] 'arose during the influenza epidemic of 1918.' As well as its general curative functions, *gyemi* was used for 'baptising children who then become immune from sickness. Women in travail are washed with it and are said to bring forth immediately.'[52] Applications to practise medicine all received the same response from the District Commissioner: there was no such thing as a licence for 'native doctors to administer native medicines.'

Archives show hints of conflict between indigenous and western methods of dealing with health problems, reproduction and fertility. In Assin in Central Province, people were suffering from 'raging desease [sic.]' in the 1930s. The District Commissioner advised them to engage a European doctor. The leaders of Assin Sibinsu wrote back thanking the Commissioner for this 'kind assistance' but informing him that they have brought 'to the town a medicine or Fetish to prevent all witchcrafts or Devils, Bad Medicines or other deceases [sic.].'[53] Others, however, began to demand state medical provision. In 1935, for example, the Omanhene of the Komenda State in Central Province wrote describing the harm done to the 'poor ignorant masses' of his state by 'pretenders' posing as medicine-men. In the same letter, the Omanhene applied to the District Commissioner for a MO to be sent regularly, as they were to other states in the area.[54]

As Deborah Atobrah has emphasised, and the above analysis shows, medicine in the Gold Coast was usually preventative.[55] Methods such as warding off witchcraft, scarring children's faces or wearing certain protective tokens, were usually meant to impede disease rather than to cure it. T. E. Kyei describes his boyhood in the 1910s and 1920s in Agogo:

> Community health was the concern of all in Agogo … the *abosom* (fetishes), the Agogohene and his Stool Elders, men and women as well as children, all contributed to keep and maintain … the highest sanitary condition. It was the practice in those days … to consult … the two state *obosom* … concerning the general welfare and progress of the town.[56]

Kyei's testimony highlights two important points: firstly, that the protection of public health was a community matter, led by shrine priests or priestesses and elders; secondly, that the maintenance of public health was essential to the *progress* of the town. As the interwar period went on, as will be documented below, alternative preventative medicine was instituted in the form of infant welfare centres. Megan Vaughan has suggested that attendance at these welfare centres in East Africa was relatively normalised by the 1930s.[57] In Ghana, recourse to colonial biomedicine was certainly not the norm but increasingly became an *option.*

Limiting Fertility

Historians of demography have also shown that societies in which children are supported by lineage lack incentive to limit births.[58] This applies to Akan society. Indeed, there is scarce evidence of attempts to limit the population or for the use of contraception or abortion in this period. Meyer Fortes reported that 'contraception is contrary to Asante ideals and sentiments.'[59] Indeed, in Ashanti, a special festival, when the tenth child was 'able to walk and go from house to house,' the mother's *abusua* provided and killed a sheep for the occasion, cooked and shared it with the community. This ritual was supposed to prevent any evil from befalling the child or its parents.[60] Higher populations were desirable to chiefs under the indirect rule as their representation in Provincial Councils was directly linked to this number. Cardinall noted that for chiefs, 'an exaggeration of the number of one's subjects adds glory and power to the monarch.'[61] A larger population meant that chiefs could claim and maintain a greater expanse of land. The idea that chiefs derived power from their populations suggests that they may have taken an interest in controlling women's sexuality and reproduction, as it was crucial to indigenous concepts of development.

Nevertheless, there is archival evidence of methods by which women could avoid or interrupt pregnancy. For example, a missionary in Central Province spoke of dark rumours of local priests who claimed they could induce abortion.[62] The Commissioner for the Central Province was asked to contribute to a report on *West Africa Materia and Toxicology* in 1930. He asserted that 'there is little doubt that Native medicine is used frequently … to produce abortions.'[63] Indeed, District Commissioners observed abortion as a common practice among the poor, especially if women became pregnant whilst still breastfeeding the previous child.[64] Edward Devaux, Assistant District Commissioner in Twifu, reported in 1930 that

> there are two ways of killing a child in the womb, provided action is taken before two months after conception. One method is to mix salt, lime juice and a herb called "nyena" and then to syringe the woman with it. Another way is to take the bark of the "TAKWADUA" tree and to crush it with eggs and then to fry the mixture and give it to the woman to eat.

He did not comment on how frequently these methods were practised.[65]

Women commonly lived separately from their husbands following childbirth. What is more, if women did sleep with their husbands, then breastfeeding acted as a contraceptive.[66] Oral testimonies mentioned knowledge of methods to control fertility such as blocking their vaginas with lime-soaked cloth before sex.[67] Women born in the 1940s and 1950s said that their mothers and grandmothers had 'something they were using to protect themselves,' which consisted of certain herbs, which they could chew to avoid conception.[68] Lime juice, mixed with salt and a particular local herb, was also used to induce abortion in the Central Province in the 1930s.[69]

However, more frequently, women denied that there was any knowledge of contraception and dismissed the idea of using any. One group of women said that their mothers and grandmothers refused to pass on their knowledge of herbal remedies to prevent conception because 'they wanted us to give birth to many children for them.'[70] This suggests that individuals' contraceptive knowledge was kept close and that the overall cultural value of having children was not altered or undermined by it. Their efficacy was probably limited, for example, lactational amenorrhoea is usually only effective for around six months after birth, meaning that women could become pregnant again within a year of giving birth. Cases of abortion or even infanticide reported by colonial officials could reflect fears and prejudices against 'native medicine' rather than widespread practices. Likely these references to abortions simply articulated colonial anxieties about 'fetish' priests and 'native doctors.'

Counting the Population

Historians have done important work highlighting that demography itself is the result of precise historical contexts and did not *prove* but emerged as a result of 'the people problem.'[71] We need to interrogate the very reasons that populations are counted and the way in which this is carried out. Colonisers' contemporary views on demographic change were often based on unreliable statistics. As rightly noted by Anne Hugon, the very definitions of infant mortality, maternal mortality and stillbirth were imprecise in this period.[72] But how and why colonisers chose to count the population is of interest, nonetheless.

They were probably informed by demographic theories that were becoming widely discussed in Europe as eugenics took hold. In his eighteenth-century, *Essay on the Principle of Population*, Malthus argued that population size was limited by food supply and territory.[73] Neo-Malthusianism was influential in the 1920s, and in 1927 the first World Population Conference was held in Geneva. It was in this context of Malthusian predominance that population and development came into conversation among British imperialists.[74] That is, the productivity, territory and international relationships of nations were linked to population. As Alison Bashford has demonstrated, those interested in population matters in the 1920s did not limit their understanding of the issues to fertility and mortality but saw it as a question of geopolitics, migration, food production, geography and international law.[75] In other words, growing interest in and theorisation of population growth had not yet taken on the narrow relationship it later would with limiting fertility.

However, in interwar Britain, there was far more concern that low birth rates were threatening the nation's prosperity.[76] Whilst the growing populations in Asia may have been seen as a threat by some, demographers in the interwar period focused on Africa's problem of underpopulation.[77] It was not until after World War II that neo-Malthusian ideology became so influential in terms of limiting the population in Africa.[78] Because of perceived underpopulation, colonial officials did have a heightened awareness of population matters in the Gold Coast. There is abundant evidence that colonial officials worried over low birth rates and child survival rates. However, these low survival rates were not explained through a lack of land or food, though, as neo-Malthusians would frame it, but as a *health* issue: women's ignorance as to their own and their children's health was most frequently blamed. Colonial officials acknowledged that the slave trade had damaged West Africa's population but reconciled this through the belief that population density had never been high on the continent.

The 1911 census stated that: 'the imagination of the Native peoples the Forest with Spirits and the imagination of the Official peoples it with men, but experience tends to dispel the fears or hopes of either.'[79] Although this official refuted the notion that the forests were full of uncounted Africans, he insinuates that this would be welcome. Despite this, fertility was 'apparently not discussed in official documents' until 1920.[80] The sudden interest after 1920 suggests that anxieties over fertility among colonial officials grew during this period. Partly because of labour demands, the government took an interest in rates of population growth. Furthermore, at a time when imperialism was coming under scrutiny, population growth was evidence of both economic and social development, mainly because its stagnation was associated with high levels of venereal disease and infant mortality.

Reflecting problems with census taking across Africa in the colonial period, data about the population of the Gold Coast, and women's fertility, was generally unavailable, incomplete or unreliable.[81] Although censuses began as early as 1891, they covered small areas and the total population was extracted from those numbers. Census taking was often very inaccurate due to inefficient enumeration methods and avoidance measures.[82] Until 1931, censuses were carried out by chiefs, who reported their numbers to District Commissioners. There were numerous reasons why reported figures might have been inaccurate. The foremost is that requirements for taxation and communal labour were linked to the number of people living under a certain chief. Inaccuracies in the 1921 census were blamed on the general 'backward' nature of the 'native.' Officials noted that only the colony had reliable returns because it was 'man for man, the most enlightened Province.'[83]

It was not until 1931 that the population was counted individually.[84] This total, 2,869,854, was not thought to be a significant understatement, though numbers for the 1948 census indicate that it probably was.[85] Dr Selwyn-Clarke, acting as Principal Registrar in 1931, commented on the 'remarkable increase in the population' of 37% since 1921. He reported that it was 'indicative of the rapid development … and the confidence shared in the ultimate prosperity' of the Gold Coast.[86] This indicates contemporary attitudes that population growth was a signifier of development. Indeed, stagnation in Africa's population growth was blamed by demographers on disease, 'native customs' and, by Julian Huxley in particular, on 'a strange distaste for living or conferring life which seized upon various primitive peoples.'[87]

In 1931 and 1948, surveys of women's fertility were also carried out. Colonial officials' perception was that African women were very fertile; a report on Togoland in 1920 said that women produced around six children each, 'as is usual with Africans.'[88] In 1924 a survey of 1,000 in Koforidua estimated the birth rate at 6.8 children per woman. However, when compared to other surveys, this was high. In 1931 it was recorded as 5.8 or 5.3 live births.[89] In 1931, the average number of 'barren' women – meaning childless – was found to be 4.62%. Throughout Cardinall's report, the percentage of 'barren' women was recorded but not commented on except to say that it was higher in more 'advanced' regions.[90] This could suggest a connection between urban life and low fertility. Emmanuel Akyaempong has argued that women in the early twentieth century began following men to towns and cities to gain wealth and autonomy and were less likely to marry and have children.[91] Whilst differences in fertility in towns could be explained by economic and social shifts, there was also reduced capacity for childcare from extended families.

Colonial officials judged that in the 1930s 'conditions on the Gold Coast [were] favourable to a high birth rate.'[92] Officials observed that both women and men were generally married in their teens. The Census Officer for 1931 noted that 'the Gold Coast … does not regard the bachelor or the spinster with favour; and the religion of animism which is so involved with ancestor-worship practically enforces not only marriage but also child-production.'[93] Observations suggest that officials neither thought Africans in the Gold Coast unwilling nor unable to produce children. Discursively, this was linked to apparently timeless religious practices rather than historical forces. This presents a different situation to that in East Africa or the Belgian Congo, where Meghan Vaughan and Nancy Hunt have argued that there was persistent fear among colonial officials over low fertility rates.[94]

There were exceptions to officials' general desire for high birth rates. Dr Cicely Williams, who worked at Kumasi infant welfare clinic, commented that women were under pressure to give birth early and repeatedly. She stated that they would go on having children 'whether they survive or not.'[95] This statement indicates that she thought women had a choice over whether they became pregnant and implicitly links their high fertility to high infant mortality. This is an interesting exception to the positive way high birth rates were interpreted in the colonial mindset. In another example, Cardinall commented on the fact that in the Volta Region, the infant mortality rate was the lowest of all regions, and the birth rate was also relatively low. He pondered whether 'a low birth-rate, might, under certain circumstances, be an advantage.'[96] This pre-dates the much later view that reducing births means more resources available for existing children. However, this comment may have been made in the hope that reducing the infant mortality rate would lead to population *increase* overall.

Certainly, infant mortality was a widespread concern among colonial officials. The infant mortality rate for 1922 was recorded as 247/1,000 in Accra. No figures were kept outside the city.[97] From 1927 it was recorded across all registration districts (Table 1.1). Overall, these figures suggest a significant drop in infant mortality. Registration areas coincided heavily with the towns where welfare clinics were established in the late 1920s, suggesting that they quickly rendered impressive results. However, data was difficult to collect because of inefficient methods and because children's deaths were a taboo topic.[98] The 1931 fertility survey showed that only 4.42 of 5.8 children born per woman survived puberty and 3.21 to adulthood.[99] This put infant mortality at 170.6/1,000 for the group surveyed, which was more randomised than those registering births and deaths. It also marked the stillbirth rate at 81/1,000 as 'high,'[100] compared to the Report on Births, Deaths and Burials for 1931, which commented that it stood at a 'remarkably low figure' of 40/1,000.[101] This suggests that figures from registration areas were an understatement.

Maternal mortality statistics were not routinely kept. Surveys such as the one above, which relied on interviewing women, necessarily excluded those who had died in childbirth. Evidence suggests that maternal mortality rates were high in the 1920s. The author of the Annual Colonial Report for 1929–1930 stated: 'it is impossible to make a true estimate of puerperal mortality, but such figures as can be obtained indicate that mortality in women at child-birth is more than four times the ratio in England and Wales.'[102] One survey in 1932 showed maternal mortality rates in five towns in the Gold Coast for the second half of the 1920s. The figures do not seem to show any trend at all, which suggests the ineffectiveness of welfare measures in this area for *women*. In fact, after a drop in Tarkwa and Sekondi in 1928, maternal mortality rose sharply in 1931.[103]

The overwhelming impression left by a survey of colonial record-keeping in the 1920s and 1930s is of extremely unreliable and generally underestimated rates of infant and maternal mortality. Statistics were based on very limited surveys of the population, often reflecting urban biases. The data suggest a highly fertile population, although less fertile than anecdotal and anthropological evidence indicates. Furthermore, the population growth was steady but limited due to high rates of mortality, particularly among infants.

Table 1.1 Infant mortality in registration areas 1927–1931

	1927	*1928*	*1929*	*1930*	*1931*
Infant mortality/1,000	121	137	113	116	114

Source: PRAAD, Accra, CSO 11/16/6: Annual Summary and Report of Principal Registrar of Births, Deaths and Burials of the Gold Coast, 1931, Government Printing Office, Accra, 1932, 9.

'Ignorant Parents ... ignorant midwives'

Maternal and infant mortality was frequently blamed on the ignorance of women: either mothers, or 'native midwives.' The colony's first survey of infant and maternal mortality, carried out in 1916, reported that there were three causes of 'excessive' infant mortality. The first was the 'ignorance of midwives,' and the 'bad treatment of mothers in confinement.' The second lay with the ignorance of parents, particularly 'faulty treatments and feeding infants.' Finally, 'bad sanitation and dwelling conditions' resulted in disease.[104]

Dr Cicely Williams described a typical childbirth at that time.[105] Beforehand, 'out of idleness and excessive advice from the grandmothers an enema may be administered', which she stated, only resulted in the spread of gonorrhoea. Then:

> The grandmother supervises the labour and delivers the baby. Her methods are ignorant and sometimes violent. If she suspects or sees trouble she gets the local medicine man. He encourages the patient with exhortations, dances and clapping or drugs, which he may drink himself, and sometimes with vigorous manipulation. The woman is delivered in the squatting position ... [T]his position has its disadvantages, and tears, postpartum haemorrhage, and to the child injuries to the head or umbilical cord are not infrequent.[106]

She presents a derogatory view of women and men attending births. Any value of indigenous knowledge is dismissed. Herbal enemas were only given out of 'idleness,' and the 'medicine man' is described in turns as violent and faintly ridiculous. Treatment is described as random and unscientific. However, oral history testimony – albeit relating mainly to later periods – suggested that birth attendants went through a kind of apprenticeship and acquired specific knowledge, usually from older generations of attendants.[107]

Two leading reasons were given for stillbirths and infant mortality. Firstly, 'many of the stillbirths are really cases of suspended respiration. Valuable lives are being lost owing to the native midwives' ignorance of artificial respiration.' Secondly, mothers were weaning infants on 'unsuitable and often injurious dishes' due to their 'ignorance' regarding food-values.[108] Cardinall wrote in 1931 that a survey on infant mortality looked into the 'diseases, diet and native customs are practices which might be contributory to the high stillbirth, infant and child mortality rates,' suggesting that 'native customs' lay on a par with disease and diet as deadly killers.[109]

In fact, childhood malnutrition was a major problem. Dr Williams commented that babies were fed inadequately with 'gruel and kenki.'[110] A general phenomenon was described: when a new baby was born to a mother, and the previous child weaned, this child suffered severe malnutrition. Williams 'discovered' the disease behind this: *kwashiorkor*.[111] According to Sybil Russell, a doctor working in the Gold Coast from the early 1920s, there was 'a general belief among the people that the unborn child exerts a direct malign influence upon his brother.'[112] Indeed, Hannah Bowah remembered that for her mother, the child 'on her back' always died when she gave birth to another.[113] Dr Williams explained that when children reached the age of about two, their 'existence [wa]s rudely awaked,' as, in her opinion, African women lost interest in older children.[114] Given these observations, Dr Williams and probably also Dr Russell advised longer periods of breastfeeding in an attempt to combat nutritional diseases. It is possible that these doctors also believed it beneficial since it delayed pregnancy. In cases of food scarcity, malnutrition was especially a problem for women given the gendered patterns of food distribution which favoured men, a factor that potentially increased the rate of stillbirths.[115] Another cause of stillbirths, infant mortality and health problems for pregnant women was malaria. Dr Russell described malaria as an inevitability for toddlers, which would determine 'whether he fares well or ill.'[116] Other potentially fatal childhood diseases included bronchitis, gastro-enteritis, dysentery and yaws.[117]

Despite this range of diet-related and other diseases, venereal disease was commonly blamed for infant mortality and unsuccessful pregnancies. Allman has explained how chiefs in the 1930s ordered that unmarried young women be rounded up and married in Ashanti. One of the main fears that prompted this action was specifically sterility, which was linked to venereal disease. Chiefs aimed to promote reproduction.[118] It was not only chiefs and colonial officials who saw the prevalence of venereal disease as a threat to fertility. T. E. Kyei remembers that mothers warned daughters to avoid them, 'emphasizing that the disease could cause barrenness.' He remembers a 'charming, fashionable, unmarried young woman' who lived in the town and was contaminated with syphilis. She was therefore known as: 'Afua, the Killer.'[119] Again, people connected the woman's marital status to disease and danger.

Fears about venereal disease were exacerbated by the movement of people, heightened by the colonial economy. In fact, gonorrhoea and syphilis were referred to as 'Kumasi Sickness,' indicating that they were associated with migration to and from that town.[120] Despite the fact that men more commonly migrated for work, *women* were perceived as sources of sexual immorality as they used sex to 'amass affluence and buy finery.'[121] In Togoland, it was reported that women commonly had six or ten miscarriages as a result of venereal disease.[122] In 1923, the government reported that 'the whole subject of [sexual] immorality and its attending diseases is of the utmost importance to the whole of West Africa, as it is one of the potent factors limiting the increase of the population.'[123] Again, this indicates a desire for population increase.

In 1930, the Director of Laboratory Services used eugenic language, warning that syphilis could lead to the 'slow disappearance of a race' in the Gold Coast. The idea that venereal disease would lead to population decline was evidently a concern in the colonial imagination. However, in reality, he noted that only about 3% of Maternity Hospital cases had contracted syphilis. This led the Census Officer, Cardinall, to once again go against the grain and conclude that venereal disease was not a leading cause of infant mortality or stillbirth.[124]

In practice, the 'wrong treatment' of mothers at childbirth and of newborns shortly after was seen as a much more serious cause of infant mortality.[125] For colonial officials, this was a much simpler solution than delving into the socio-economic conditions that might be causing the high levels of infant mortality.[126] Requiring African women to reform their approaches to health and reproduction was far easier than tackling malnutrition, endemic disease or poverty.

Anxieties over stillbirths, infant mortality and poor maternal health were felt by the colonial government partly due to concern over the availability of labour for colonial and foreign industries.[127] In 1922, for example, it was reported that 'the available labour was barely sufficient' in the mining industry and had dropped by 314 labourers from the previous year.[128] The following year the so-called 'labour problem' was somewhat relieved by 'boys' 'obtained' from Nigeria. However, shortages still seriously inhibited the production of gold in the colony.[129] By 1926, mines were experimenting with wet hammer machine drills to compensate for labour shortages, but this 'by no means' solved the problem.[130] Cardinall put 1920s labour shortages down to a 'general post-war lassitude,' the influenza epidemic of 1918, as well as alternatives such as government jobs or cocoa production.[131] Evidently, the reproduction of the labour force was an issue for colonial officials.

Imperial Trusteeship, Internationalism and Health

The establishment of imperial 'trusteeship' also played its part in colonial desires for the reduction of maternal and especially infant mortality. Low infant mortality was 'a useful index of local health conditions.'[132] Its reduction was evidence of the provision of welfare services and improvements in sanitation by the British colonial government or their lack.[133] Alongside population increase, it was an indicator of development. As Corinna Unger has argued, the 'civilizing mission' of the nineteenth century became an internationalist movement.[134] Imperialism was under national and international pressure to evolve during the interwar period, and maternal and infant healthcare became a way of signposting a move to a more 'welfare'-focused regime.

Colonial officials' motivation to delve into the reproductive lives of Gold Coast women in the 1920s and 1930s was inspired by a balance of humanitarianism and economics. Trusteeship was founded on a conceptualisation of development that assumed every country had the capacity to evolve, but western nations had evolved first, as evidenced by higher levels of production.[135] Imperial trusteeship was a method by which 'backward' nations would 'catch up.' The way to do this was through production and growth. This 'economic approach' extended into domestic space, fertility and domestic production.[136] Given this understanding of development, connecting production with reproduction, social services came under the remit of the colonial state. This brought women and children under its sphere of influence.

Much of the drive for development on the part of the colonial government, and non-governmental actors, stemmed from the humanitarian discourse which had been evolving throughout the nineteenth century. Africa and Africans held a central place in the European imagination and debates over humanity. Africa was known as the 'dark continent,' 'other' in all possible ways. Europeans' humanity was based on the perceived 'otherness' of Africans: enlightenment versus ignorance, Christianity versus heathenness, cleanliness versus disease and filth.[137] 'Discourses of difference' the need for a civilising process that would aid the colonised with their evolution into reasonable, Christian, capitalist, people.[138] By the 1920s colonial development became recognisable as such for the first time as a number of factors came together to transform this 'civilizing mission' into colonial state policy.

World War I triggered systematic economic exploitation of colonies.[139] Interventionist and institutionalised colonial governance began in Africa in the interwar period.[140] This included widespread censuses, registration of births and deaths, the provision of certain social services, and more efficient exploitation of recourses. Imperialist Lord Lugard declared in *The Dual Mandate* 1922 that 'to the twentieth century belongs the heritage of the tropics and the tasks of their development.' This *development* concerned not only 'material output' but also the 'welfare of the subject races.'[141] Within this doctrine of 'welfare,' imperialism was supposed to benefit both the colonised and the coloniser. Improvements in Africans' standards of living would allow for industrialisation and exploitation of Africans' natural resources. Many saw the contradiction in this policy, fearing that industrialisation would lead to the exploitation of colonised workers.[142]

'Indirect rule' became a necessary mode of governance given the scanty presence of British officials on the Gold Coast. Traditional leaders were assumed to guarantee law and order and control over land and labour, essential to the Gold Coast economy.[143] Indirect rule also allowed for colonisers to gain control over domestic spaces, 'the world of marriage, divorce, adultery, childbirth and death,' since chiefs oversaw customary law.[144] Indirect rule depended on the maintenance of 'tribal' structures, clashing in many ways with the principles of the civilising mission, which called for the Christianisation of domestic spaces.[145] A distinction can be made here between the aim of Christianising *families* and domestic space, whilst maintaining 'native' structures of government.

One reason that 'welfare' provision became state policy was, as Joseph Hodge argues, the agenda of the League of Nations. Humanitarian critiques of colonialism could no longer be ignored by imperialists.[146] How much influence the League, and specifically the Permanent Mandates Commission (PMC), had on imperialism has been a subject of considerable scholarly debate. The covenant of the League stated that 'the well-being and development of … peoples not yet able to stand by themselves under the strenuous conditions of the modern world was the "sacred" duty of the international community.'[147] This statement invokes the possibility of progress in its qualifying words, 'not *yet* able.' It refers to modernity as both a challenge and an aspiration. This was a clear prompt for imperial rulers of 'peoples not yet able to stand by themselves' to promote development. Paul Nugent called the PMC a 'watershed,' which saw the beginning of the discourse of 'trusteeship,' whereby African *people*, as well as resources, had to be considered by imperialists.[148] Others are less positive. In terms of health, Bourmaud argues that although the League of Nations Health Organisation (LNHO) insisted on getting health information from the mandates, this information reflected the 'abstract concerns of pressure groups in Europe' more than the needs of those living there.[149]

Whilst agreeing that the PMC did not oblige colonial powers to change anything 'on the ground,' Susan Pedersen concludes that imperialism was brought under international oversight and discursively undermined in this period.[150]

Indeed, the League impacted British imperialism in three important ways. The first was its role at the centre of a global humanitarian outcry for women and children.[151] It cooperated with a series of individuals and organisations regarding infant mortality, which received unprecedented interest.[152] The majority of statistics and reports related to Europe, although a 1936 Commission on Infant Mortality included investigations in French West African colonies and India.[153] The idea of this Commission's report was to 'formulate international doctrine regarding infant mortality and its prevention.'[154] Although we perhaps see here one of the 'pressure groups' implied in Bourmaud's argument, it is also true that infant mortality remained extremely high throughout the world. It was certainly a concern of Africans living in the Gold Coast, not just Europeans.

Secondly, the PMC gave the League opportunity to pass judgement on Britain's activities in Africa. Tanganyika and parts of Togoland and Cameroon were mandated to Britain following the war. In 1925, *A Note on the Report of the East African Commission* made it clear that Britain had a 'moral obligation' to ensure the economic development of East Africa. It stated, 'along with the moral obligation to make available the potential wealth of these territories, there exists a parallel and equal obligation … to promote the physical, mental, moral and social advancement of their native inhabitants.'[155] Economic development was made to go hand in hand with *social* development. In East Africa, this was in the context of fears over population decline, which the *Note* stated was a direct threat to 'economic development and prosperity of these territories.'[156] Population decline, according to the report, was caused by changing labour patterns and social habits, which took men away from home for long periods and left women overburdened. This also encouraged the spread of venereal disease, which damaged the birth rate.[157] Population decline was specifically linked to economic development. Furthermore, its causes were *social*. A triangular relationship evolved between fears over population decline, hopes for economic development and social solutions.

In 1922, the Gold Coast government, now responsible for the Togoland mandate, reported to the PMC that the spread of venereal disease and 'immorality' on the part of women was preventing an increase in the population there.[158] It argued that improvement in women's socio-economic condition and provision of prenatal and obstetric services would lessen infant and maternal mortality.[159] Similar findings were reported to the LNHO about Latin America, although here as well as poor socio-economic conditions, abandonment, unqualified midwives and the 'persistence of prejudices' were highlighted.[160] Research on infant mortality did not investigate British colonies in Africa directly but prompted discussion of the need for medicalisation, socio-economic improvements and women's education among the international community. The fact that it was Gold Coast government officials who were obliged to report on these matters to the PMC illustrates its closeness to imperial networks.

Thirdly, LNHO organised two conferences regarding health in Africa. Dr Selwyn-Clarke, who was instrumental in establishing maternal and infant welfare services in the Gold Coast, attended these conferences in 1932 and 1935. The overarching theme of the first conference was sleeping sickness and aviation laws. However, attendees concluded that:

> most important in the amelioration of health conditions are measures directed towards the raising of the economic status of the population; this automatically results in the improvement of … national health.[161]

This indicates that health improvements were seen as a potential result of economic and social development. One of the key aspects of social development that would lead to better health standards, according to the conference, was the education of 'female natives.'[162]

At the second conference in 1935, it was again expressed that 'no notable advance in the improvement of the health of the population … will be achieved until the economic status of the African population is raised very considerably.'[163] Reflecting on this, the focus of the second conference was on 'hygiene and medical services in rural areas.'[164] 'Public health and 'social medicine' were defined as applying preventative measures to the entire population rather than curing diseases individually.[165] The idea of public health originated as LNHO's interest in rural hygiene and moved across 'colonial and international frontiers.'[166] At the conference, colonial health officials described expansions in rural health: new hospitals and dispensaries, the latter equipped with maternity beds and midwives. These were supposed to act as propaganda aimed at educating 'the native' on proper diet and hygiene.[167] Other propaganda methods were mentioned: Dr Selwyn-Clarke said that film was 'sugar coating round the pill which we try to get the natives to swallow.'[168] The representative for Nyasaland also emphasised that MOs should ultimately be taking an interest in 'development of rural areas.'[169] He stated that 'this question is not only a medical and sanitary one, but the whole problem has moral, social and economic aspects, and is linked up with the ultimate prosperity and economic development of the native population.'[170] In the field of health and population, development was bound up with social and moral concerns.

Colonial Development and Population Anxiety

During the interwar period, the establishment of colonial maternal and infant welfare infrastructure began. Dr Nanka-Bruce, who sat on the Legislative Assembly, was one of the first African doctors with formal medical training to work in the Gold Coast. In 1915, he alerted the Assembly to high levels of infant and maternal mortality. Nothing was immediately done about the problem. The lack of health provision for women and children mirrored the minimal colonial infrastructure. Governor Guggisberg explained that a successful programme of 'development' had been cut short by the war, which had imposed 'rigid economies.'[171] However, in 1919 he expressed a desire to return to promoting the '"development and well-being of peoples not yet able to stand by themselves,"' quoting from the League of Nations covenant.[172] The development programme in the 1920s was part of policy geared towards making the colony a 'viable social and economic' entity.[173] This included the building of a harbour at Takoradi, Achimota College and other public buildings and roads. The new African hospital in Accra was opened in 1923, a symbol of modernity and progress in West Africa.[174] In 1923 Guggisberg claimed that 'the most important point in Government's medical programme is the lessening of infant mortality.'[175] The Governor worried about underpopulation in the colony.[176] In this context, a series of health interventions specifically geared towards women and children were instigated from the mid-1920s.[177]

A number of historians have linked interwar provision of maternal healthcare to colonial governments' desires for effective labour forces.[178] Invested interest in Africans' reproduction necessitated provision for women's as well as men's health. Nancy Hunt has argued that little interest was taken in maternal and infant welfare, run by European women in the Belgian Congo, until 'the emergence of colonial concern about the impact of population loss, infertility, and low birth-rates on industrial labour requirements in the early 1920s.'[179] Medical services for women were linked to economic development from the outset. Indeed, the philosophical understanding of development dating back to the eighteenth century saw entry into the world market through productive labour as essential for societies to move from 'primitive' to 'advanced' status.[180] In this sense, economic growth was essential to developmental humanitarianism. Indeed, the humanitarian side of the empire was focused on creating healthy, productive subjects. However, Margaret Jones argued that humanitarian work for women and children throughout the British Empire was not necessarily negated or subsumed by the larger imperial project.[181] Maternal and child welfare workers were frequently motivated by compassion. Interventions certainly attempted to change social practices in the name of Christianity.

Health was linked to social and moral 'progress.' The 1931 census aimed to measure the 'general health' of Africans in the Gold Coast and their attitudes to 'European customs,' including higher education and, significantly, infant welfare and ante-natal centres.[182] In 1923, Governor Guggisberg expressed disappointment that 'the more enlightened citizens, both African and European' had not founded child welfare associations.[183] The 'progress' of Africans on the Gold Coast was judged by their openness to healthcare for women and children.

In 1922, the Deputy Director for Health Services in Accra published a pamphlet entitled 'Simple Advice on Personal Hygiene,, specifically 'Addressed to Young Africa,' The Director states that '*health* is the worker's best asset.' What is more, 'people who bring illness on themselves by … laziness, bad habits, sexual indulgence … are to be despised as unworthy citizens.' In this sense, health also became a basis for moral judgement in colonial Africa. The Director argued that 'the formation of all personal qualities and habits is the home.'[184] By situating the origins of disease and bad habits 'in the home,' domesticity, and therefore women, are blamed. At the time, new 'African' hospitals were being built, and attention was given to infant and maternal welfare. Despite this, responsibility for good health was an individual matter. Particularly relevant, given the contemporary fear of venereal disease, is the link between health, morality and 'sexual indulgence.'

Institutionalising Women's Health

Dr Selwyn-Clarke argued that mothers in the late 1920s Gold Coast were missing out on the 'advice, treatment and teaching in mothercraft' from welfare centres because of their own 'suspicions.'[185] This reflected the more general belief across the British Empire that it was women's temerity and attachment to tradition that prevented them from seeking medical help.[186] In fact, until the 1920s, the colonial government did not provide any systematic reproductive healthcare for women. Even after Dr Nanka-Bruce drew attention to appalling rates of maternal mortality in 1915, the response was apathetic.

Health services in the 1920s were extremely limited: those served by the small number of 'African' clinics and hospitals were men working for European employers or the colonial government. Usually, hospitals were situated alongside mines or other sites of production.[187] In the Gold Coast colony, there were around four times as many men as women attending hospitals as inpatients in the early 1930s.[188] Whereas in the 1920s, men were already seen by the colonial government as an essential part of economic development thanks to the labour they provided, women, despite the obvious role they played in production for the market, came to be associated with 'welfare.'[189] Men were associated with production and women with reproduction, and this was mirrored in health services expanded to women.

In 1930, the Gold Coast Governor expressed his 'hope' to Lord Passfield, the Colonial Secretary, that the training and registration of midwives would soon extend to all towns.

> In this way will be ousted gradually the 'Sairey Gamps' who through ignorance and not because they practice any injurious rite are, to a large extent, responsible for the heavy death rate among women at childbirth and thus for preventing a satisfactory increase in the Colony's population.

Here, the 'Sairey Gamp' figure, an incompetent nurse taken from the pages of Dickens, is linked directly to the colony's failure to increase its numbers. As Governor Slater indicated in his letter, however, this was something that the colonial government was actively challenging. Interestingly though, it was not 'Sairey Gamps,' that is, birth attendants without formal education, that were targeted directly. Instead, colonial policies mainly involved educated, urban young women.

The response to rising awareness of high infant and maternal mortality began in the early 1920s. Jessie Beveridge, a Scottish missionary, opened an infant welfare clinic in Christiansburg in 1921. Although it was attached to the mission school and intended mainly to treat children, women also came for ante-natal care.[190] According to government medical reports, it grew popular and was well attended.[191] In 1924, the government took over the clinic and opened another in Jamestown.[192] Interestingly, infant mortality for the city of Accra dropped from 405/1,000 to 247/1,000 from 1921 to 1922 and then remained stable until the early 1930s, suggesting that clinics were effective.[193]

The 1920s saw organised volunteerism among European and African civil society to combat infant mortality and encourage British values in child-rearing. For example, 'Baby Shows' awarded prizes to babies that were healthy and properly vaccinated. Babies were judged in categories by age and by ethnicity.[194] In Dunkwa in 1927, a local town committee held a Baby Show as part of a Health Week in October of that year. Winning babies were given prizes of gold bangles. The government organised Baby Shows in Accra. Mothers were encouraged to bring their babies and given prizes if they were healthy and growing well.[195] A letter in 1924 petitioned organisers in Accra to have a separate category for babies from Ashanti for fairness. The fact that the matter was discussed between the Acting Colonial Secretary and Ashanti's Chief Commissioner signals its proximity to government and its imperialist tone.[196] Indeed, the 1924 Show in Accra was endorsed by Queen Mary herself, who sent a silver cup as a prize for the winner.[197]

Whilst on a visit to West Africa in April 1925, Princess Marie Louise of Schleswig-Holstein laid the foundation stone for a children's hospital in Derby Avenue, Accra.[198] In 1926, the Princess Marie Louise Hospital (PML) was opened. Although this was a children's hospital, its establishment was significant for women's health. In its first year, there were over 12,000 attendances at PML's outpatient clinic, which 'absorb[ed] most of the time of the Lady Medical Officer.'[199] A Woman Medical Officer was specifically employed according to the prevailing attitude towards the gendering of staff in hospitals. Women doctors were seen as necessary to make African women comfortable in medical spaces. Indeed, women have historically been associated with preventative medicine and caregiving.[200] We can read the choice of a woman as an indication that mothers, rather than fathers, were assumed to be responsible for children's health. PML also held three or four beds specifically for 'mothers with sick infants' to stay with their children on the wards.[201] Indeed, women often travelled from outside the city to bring their children to the hospital and stayed nearby for several weeks whilst their children underwent treatment.[202] Arguably, women's presence at PML meant exposure to biomedical approaches.

In 1928 the Accra Maternity Hospital was opened with a great ceremony. It was the first government institution built specifically for women's health. It would be easy to argue that the Maternity Hospital did not have a significant effect on Gold Coast women. In 1930, there were 678 women admitted from a population of around 2 million. The vast majority of women would never have heard of the new hospital. However, 678 women accounted for 31% of all women's attendances across health posts and hospitals throughout the colony that year. It also accounted for 64% of all women attending hospitals with obstetric or gynaecological problems.[203] Furthermore, attendances grew quickly, and outpatient

Table 1.2 Attendance at Maternity Hospital 1928–1932

					Deaths		
	Admissions	*Outpatients*	*Deliveries*	*Stillbirths*	*Mothers*	*Infants*	*Live births*
1928–1929	183	3,599	107	25	11	9	82
1929–1930	418	6,224	260	52	25	23	208
1930–1931	678	9,968	452	63	13	15	389
1931–1932	972	12,722	553	68	13	32	485
April–Dec 1932	1,024	10,475	582	86	24	33	518

Source: PRAAD, Accra, CSO 11/4/9: 'Maternity Hospital, Accra' Enclosed in Letter to Acting Director of Medical and Sanitary Service, 13 January 1933.

services were popular. Despite fears that African women would be inclined to avoid hospitals and would need persuading to enter, the figures for attendance at the Maternity Hospital show a significant climb (Table 1.2). Furthermore, following the hospital's inauguration, maternal mortality in Accra is recorded as dropping from 14/1,000 in 1929 to 6/1,000 in 1930 and 7/1,000 in 1931.[204]

The Maternity Hospital had 20 beds when it opened, which increased to 28 when the two verandas were enclosed in 1932 to allow more patients.[205] At this point, the hospital's staff consisted of one Woman Medical Officer (WMO), Dr Lawlor, who oversaw the hospital for many years. There were two nursing sisters as well as two midwives in training, seven nurses in training and three unpaid pupil midwives.[206] This staff list indicates how vital the hospital was for training female nurses and midwives in the colony. It also draws attention to the low numbers of qualified staff. Dr Lawlor was the only doctor stationed there for 28 women and their infants. Not only did she care for women that needed 'immediate, urgent attention and unceasing care,' but she was also in charge of administration, emergency operations and midwifery training.[207] Dr Lawlor commented that the work of the doctors and nurses could not be satisfactory given increasing demand.[208]

As well as the Maternity Hospital, a new Midwifery School was opened. Its first cohort of students joined in 1928, graduating two years later. Officials perceived the training of African female nurses as an incentive for women to enter hospitals. Dr Selwyn-Clarke wrote in 1934 that 'it is only within recent years that women patients have cared to become in-patients in outstation hospitals – partly, no doubt as a result of the training of female nurses.'[209] In 1926, Dr Peacock, working in Sierra Leone, noted that training midwives 'indicate[d] a clear appreciation of the infant mortality question.' Because most infants die very 'shortly after birth,' he argued, the rate could not be lowered by community nurses or welfare centres. Combatting infant mortality and stillbirths relied on midwives and 'the education of the parents to make use of them.'[210] Dr Peacock strongly advocated the presence of midwives at every birth because this would combat *infant* mortality. Midwifery in West Africa was not introduced and encouraged first and foremost for its benefits to women.

By 1932 the School was training 25 students per year, and by 1933, its hostel was oversubscribed.[211] Similarly to the Maternity Hospital, the demand for services was underestimated. Young women trained at the Midwifery School were generally taken from a small but growing population of educated girls in the Gold Coast.[212] Between 1921 and 1931 only 967 girls sat the Standard VII exam required to enter midwifery training, and 401 passed.[213] This left a small pool of eligible young women. Anne Hugon has emphasised the significance of the identity of these women as young professionals, studying, working and living in a women-only environment.[214] The midwives' blue uniforms became a 'status symbol' in the hierarchy of colonial life. Arguably, their status acted to disassociate them from the women blamed for high levels of infant mortality and stillbirths. However, Hugon found that many midwives saw themselves as inheriting the roles of mothers or grandmothers who had worked as 'traditional' midwives. As she notes, it exhibits a fundamental difference in attitude towards modernity between coloniser and colonised. Colonial officials saw their role as tearing down and replacing African social and medical systems, whilst Africans themselves looked to build upon existing knowledge.[215] We see time and again that African women sought to access plural healthcare options, whilst governments accorded moral and legal status only to biomedical institutions.

Indeed, 1931 saw the Midwives Ordinance passed, which forbade unqualified women from practising midwifery. It was written in consultation with MOs, Dr O'Hara May and Dr Duff.[216] The Ordinance was only applicable to four towns: Accra, Sekondi, Cape Coast, and Koforidua.[217] This reflected a realistic admission that the effect of colonial maternal and infant health methods was not much felt beyond these towns. Indeed, some chiefs sitting on the Legislative Council suggested that the Bill be delayed to educate people, and avoid 'suspicion in the minds of the illiterate mass.'[218] However, the Ordinance was greeted positively by others. The Provincial Council of the Central Region thanked the government for this 'most desirable step' and proposed announcing it by gong-gong far and wide to encourage midwives to take advantages of new 'opportunities' it would bring.[219] The Omanhene of Nzima expressed regret that given the 'appalling rate of our infant mortality,' such a Bill had not been passed earlier. In fact, he suggested extending it to enrol all those involved in attending births so that it be ascertained that they had adequate 'experience and good character.'[220] This would not be done systematically for another 70 years. These responses suggest that chiefs connected midwifery with an improvement in infant mortality, something that was clearly worrying them; from these quarters came suggestions to push the colonial government's plans further.

The Gold Coast League for Maternal and Infant Welfare

The same year as construction began for the Maternity Hospital, the Gold Coast League for Maternal and Infant Welfare was established. It was made up entirely of women – both European and African – excepting its secretary Dr Selwyn-Clarke.

The Gold Coast League had access to women's homes and bodies. Their work was divided into three spheres. They volunteered at the Maternity Hospital and carried out 'hundreds of house-to-house visits' in Accra and Sekondi.[221] Weighing clinics were established in Accra by Dr Williams and Mrs Cranston, the Deputy President of the League.[222] League Members persuaded women whose homes were 'not suitable for confinement,' or whose medical histories indicated possible problems to enter the Maternity Hospital for delivery. Failing that, they persuaded them to attend ante-natal clinics, where doctors could press the need for them to attend hospital.[223] In other words, this group pushed for medicalisation of childbirth and pregnancy. Within five years of their establishment, there were nearly 16,000 attendances at weighing centres held by the League in Accra.[224]

Conclusion

The 1920s were a time of rapid economic and social change in the Gold Coast. We have seen that concerns over reproduction and fears connected to infant mortality were common among diverse actors and were linked to development aspirations. In the 1920s, a range of actors from chiefs, mothers, colonial officials, medical officers, to humanitarians in Geneva saw reproductive health as a cornerstone of social and economic progress.

Economic and social pressures governed African's attitudes to reproduction whilst more intensive colonial governance brought about massive change. Measurements for people and productivity led to widespread interventions, albeit based on statistics shaped by preconceived attitudes. Finally, international pressure for 'trusteeship' meant that maternal and infant welfare became a measure by which colonial governments were judged. These strands came together to create an atmosphere in the 1920s in which healthy reproduction and population increase were viewed both as signs of and as essential to economic, social and moral development.

Early colonial development was inherited from the 'civilising mission' and was tied up with internationalist humanitarianism as well as imperialist economic goals. It drove production as well as state provision of social services. It took on a moral meaning when infant mortality was blamed on the ignorance of women and progressive status linked to those adopting colonial solutions. Despite this, reflecting the fact that there were numerous pressures on a range of actors regarding maternal and infant health, there were also multiple solutions in play. Women utilised family, spiritualists, herbalists, welfare centres and hospitals. Some even became volunteers or midwives and part of a movement for maternal and infant welfare.

Notes

1 Interview with Mary Boanno and Martha Abena, Abrafo, Central Region, 23 July 2019 and Interview Efua Ata, Abrafo, Central Region, 23 July 2019. Also see: Christine Oppong, 'Notes on Cultural Aspects of Menstruation in Ghana' (Geneva:

Task Force on Acceptability of Fertility Regulating Methods, 1974), 33–38; T. E. Kyei, *Marriage and Divorce among the Asante: A Study Undertaken in the Course of the Ashanti Social Survey (1945)* (Cambridge: African Studies Centre, 1992), 122–32.

2 Kyei, *Marriage and Divorce*, 44. Interview Efua Ata, Abrafo, Central Region, 23 July 2019. This is in the context of Ghanaians 'houses' being made up of multiple separate structures usually already divided by gender.

3 Many of the interviews I conducted referred to different herbal remedies that should be given at each month of pregnancy. Interviews conducted between October 2017 and July 2019. For more detail see the introduction to this book.

4 Wellcome, PP/CDW/B.1/1: 'Maternal and Child Health in Kumasi' by Dr C. D. Williams, 1935, 31. This was also testified to in many oral history interviews.

5 I am grateful to Cerdick Ofori Antoh for distinguishing between the translation of these two terms, which interviewees used in Akan. Frequently, both categories of birth attendant are referred to in English as 'traditional birth attendant.'

6 Kyei, *Marriage and Divorce*, 43.

7 Kofi Appiah-Kubi, *Man Cures, God Heals: Religion and Medical Practice among the Akans of Ghana* (Totowa, NJ: Allanheld, Osmun & Co. Publishers, 1981), 51.

8 Interview with Adjoa Ewusiwa, New Ebu, Central Region, 22 July 2019. Also see for Ga methods: M. J. Field, *Religion and Medicine of the Ga People* (Oxford: Oxford University Press, 1961), 161.

9 Cheikh Mbacké and National Research Council, 'Family Planning Programs and Fertility Transition in Sub-Saharan Africa', *Population and Development Review* 20, no. 1 (March 1994): 190.

10 CUL, Add.9359/14/8: Meyer Fortes, file of notes on 'African workers, Marriage. Summaries of ethnography on marriage', notebook 34: 'Miscellaneous Questionnaires'.

11 Appiah-Kubi, *Man Cures*, 10; Field, *Religion and Medicine*, 177.

12 Jean Allman and John Parker, *Tongnaab: The History of a West African God* (Indianapolis, IN: Indiana University Press, 2005), 50.

13 *Colonial Reports-Annual, No. 1386, Gold Coast Report for 1926–1927*, Government Press, Accra, 1927, 16.

14 Geoffrey Kay and Stephen Hymer, eds., *The Political Economy of Colonialism in Ghana: A Collection of Documents and Statistics, 1900–1960* (Cambridge: Cambridge University Press, 1972), 334–35.

15 John Daniel Nott, 'Between Famine and Malnutrition: Spatial Aspects of Nutritional Health during Ghana's Long Twentieth Century, c. 1896–2000' (PhD Thesis, University of Leeds, 2016), 76.

16 See chapters 16 and 19 of: Gareth Austin, *Labour, Land and Capital in Ghana: From Slavery to Free Labour in Asante, 1807–1956* (New York: University of Rochester Press, 2009).

17 Jean Allman and Victoria B. Tashjian, *I Will Not Eat Stone: A Women's History of Colonial Asante* (Portsmouth, NH: Heinemann, 2000), 8.

18 Interview with Efua Ata, Abrafo, Central Region, 23 July 2019.

19 CUL, Add.9359/14/8: Meyer Fortes, file of notes on 'African workers, Marriage. Summaries of ethnography on marriage', notebook 40: 'Courtship and Marriage (2 notebooks).'

20 CUL, Add.9359/14/8: Meyer Fortes, file of notes on 'African workers, Marriage. Summaries of ethnography on marriage', notebook 38: 'Mainly Marriage Payment Details.'

21 Jean Allman, 'Fathering, Mothering and Making Sense of "Ntamoba": Reflections on the Economy of Child-Rearing in Colonial Asante', *Africa: Journal of the International African Institute* 67, no. 2 (1997): 296–321.

22 Sarpong, Peter, *Girls Nubility Rites in Ashanti* (Accra: Ghana Publishing Co., 1977), 7.

23 Sjaak van der Geest and Kristine Krause, 'Introduction: Studying Health and Health Care in Ghana', *Ghana Studies* 15/16 (2012/2013): 18.
24 Field, *Religion and Medicine*, 161.
25 Kyei, *Marriage and Divorce*, 106.
26 CUL, Add.9359/14/8: Meyer Fortes, file of notes on 'African workers, Marriage. Summaries of ethnography on marriage.'
27 Kyei, *Marriage and Divorce*, 40.
28 For examples see: PRAAD, Cape Coast, ADM 23/1/441: 'Confidential Memorandum of West African Materia and Toxicology', 30 September 1930, 2; ADM 23/1/213: 'Petition to the District Commissioner, Central Province', 3 June 1938; ADM 23/1/452: 'Memorandum No. 50/29/10', n.d.
29 PRAAD, Koforidua, ADM 29/6/38: 'Subject: Bompata Fetish', 13 February 1918, 2.
30 Patrick Twumasi, *Medical Systems in Ghana: A Study in Medical Sociology* (Tema: Ghana Publishing Corporation, 1975), 41.
31 PRAAD, Cape Coast, ADM 23/1/441: 'Native Drugs', 10 December 1930.
32 Field, *Religion and Medicine*, 169.
33 PRAAD, Cape Coast, ADM 23/1/213: Letter from Kobina Anan to District Commissioner, Central Province, 16 March 1936.
34 Allman and Parker, *Tongnaab*, 117.
35 PRAAD, Kumasi, ADM 1/30/1/11: 'Report from Commissioner's Office', 1 May 1912.
36 PRAAD, Kumasi, ADM 1/30/1/11: 'Fetish Custom in Wenchi. Enclosure B', 2 May 1912.
37 All of the quotes above are taken from BDL, Mss.Afr.s.849: Papers of Walter Kilby: 'The Witches of Jenase' dated between 1919 and 1923.
38 Allman and Parker, *Tongnaab*, 121.
39 T. C. McCaskie, 'Anti-Witchcraft Cults in Asante: An Essay in the Social History of an African People', *History in Africa* 8 (1981): 125–54.
40 PRAAD, Koforidua, ADM 23/6/38: Letter from J. P. Gildes, Assistant Police Commissioner, 16th June, 1926, 3.
41 McCaskie, 'Anti-Witchcraft Cults', 143.
42 PRAAD, Cape Coast, ADM 23/1/452: 'Meeting with Commissioner for Central Province', 20 October 1921.
43 McCaskie, 'Anti-Witchcraft Cults'; Allman and Parker, *Tongnaab*, 129–31.
44 A. W. Cardinall, *The Gold Coast, 1931* (Accra: Government Printer, 1933), 215.
45 PRAAD, Cape Coast, ADM 23/1/452: 'Meeting with Commissioner for Central Province', 20 October 1921.
46 PRAAD, Cape Coast, ADM 23/1/213: Letter from Native Tribunal Office, 26 December 1941.
47 PRAAD, Cape Coast, ADM 23/1/213: Letter from Fanti Yankumasie to District Commissioner, 1 December 1923.
48 PRAAD, Cape Coast, ADM 23/1/213: Letter from Kofi Andzi and the Omanhene of Moree to the District Commissioner, 31 May 1924.
49 PRAAD, Cape Coast, ADM 23/1/213: Letter from Omanhene Kwessie Offori II to the District Commissioner, 8 July 1924.
50 Cardinall, *The Gold Coast, 1931*, 243.
51 This meaning is also recorded in *Asante Twi Dictionary & Phrasebook* (New York: Hippocrene Books, 2015), 24. The verb 'gye' is translated as 'collect, save.'
52 PRAAD, Cape Coast, ADM 23/1/213: 'The Foso and Baduwa I. Fetishes, 10 August 1926, 1.
53 PRAAD, Cape Coast, ADM 23/1/213: 'Letter from Fanti Yankumasie to District Commissioner Central Province', 28 June 1938.
54 PRAAD, Cape Coast, ADM 23/1/213: 'Letter from Omanhene of Komenda State', 8 August 1935.

55 Deborah Atobrah, 'Caring for the Seriously Sick in Ghanaian Society: Glimpses from the Past', *Ghana Studies* 15/16 (2012/2013): 76.
56 T. E. Kyei, *Our Days Dwindle: Memories of My Childhood Days in Asante*, ed. Jean Marie Allman (Portsmouth, NH: Heinemann, 2001), 91.
57 Megan Vaughan, *Curing Their Ills: Colonial Power and African Illness*, 1st edition (Cambridge: Polity, 1991), 69–70.
58 E Hillbom, 'African Demographics: How Many People Are Too Many People?', in *The History of African Development. An Online Textbook for a New Generation of African Students and Teachers*, ed. E Hillbom et al. (African Economic History Network, 2018), 8.
59 Nott, 'Between Famine and Malnutrition', 83.
60 CUL, Add.9359/14/8: Meyer Fortes, file of notes on 'African workers, Marriage. Summaries of ethnography on marriage', notebook 4: 'The Baduguan Festival.'
61 Cardinall, *The Gold Coast, 1931*, 124.
62 PRAAD, Cape Coast, ADM 23/1/452: 'Letter from Wesleyan Missionary Society', 16th February, (year illegible 192-).
63 PRAAD, Cape Coast, ADM 23/1/441: 'Letter from District Commissioner', 3 October 1930.
64 E. V. T. Engmann, *Population of Ghana, 1850–1960* (Accra: Published for the University of Cape Coast by Ghana Universities Press, 1986), 149.
65 PRAAD, Cape Coast, ADM 23/1/441: 'Native Poisons', 16 October 1930.
66 Beatrice A. S. Russell, 'Malnutrition in Children under Three Years of Age in Ashanti, West Africa', *Archives of Disease in Childhood* 21, no. 106 (1 June 1946): 110–12.
67 Interview with Sabina Mensah, Anaji, Western Region, 2 February 2018.
68 Interview with Ekua Esawa, Mary Edu, Aba Donky, Asko Nkrumah, Mary Ahin, Barabadze, Central Region, 30 November 2017.
69 PRAAD, Cape Coast, ADM 23/1/441: Native Poisons', 16 October 1930.
70 Interview with Ekua Mensah, Ekua Amah, Efua Kaya, Esi Adjumah, Comfort Kwenu, Barabadze, Central Region, 30 November 2017.
71 Emily Klancher Merchant, *Building the Population Bomb* (Oxford: Oxford University Press, 2021), 26.
72 Anne Hugon, *Être mère en situation coloniale: Gold Coast, 1910–1950*, (Paris: Éditions de la Sorbonne, 2020), 38.
73 Thomas Robert Malthus, *An Essay on the Principle of Population as It Affects the Future Improvement of Society with Remarks on the Speculations of Mr. Godwin, M. Condorcet and Other Writers* (London: J. Johnson, 1798).
74 Karl Ittmann, *Problem of Great Importance* (Berkeley, CA: University of California Press, 2013), 22.
75 Alison Bashford, *Global Population: History, Geopolitics, and Life on Earth* (New York: Columbia University Press, 2014), 3.
76 Ittmann, *Problem of Great Importance*, 18–19.
77 Ibid., 21.
78 Marc Frey, 'Neo-Malthusianism and Development: Shifting Interpretations of a Contested Paradigm', *Journal of Global History* 6 (2011): 79.
79 Kuczynski, *Demographic Survey*.
80 Ibid., 468.
81 Shane Doyle, *Crisis & Decline in Bunyoro: Population & Environment in Western Uganda 1860–1955*, Eastern African Studies (Oxford: James Currey, 2006), 135.
82 Ewout Frankema and Morten Jerven, 'Writing History Backwards or Sideways: Towards a Consensus on African Population, 1850–2010', *The Economic History Review* 67, no. 4 (2014): 912.
83 Kuczynski, *Demographic Survey*, 402.

84 PRAAD, Accra, ADM 5/2/9: *The Gold Coast Census of the Population 1948. Records and Tables.* Government Printing Dept., Accra, 1950, 7.
85 Kuczynski, *Demographic Survey*, 417.
86 PRAAD, Accra, CSO 11/16/6: *Annual Summary and Report of Principal Registrar of Births, Deaths and Burials of the Gold Coast, 1931*, Government Printing Office, Accra, 1932, 1.
87 Quoted in: Ittmann, *Problem of Great Importance*, 22.
88 Kuczynski, *Demographic Survey*, 468.
89 Ibid., 468–69.
90 Cardinall, *The Gold Coast, 1931*, 219.
91 Emmanuel Kwaku Akyeampong, '"Wo Pe Tam Won Pe Ba" ('You Like Cloth but You Don't Want Children') Urbanization, Individualism and Gender Relations in Colonial Ghana', in *Africa's Urban Past*, ed. David Anderson and Richard Rathbone (Oxford: James Currey, 2000), 228.
92 Cardinall, *The Gold Coast, 1931*, 223.
93 Kuczynski, *Demographic Survey*, 438.
94 Vaughan, *Curing Their Ills*, 68; Nancy Rose Hunt, *A Nervous State: Violence, Remedies, and Reverie in Colonial Congo* (Durham, NC: Duke University Press, 2016); Nancy Rose Hunt, *A Colonial Lexicon: Of Birth Ritual, Medicalization, and Mobility in the Congo* (Durham, NC: Duke University Press, 1999).
95 Wellcome, PP/CDW/B.1/1: C. D. Williams, 'Mortality and Morbidity of Children of the Gold Coast', Thesis for Doctorate of Medicine, Oxford, 1936, 47.
96 Cardinall, *The Gold Coast, 1931*, 214.
97 PRAAD, Accra, CSO 11/16/6: *Annual Summary and Report of Principal Registrar of Births, Deaths and Burials of the Gold Coast, 1931*, Government Printing Office, Accra, 1932, 2.
98 League of Nations, R20/54416/3099: *Report by His Majesty's Government to the League of Nations on the Administration of the British Sphere of Togoland for the year 1925*, Non-Parliamentary Publication, Colonial No. 14, London, 1925, 62.
99 Cardinall, *The Gold Coast, 1931*, 212–13.
100 Ibid., 219.
101 PRAAD, Accra, CSO 11/16/6: *Annual Summary and Report of Principal Registrar of Births, Deaths and Burials of the Gold Coast, 1931*, Government Printing Office, Accra, 1932, 6.
102 *Colonial Reports-Annual No. 1504, Gold Coast Report for 1929–1930*, Government Press, Accra, 1930, 36.
103 PRAAD, Accra, CSO 11/4/9: 'Maternal Morality' Enclosed in Letter to Acting Director of Medical and Sanitary Service, 13 January 1933. This could be linked to the global depression which hit this area badly.
104 PRAAD, Accra, CSO 11/4/9: 'Synopsis of the Maternity and Infant Welfare Movement in Accra' Enclosed in Letter to Acting Director of Medical and Sanitary Service, 13 January 1933, 1.
105 For more information on Dr Cicely Williams see: J. Stanton, 'Listening to the Ga: Cicely Williams' Discovery of Kwashiorkor on the Gold Coast,' in *Women and Modern Medicine*, ed. Anne Hardy and Lawrence Conrad (Leiden: Brill, 2001), 149–71.
106 Wellcome, PP/CDW/B.1/1: C. D. Williams, 'Mortality and Morbidity of Children of the Gold Coast' (PhD Thesis, Oxford), 1936, 31.
107 In particular: Esi Koffuah. Gyabenkrom, Western Region, 27 October 2017; Aunty Moses, Adjumako, Western Region, 23rd October, 2017; Araba Yedua, Gyabenkrom, Western Region, 27th October, 2017. This will be explored further in later chapters.
108 Cardinall, *The Gold Coast, 1931*, 219.
109 Ibid., 213.
110 Wellcome, PP/CDW/B.1/1: C. D. Williams, 'Mortality and Morbidity', 29.

111 BDL, MSS.Afr.s.1872/154, Box 43: Williams, C. 'Kwashiorkor', reprinted from *The Lancet*, 16th November, 1935, 1151. See also Nott, 'Between Famine and Malnutrition', 41–43.
112 Russell, 'Malnutrition in Children', 110.
113 Interview with Ama Fosua, Adua Bensua, Nana Esebu and Esi Mensema, Barabadze, Central Region, 30 November 2017.
114 Wellcome, PP/CDW/B.1/1: C. D. Williams, 'Mortality and Morbidity of Children of the Gold Coast', Thesis for Doctorate of Medicine, Oxford, 1936, 35.
115 Nott, 'Between Famine and Malnutrition', 92.
116 Russell, 'Malnutrition in Children', 110.
117 Cardinall, *The Gold Coast, 1931*, 220.
118 Jean Allman, 'Rounding Up Spinsters: Gender Chaos and Unmarried Women in Colonial Asante', *The Journal of African History* 37, no. 2 (1996): 212.
119 Kyei, *Our Days Dwindle*, 99.
120 Cardinall, *The Gold Coast, 1931*, 220.
121 LN, R20/29429/3099: *Report on the British Mandated Sphere of Togoland for 1922*, Accra, 1923, 17.
122 LN, R20/44616/3099: *Report by His Majesty's Government on the Administration under Mandate of British Togoland for the Year 1924*, Non-Parliamentary Publication Colonial No. 14, London, 1925, 55.
123 LN, R20/29429/3099: *Report on the British Mandated Sphere of Togoland for 1922*, Accra, 1923, 17.
124 Cardinall, *The Gold Coast, 1931*, 221.
125 See for example LN, R20/44616/3099: *Report by His Majesty's Government on the Administration under Mandate of British Togoland for the Year 1924*, Non-Parliamentary Publication Colonial No. 14, London, 1925, 58.
126 Hugon, *Être mère en situation coloniale*, 144.
127 Cardinall, *The Gold Coast, 1931*, 243.
128 *Colonial Reports-Annual No. 1207 Gold Coast Report for 1922–1923*, Government Press, Accra, 1924, 35.
129 *Colonial Reports-Annual No. 1255 Gold Coast Report for 1923–1924*, Government Press, Accra, 1925, 54.
130 *Colonial Reports-Annual No. 1333 Gold Coast Report for 1926–1927*, Government Press, Accra, 1927, 25.
131 Cardinall, *The Gold Coast, 1931*, 243.
132 PRAAD, Accra, CSO 11/16/6: *Annual Summary and Report of Principal Registrar of Births, Deaths and Burials of the Gold Coast, 1931*, Government Printing Office, Accra, 1932, 6.
133 Philippe Bourmaud, 'Internationalizing Perspectives: Re-Reading Mandate History through a Health Policy Lens', *Canadian Bulletin of Medical History* 30, no. 2 (2013): 13.
134 Corinna Unger, 'Histories of Development and Modernization: Findings, Reflections, Future Research', *H-Soz-Kult. Kommunikation Und Fachinformation Für Die Geschichtswissenschaften* (2010), 7.
135 Gilbert Rist, *The History of Development: From Western Origins to Global Faith*, trans. Patrick Camiller (London: Zed Books Ltd, 2008), 40.
136 Ibid., 14.
137 Jean Comaroff and John Comaroff, 'Homemade Hegemony: Modernity, Domesticity, and Colonialism in South Africa', in *African Encounters with Domesticity*, ed. Karen Tranberg Hansen (New Brunswick, NJ: Rutgers University Press, 1992), 40.
138 Michael N. Barnett, *Empire of Humanity: A History of Humanitarianism* (Ithaca, NY: Cornell University Press, 2011), 62.

139 Richard Rathbone, 'World War I and Africa: Introduction', *The Journal of African History* 19, no. 1 (1978): 1–9.
140 Joseph M. Hodge and Gerald Hodl, 'Introduction', in *Developing Africa: Concepts and Practices in Twentieth-Century Colonialism*, ed. Joseph M. Hodge, Gerald Hodl, and Martina Kopf (Manchester, MA: Manchester University Press, 2014), 7.
141 Frederick John Dealtry Lugard, *The Dual Mandate in British Tropical Africa* (London: W. Blackwood and Sons, 1922), 6.
142 Emily Baughan, *Saving the Children: Humanitarianism, Internationalism, and Empire*, Berkeley Series in British Studies 19 (Oakland, CA: University of California Press, 2022), 82.
143 Richard Rathbone, *Nkrumah and the Chiefs: Politics of Chieftaincy in Ghana 1951–1960*, 1st ed. edition (Oxford: James Currey, 2000), 14.
144 Allman, 'Rounding Up Spinsters', 211.
145 Comaroff and Comaroff, 'Homemade Hegemony', 64.
146 Joseph M. Hodge, *Triumph of the Expert: Agrarian Doctrines of Development and the Legacies of British Colonialism* (Athens, OH: Ohio University Press, 2007), 117.
147 Covenant of the League of Nations. Accessed: http://avalon.law.yale.edu/20th_century/leagcov.asp [Last accessed 22/02/2022].
148 Paul Nugent, *Africa since Independence*, 2nd edition (New York: Palgrave Macmillan, 2012), 12.
149 Philippe Bourmaud, 'Internationalizing Perspectives: Re-Reading Mandate History through a Health Policy Lens', *Canadian Bulletin of Medical History* 30, no. 2 (1 October 2013): 13.
150 Susan Pedersen, *The Guardians: The League of Nations and the Crisis of Empire* (Oxford: Oxford University Press, 2015), 4–13.
151 Lara Putnam, 'Global Child-Saving, Transatlantic Maternalism, and the Pathologization of Caribbean Childhood, 1930s–1940s', *Atlantic Studies* 11, no. 4 (2 October 2014): 491–514; Susan Pedersen, 'The Maternalist Moment in British Colonial Policy: The Controversy over 'Child Slavery' in Hong Kong 1917–1941', *Past & Present* 171 (2001): 161–202.
152 Iris Borowy, *Coming to Terms with World Health: The League of Nations Health Organisation 1921–1946* (Frankfurt am Main: Lang, 2009), 184.
153 LN, see file 8A/24734/247/34.
154 LN, 8F/13300/321: 'Memorandum Relating to the Enquiries into the Causes and Prevention of Still Births and Mortality during the First Year of Life', 1929, 1.
155 LN, 12B/44130/15313: 'A Note on the Report of the East Africa Commission', n.d. but July 1925, 2–3.
156 Ibid., 5–6.
157 Ibid., 6–7.
158 LN, R20/29429/3099: *Report on the British Mandated Sphere of Togoland for 1922*, Accra, 1923, 17.
159 LN, A.9.1927.III: 'Annual Report for the Health Organisation for 1926', 4 February 1927, 24; A.8.1929.III, 'Annual Report for the Health Organisation for 1928', 18 April 1929, 46.
160 See: Juanita De Barros, *Reproducing the British Caribbean: Sex, Gender, and Population Politics After Slavery* (Chapel Hill: UNC Press Books, 2014), 88–89. on the perception of 'grandmothers' in the colonial Caribbean.
161 *Quarterly Bulletin of the Health Organisation. Vol II*, Geneva, June 1933, 102.
162 Ibid., 106.
163 LN, 8A/22248/12886: 'Conference Panafricaine Novembre 1935 Procès-verbaux', 23 November 1935, 4.
164 Ibid.

165 League of Nations, A.9.1930.III: 'Annual Report for the Health Organisation for 1929', July 1930, 35.
166 Sunil S. Amrith, *Decolonizing International Health: India and Southeast Asia, 1930–65*, Cambridge Imperial and Post-Colonial Studies Series (Basingstoke: Palgrave Macmillan, 2006), 27–29.
167 LN, 8A/22248/12886: 'Conference Panafricaine Novembre 1935 Procès-verbaux', 23d November 1935, 9–19.
168 Ibid., 22.
169 Ibid., 8.
170 Ibid., 9.
171 SOAS, CBMS/IMC, Box 264: 'Legislative Council of the Gold Coast Message Addressed by His Excellency the Governor, to the Legislative Council', 1919, 1.
172 SOAS, CBMS/IMC, Box 264: 'The Post-War Gold Coast. A Review of the Events of 1923' by Sir Gordon Guggisberg, Governor, 1924, 65.
173 David E. Apter, *Ghana in Transition* (New York: Atheneum, 1963), 73.
174 Jonathan Roberts, 'Remembering Korle Bu Hospital: Biomedical Heritage and Colonial Nostalgia in the "Golden Jubilee Souvenir"', *History in Africa* 38 (2011): 197.
175 SOAS, CBMS/IMC, Box 264: 'The Post-War Gold Coast. A Review of the Events of 1923' by Sir Gordon Guggisberg, Governor, 1924, 87.
176 Hodge, *Triumph of the Expert*, 123.
177 Boddy argues that a similar dynamic occurred in Sudan at the end of the First World War as demographic concerns and the end of the war led to a resumption of development goals in the colonies. Janice Boddy, *Civilizing Women: British Crusades in Colonial Sudan* (Princeton, NJ: Princeton University Press, 2007), 184–85.
178 Jean-Germain Gros, *Healthcare Policy in Africa: Institutions and Politics from Colonialism to the Present* (London: Rowman & Littlefield Publishers, 2015), 45; Anne Hugon, 'La Redéfinition de La Maternité En Gold Coast, Des Années 1920 Aux Années 1950: Projet Colonial et Réalités Locales", in *Histoire Des Femmes En Situation Coloniale Afrique et Asie, XXe Siècle*, ed. Anne Hugon (Paris: Editions Karthala, 2004), 147; Karl Ittmann, *Problem of Great Importance,* 58.
179 Nancy Rose Hunt, '"Le Bébé En Brousse": European Women, African Birth Spacing, and Colonial Intervention in Breast Feeding in the Belgian Congo', in *Tensions of Empire: Colonial Cultures in a Bourgeois World*, ed. Frederick Cooper and Ann Laura Stoler (London: University of California Press, 1997), 288.
180 Shahrukh Rafi Khan, *A History of Development Economics Thought: Challenges and Counter-Challenges* (New York: Routledge, 2014), 2.
181 Margaret Jones, 'Infant and Maternal Health Services in Ceylon, 1900–1948: Imperialism or Welfare?', *Social History of Medicine* 15, no. 2 (2002): 263–89.
182 Ibid., 143.
183 SOAS, CBMS/IMC, Box 264: 'The Post-War Gold Coast. A Review of the Events of 1923' by Sir Gordon Guggisberg, Governor, 1924, 87.
184 BDL, MSS.Brit.Emp.s.470, Box 10: 'Simple Advice of Personal Hygiene' by A. Chas Lorena, Acting Deputy Director of Sanitary Services, 10 October 1922, 8.
185 PRAAD, Accra, CSO 11/6/8: 'British Red Cross Society Gold Coast Branch', 26 June 1932.
186 See Chapter 2 of this book.
187 Apter, *Ghana in Transition*, 73.
188 PRAAD, Accra, ADM 7/1/65: 'Blue Book 1931–32', Government Printer, Accra, 1932 and ADM 7/1/66:'Blue Book 1932–33', Government Printer, Accra, 1933.
189 Gareth Austin, 'Cash Crops and Freedom: Export Agriculture and the Decline of Slavery in Colonial West Africa', *International Review of Social History* 54, no. 1 (April 2009): 26.
190 NA, CO 96/702/1: 'Infant Welfare Centres: General Principles', 21 March 1932, 7.
191 Ibid.

192 PRAAD, Accra, CSO 11/4/9: 'Synopsis of the Maternity and Infant Welfare Movement in Accra' Enclosed in Letter to Acting Director of Medical and Sanitary Service, 13 January 1933, 2.
193 It is also possible that the figure from 1921 is higher than it would usually be due to the consequences of a temporary trade depression lasting from late 1920 – late 1921. See: *Colonial Reports Annual No. 1154. Gold Coast Report for 1921*, London, 1923, 6.
194 Anne Hugon, *Être mère en situation coloniale: Gold Coast, 1910–1950*, Histoire contemporaine 28 (Paris: Éditions de la Sorbonne, 2020), 135–36.
195 SOAS, CBMS/IMC, Box 264: 'The Gold Coast: A Review of the Events 1924–25 and the prospects of 1925–26' by His Excellency Brigadier-General Sir Frederick Gordon Guggisberg, Accra, 1925, 112.
196 PRAAD, Kumasi, ARG 1/14/15: Letter from John Maxwell, Chief Commissioner Ashanti, to Acting Colonial Secretary, 19 April 1924.
197 Hugon, *Être mère en situation coloniale*, 136–38. Hugon describes the event in detail including photographs of the winner and her mother. Interestingly, the proud mother is alternatively dressed in European clothing and then in very impressive *kente* illustrating her elite status.
198 'Princess Marie Louise', *Gold Coast Independent*, 25 April 1925, 830.
199 NA, CO 96/679/2: 'Report of the Medical and Sanitary Department for the year ended April 1926 – March 1927', Government Printer, Accra, 1927, 36.
200 Hugon, *Être mère en situation coloniale*, 85.
201 NA, CO 96/679/2: 'Report of the Medical and Sanitary Department for the year ended April 1926 – March 1927', Government Printer, Accra, 1927, 36.
202 PRAAD, Accra, CSO 11/1/315: 'Letter: Dr Duff, Director Medical and Sanitary Service, to the Colonial Secretary', 12 July 1933.
203 PRAAD, Accra, ADM 7/1/64: 'Blue Book of Statistics, 1929–1930', Government Printer, Accra 1931, 829–1037.
204 PRAAD, Accra, CSO 11/4/9: 'Maternal Mortality' Enclosed in Letter to Acting Director of Medical and Sanitary Service, 13 January 1933.
205 PRAAD, Accra, CSO 11/2/3: Letter from Acting Secretary of Native Affairs, Chairman of the Board of Visitors to Acting Colonial Secretary, 3 October 1933, 3.
206 PRAAD, Accra, ADM 5/1/128: *Report of the Medical Department for the Year 1932–1933*, Government Printer, Accra, 84.
207 PRAAD, Accra, CSO 11/2/10: 'Board of Visitors to the Gold Coast Hospital and the Maternity Hospital', 25 May 1939, 8.
208 PRAAD, Accra, CSO 11/2/3: Letter from Acting Secretary of Native Affairs, Chairman of the Board of Visitors to Acting Colonial Secretary, 3 October 1933, 3–4.
209 PRAAD, Cape Coast, ADM 23/1/2088: 'Notes on Visit to Winneba', 22 May 1934.
210 PRAAD, Accra, ADM 5/3/26: 'Dr Inness Report on the Scheme for the establishment in British West Africa of a college for the training of medical practitioners', 1926, 48.
211 PRAAD, Accra, CSO 11/2/3: Letter from Acting Secretary of Native Affairs, Chairman of the Board of Visitors to Acting Colonial Secretary, 3 October 1933, 4.
212 PRAAD Accra holds the personal files of many of the women who trained as midwives at this school. However, at present the majority of their files do not appear in the PF finding aid. Those files that were available indicated that women usually attended government or mission schools up to Standard VII before applying to train as midwives. For example, Margaret Eva Nachoi Addy was 18 when she began training in 1928 having completed her education at Accra Government Girls' School (see PF 3/32/49). Miss Randolph also attended this school and her reference, like Margaret's came from Ruby Quartey Papafio, who was involved with the Gold Coast League. She applied at age 19 (see PF 3/32/842). Constance Acolaste was 17 and had just completed her education at Ewe Presbyterian Senior School (see PF 3/32/14). Others did not fit this pattern, for example Hepzibah Henrietta Quartey, who came

from Belgian Congo and was 26 when she began training in 1931 having previously worked as a seamstress (see PF 3/32/820).

213 Cardinall, *The Gold Coast, 1931*, 190.

214 Hugon, *Etre mère en situation coloniale,* chapter 5. Anne Hugon, 'Korle Bu and the Midwives Hostel as a Site of Memory for Ghanaian Pupil Midwives, 1930s–1950s', *Ghana Studies* 7 (2004): 43–58.

215 Hugon, *Être mère en situation coloniale*, 154–57.

216 PRAAD, Accra, CSO 5/1/327: 'Extract from file 1488/30', 5 March 1931.

217 PRAAD, Accra, CSO 5/1/327: 'The Midwives Ordinance', 1931.

218 PRAAD, Accra, CSO 5/1/327: See extract from Legislative Council Minutes, n.d.

219 PRAAD, Accra, CSO 5/1/327: Letter from Provincial Council of Chiefs, Central Province, to the Acting Commissioner of Cape Coast, 22 September 1931.

220 PRAAD, Accra, CSO 5/1/327: Letter from Nana Annor Adjaye, Omanhene in Nzima, to Commissioner of the Western Province, 10 September 1931.

221 PRAAD, Accra, CSO 11/6/4: Letter from Dr. Selwyn-Clarke to the Colonial Secretary, Accra, 28 June 1932.

222 NA, CO 96/702/1: 'Appendix K: Illustrating various opinions on Infant Welfare showing the history of local movement, etc.', 1932, 5.

223 PRAAD, Accra, CSO 11/6/8: 'British Red Cross Society Gold Coast Branch', 26 June 1932.

224 BDL, MSS.Brit.emp.s.470, Box 9: 'Report on the British Red Cross Society on the Gold Coast', 1932.

2 Humanitarianism in the Gold Coast 1932–1939

The Establishment of Maternal and Infant Welfare

Introduction

In the 1930s Gold Coast, it was humanitarian organisations rather than the colonial government that pushed for the expansion of maternal and child welfare services. These included the Gold Coast League for Maternal and Child Welfare (GCLMCW), Save the Children and, most significantly, the Red Cross. They did so in the name of 'developmental humanitarianism' that championed women and children. During this period, humanitarian organisations began to institutionalise and find peace-time roles based on developmental humanitarianism, which sought long-term progress in social and economic terms.[1] Compassion for African women and children was evoked globally, and this rhetoric became powerful locally on the Gold Coast as Africans fought for maternal and child welfare services to remain. Activists working between metropoles and colonies, not just in the British Empire, 'made child welfare a common language across multiple sites.'[2]

Narratives of victimised and ignorant women, unable to tend to their own health needs, were transposed onto Gold Coast women. The establishment of this trope was dependent on the emergence of another category of woman though, the developed and 'progressive' mother. Maternal and child welfare was adopted as a signifier by an elite group of Africans and Europeans living in Gold Coast towns. Susan Pedersen characterised the interwar period as a time when 'women's organisations began to claim colonial policy as their own, insisting on their responsibility as equal citizens, for the management and "uplift" of women and children across the colonial Empire.' Labelling this the 'maternalist moment' in imperial humanitarianism, Pedersen shows how women became both activists and recipients under humanitarian internationalism.[3] Whilst Pedersen is referring to European women, through maternal and child welfare, African women on the Gold Coast also found ways to perform their progressive status. Humanitarian development during the late 1920s and 1930s was crucial in forming two strata of Gold Coast women: firstly, the 'African woman' as an 'underdeveloped' victim; secondly, maternal and child welfare organisation fixed African women's position in a burgeoning civil society within the colony, giving them a role that defined them as 'progressive' in opposition to their 'backward' sisters.

DOI: 10.4324/9781003274162-3

Many of these women were part of the GCLMCW. This organisation was an important agent in the medicalisation of childbirth and rearing in 1920s Accra. It was supported by government-funded clinics and hospitals. However, the colonial state's provision of welfare centres was quickly threatened in two ways. Firstly, centres were heavily criticised by the medical department, which saw them as overly curative, neglecting preventative work.[4] Whilst this might have been overcome in different circumstances, the beginning of the 1930s saw a global economic depression. This was exacerbated locally by a resumption of a series of cocoa hold-ups, during which farmers refused to sell their beans in response to buying cartels, which had pushed prices down. Welfare clinics were marked for immediate closure. Outraged by this, Dr Selwyn-Clarke, the Deputy Director of Health Services, applied to London to set up a Branch of the British Society of the Red Cross in the Gold Coast (GCRC), which was established in 1932.

This Red Cross Branch had the express aim of safeguarding and eventually expanding maternal and child health services. Although general histories of medicine in Ghana treat it as unremarkable, the history of the almost comprehensive takeover of maternal and child welfare by a humanitarian organisation in the 1930s is important. Historians have not dwelt on the fact that the state could not, or did not care to, continue these services but that *they survived anyway*.[5] Intervention into what had developed as a state responsibility, by a transnational humanitarian organisation, was significant. As the Red Cross took over the state's role in providing these health services, we arguably see a much earlier precedent for the prominent role of NGOs in global health from the 1980s onwards. Anne Hugon has also noted that this takeover was framed as positive since it allowed Africans to take responsibility for their own healthcare.[6] Indeed, Gold Coasters implemented maternal and child welfare *themselves* by fighting against clinic closures at this time and through the formation of the Red Cross. This is an important part of a longer history of development discourses that affected the implementation of health in Ghana.

Shaping Maternal and Child Welfare Centres

Attendances at welfare centres and hospitals point to a shift in social norms. The establishment of biomedical healing systems in Africa has been understood as a clash between healing systems, with biomedicine supposedly alienating Africans – particularly women – from their social networks.[7] As hospitals were established for Africans' use, officials often complained that they would only attend, having exhausted all alternative options. In 1930, the Commissioner for the Central Province noted that 'even the most enlightened African will leave the qualified man and seek the advice of a native practitioner if he considers his progress is not sufficiently speedy.'[8] However, the rapid uptake of services belies the view that women avoided biomedical options. Instead, women who had the chance to attend maternal and infant welfare clinics usually opted to do this *as well* as turning to more established methods. Interviewees testifying about their own, and earlier generations', experiences of childbirth almost never reported that women chose a single option for their healthcare at the exclusion of others.[9] It is therefore unsurprising that somebody might 'leave the qualified man' in search of other options, especially since pregnant women frequently had recourse to family members or to a spiritual healer or herbalist.

In other words, women were proactive figures in a pluralistic medical system and shaped it to their own needs. When maternal and infant welfare centres were established, they quickly became popular, according to colonial records. In Koforidua and Cape Coast for example, Dr Selwyn-Clarke noted that 'the popularity of the centres was so great that new Centres had to be constructed,' expanding the temporary buildings that were established in 1929 and 1928, respectively. Similarly, the temporary clinic established in Kumasi in 1927 was expanded to include 24 cots and beds by 1928.[10] This was driven by demand. Figures show a dramatic rise in attendance at maternal and infant welfare centres between 1927 and 1932 when services were disrupted due to closures (Figure 2.1). Interestingly, although the clinics began by treating infants almost exclusively (there is no record for the number of expectant mothers seen in 1927), the proportion of expectant mothers to infants treated rose sharply from 3% of the total in 1927 to 15% by 1931.

Despite fears that Africans would avoid western medicine, the Gold Coast governor wrote in 1930 that 'the benefits of … clinics are now fully appreciated by the mothers, who readily bring their children to them for examination and treatment immediately when they show signs of illness.'[11] This call for *treatment* from mothers though was not seen positively by all concerned. Dr Duff complained bitterly that services had become 'curative' rather than 'preventative' as they were originally envisaged. Indeed, it was hoped to '[cut] out all treatment

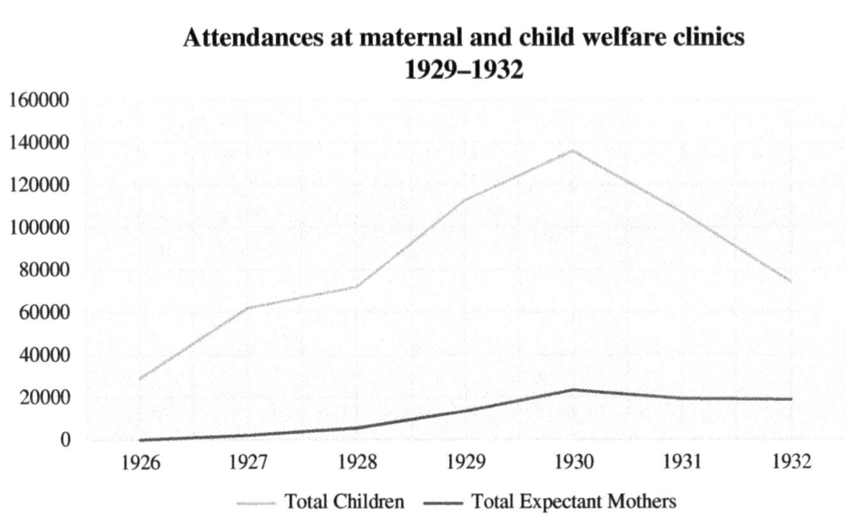

Figure 2.1 Attendances at maternal and child welfare clinics 1927–1933. Gold Coast Government reports on the Medical and Sanitary Department, 1927 through to 1933.

… and [stress] their educational and advisory aspects.' However, by the early 1930s, they had become '99% curative.'[12] He blamed this partially on Women Medical Officers (WMOs), who had been employed to focus solely on welfare work but found it 'too dull,' according to Dr Duff.[13] In defence of the clinics and their women doctors, Drs Quin and Selwyn-Clarke stressed the practicalities of offering treatment in communities where infectious diseases such as yaws and malaria were rife.[14]

Indeed, mothers came to centres seeking treatment for their children, and, to a lesser extent, for themselves. Dr Mackay, Assistant Director of the Health Service, argued that clinics were a 'powerful means of health propaganda' and that soon the educational side would gain ground over the purely curative. Although 'the idea of [not] giving any treatment whatever' was, he said, 'ideal,' it just wasn't feasible at this time.[15] Dr Vane Percy, WMO, wrote:

> the African mother is too uneducated to appreciate advice unless it is backed by a bottle of medicine. To encourage this in her may be wrong, but in her present state of ignorance and superstition, it is in my experience the only way of attaining improvement in the health of her children.[16]

Looking beyond this derogatory language, we can re-interpret the situation. Mothers were demanding medicines and treatment as their principal, or only, reason to go to clinics. Dr Cicely Williams described a similar situation in which mothers were supposed to attend weekly with 'well babies.' However, she said, 'there are only two or three mothers who understand the importance of attending every week.'[17] This might be less to do with mothers' 'understanding' though, and more to do with their using clinics differently than was envisaged, that is, only when treatment was needed.

Since clinics became 99% curative, mothers were evidently successful in tailoring them to their needs. Incidentally, this was not only a matter of 'treatment.' Mothers also took away 'soap liniment or a few grey powders' from clinics' mothercraft lessons and only attended when these commodities were offered.[18] Dr Selwyn-Clarke gave the emotive example of a woman who might come to the clinic for 'salts' for a child suffering from malnutrition and be discovered to have a small pelvis. 'Who,' he demanded, 'will say that the possible saving of a life of mother and child does not justify such "treatment"?' The scorn in the use of this last word is almost palpable from the paper it is written on. He pointed out that over one-fifth of all outpatient attendances in the Gold Coast was to welfare clinics, representing 7,866 women for ante-natal care in 1930–1931. In the same period, Dr Selwyn-Clarke stressed the effectiveness of WMOs by highlighting that the average number of patients seen by WMOs and their male counterparts were 8,818 and 2,581, respectively.[19] These figures suggest that although in proportion to the general population, attendance at clinics might appear low when it came to those seeking medical attention, maternal and child welfare represented a large proportion. Indeed, Dr Piegrome, WMO argued that the welfare clinics were 'the most popular or all the medical establishments' in the colony.[20]

Closing the Centres

The Governor wrote in 1931 that 'it is unavoidable but unfortunate that the serious diminution of the Colony's resources during the present and forthcoming financial years will entail further drastic reductions in the expenditure of all branches of the Medical Department.'[21] Due to a global economic depression, colonial governments had less money to spend, which led to the retrenchment of certain colonial officers. Dr Duff, Director of Medical and Sanitary Services, had to decide where to make cuts. It was partly their curative nature that made Dr Duff see maternal and infant welfare clinics as superfluous. He did not consider ante-natal work economically advantageous since the majority of cases of childbirth were 'normal,' so it seemed a waste to keep checks on women's health. Furthermore, he made the (sadly, realistic) point that: 'when a serious ante-natal diagnosis is made what have we to offer? Accra is the only place where a Maternity Hospital exists.' Therefore, he argued that ante-natal and post-natal work carried out by WMOs did not justify their employment by the colonial government.[22] Dr Cicely Williams, one of these WMOs, observed that, at this time, maternal and child health was seen as a 'fancy trimming' of the medical service.[23] In 1931, the first clinic at Christiansborg was closed and handed over to a private practitioner. By 1932, the number of WMOs had been halved, from eight to four,[24] and the clinics at Cape Coast and Sekondi were closed.[25]

The closure of clinics is significant because of the response it elicited from African leaders. The chiefs' and municipalities' adverse reaction to welfare centres' closure, in the context of anxiety over infant mortality explored in the previous chapter, appears to support Thomas Spear's point that 'by appealing to [Africans'] own values and institutions' relations with colonial authorities were built on 'mutual attractions.'[26] Dr Selwyn-Clarke declared, in his typically emotive fashion, that when the colonial government cut maternal and child welfare services in 1932, '[t]he African mother had learned to put her complete faith in the advice obtainable at the centres and looked forward with dismay to these services being considerably curtailed or stopped altogether.'[27] This evokes African women's supposed vulnerability. Although it is entirely untrue that women in the Gold Coast had put their 'complete faith' in clinics, women *were* engaging with and shaping services. This was especially true of elite and urban women.

A letter from the Kumasihene's office in 1932, signed by 12 local chiefs, expressed 'great disappointment' to hear rumours that the infant welfare clinic would be closing. He emphasised that this would show 'lack of sympathy on the part of the government to the children and women of this country.' In fact, many petitions and protests to the government emphasise how dependent women and children had become on government clinics. This complaint from Kumasi is particularly interesting: that before the establishment of a clinic, 'there were women who practiced obstetrics, however unqualified they might have been, and who have given up this practice at the expense of scientific methods introduced by the Whiteman.' The implication here is that the government cannot undo the irrevocable changes that it had made to Kumasi's health landscape. Although this is surely an exaggeration, it highlights the government's hypocrisy. The petition then states that people feared a return to 'considerably high' rates of infant mortality and that the closure of the clinic would go against the 'interests of the present generation and the prosperity.' This evokes a connection between a healthy and increasing population and the colony's prosperity. In sum, it argues, the clinic should remain open to prove that the British government was 'indeed a *paternal* government.' The Kumasihene pleaded that it 'continue to supply the needs of suffering humanity and especially of the children upon whom the future of this country depends.'[28] The language employed here undeniably taps into humanitarian discourse and imperial trusteeship.

Similarly, in February 1932, the Town Council of Cape Coast wrote to the Province's Commissioner to complain that the 'Lady' MO was to be removed and not replaced. They wrote that the clinic's 'good work had already spread over all the neighbouring towns and villages and its benefits are now realized even by those who were at first sceptical.' The petitioners note that infant mortality in the town had been reduced by 50%, which they attributed to the work of the clinic. Furthermore, the clinic helped local people, according to the petition, to appreciate 'scientific methods of treatment.' Finally, they stress that maternity work is of 'supreme importance' and request that the clinic be kept open.[29] Like Prempeh II and his fellow petitioners, the Council stressed the introduction of 'scientific methods.'

It was envisaged by the colonial government that Native Authorities would eventually re-open clinics. In a memorandum to the Governor, one official wrote: 'if the enthusiasm for Infant Welfare work … is genuine – and I have no reason whatever to doubt that it is – the native authorities will … devote some of the proceeds of the levy to [staffing clinics].'[30] Indeed, there were a number of examples of chiefs providing funds for clinics to be opened or to remain open. For example, in Dzodze in Keta District, chiefs raised £100 towards the building of a clinic and associated buildings for infant welfare. Since the 'people of Dzodze' had collected the money, they then demanded that the government play its part in providing the rest of the building expenses.[31] When making a donation to Cape Coast clinics, the Omanhene of Asebu employed humanitarian discourses of the time by emphasising that the 'children of the District' were dependent on the 'noble work' of 'natural ruler[s]' such as himself. He argued that he was obligated to support the Cape Coast welfare clinic and its work because of his duty to his people.[32]

Meanwhile in Sekondi, the Municipal Council also responded to clinic closures with disappointment. They proposed a practical scheme to keep theirs open, led by African women members of the local Gold Coast League.[33] They proposed that the Council, the local branch of the Gold Coast League, and the Government all pay a proportion of the amount that would be needed to keep the clinic open. In return for this ongoing, but much reduced, support from the government, it would keep all of the clinic's profits so that the government would pay £17 annually and could expect a revenue of £40. The clinic would be staffed by a WMO and volunteers: Mrs Dawson, from the League, alongside two, unnamed, 'African ladies.'[34] The WMO, Dr Piegrome, proposing to take over the clinic, emphasised that ante-natal work should be preserved since it was 'very popular and beneficial' and offered her services free to certain mothers so long as she be allowed to carry out her private practice.[35] In the end, the scheme did not go ahead as the Red Cross stepped in. What the episode shows, though, is that there was an active community, with access to government officials and funds, engaged in welfare work in the town. Furthermore, the question of maternal and infant welfare elicited a strong response from a range of actors, who clearly saw it as an important service in the town. The fact that senior, male political leaders were allocating funds and passing on demands for centres to stay open suggests that they were widely seen as positive. Dr Piegrome noted that '[t]his is the first time that the Africans have been sufficiently keen on any Government service to come together and collect money for its continuance.'[36] It was in this context of general opposition to the closure of clinics, and search for solutions, that the Red Cross was proposed.

Humanitarianism and African Women in the 1930s

The establishment of the League of Nations coincided with, and fuelled, a global humanitarian movement for maternal and infant welfare. Infant welfare had an 'emotional appeal' and in African colonies was an extension of nationalist efforts in metropoles.[37] International groups – increasingly led and populated by women– proliferated in this period and encouraged medicalisation of women's lives.[38] As colonisers and humanitarians began to focus on women and their health in the late 1920s, their aim was to bring about a change in women's practices and attitudes. Women's role in social reproduction was recognised by colonial officials and missionaries, who saw the 'pressing need for Christian wives' and began intervening ever more in women's lives from the 1920s.[39] African health practices were often depicted as timeless and the world of African women untouched by the agents of change. However, as Allman and Tashjian have shown, this was actually a period of extreme change in women's lives. In a world increasingly focused on production for trade and export, women's labour put them at the 'centre of material and economic developments,' but left them marginalised in the colonial political system, which prioritised the authority of male chiefs, and by the colonial economy.[40] Meanwhile, Christianity, new transport methods and increased medicalisation were changing the way women gave birth.

The GCLMCW was instrumental in the functioning of maternal and child welfare in the colony. Its first president was Lady Slater, wife of the governor. This reflected a pattern in imperial welfare work, in which women's public roles reflected their husbands,' but in a social capacity, usually connected with women and children. It was assumed that elite women held the solutions to the problems of their less fortunate sisters, simply by sharing their gender. Nancy Hunt has shown that in the Belgian Congo, the state, fearing depopulation 'saw a solution in European women.'[41] In humanitarianism, care is gendered and regarded as fcmininc.[42] This observation is even more pertinent in the context of activities related to childbirth and child-rearing. Voluntary work allowed European women to enter the masculine domain of imperial politics.[43] These European women were influential among networks of colonial officials in Accra. One official noted that he was discussing infant welfare centres at the Rodger Club, where Lady Slater was able to advise him about establishing committees for a new scheme.[44]

Most of the Gold Coast League's work was carried out in Accra, but there was also a very active group in Sekondi. Dr Quin, the town's Senior MO, described:

> the Welfare League was really doing some useful work in Sekondi. Lady Slater's visits were stimulating, meetings well attended, and some European ladies in company with Africans did domiciliary visiting in their allotted districts every week regularly.[45]

The League aimed to 'carry the doctrine of good personal and domestic hygiene into the compounds.'[46] Significantly, practices of medicalisation and reforms to both biological and social reproduction entered people's homes through the League. There is something invasive about attempting to alter 'personal and domestic' practices inside the home rather than providing services in spaces outside the home.

In some ways, European campaigns to improve motherhood and provide infant welfare travelled from metropole to colony. During the interwar period in Britain, a renewed sense of civic responsibility linked to increased voting rights, strengthened voluntarism.[47] Welfare associations, particularly for mothers and children, were reinforced by eugenic concerns after World War I. That the ill health of infants was mothers' responsibility because of their 'ignorance' was central to debates in Britain.[48] Lara Putnam writes that voluntary and municipal organisations formed to 'rescue working class children from poor home environments' from the late-nineteenth century.[49] In other words, we see similar practices and discourses in Britain to those which manifested in Gold Coast humanitarian organisations. However, Ulrike Lidner demonstrates that in Britain, the 1918 Maternity and Child Welfare Act meant that local authorities were forced to provide maternity services.[50] In contrast, on the Gold Coast, pressure came from an elite, non-governmental, section of society.

However, we certainly see a similar attitude in terms of European women coming to the aid of their African sisters. In Britain-, middle- and upper-class women volunteered in an attempt to reform motherhood for lower-class women. In the Gold Coast, it was the 'Mammies' – ordinary African mothers – who were the target. For example, Sylvia Ward, a music teacher who travelled to the Gold Coast alongside her husband,

> visited mothers and babies in the back streets of Accra, cases indicated to me by the medical authorities. Many mothers had very little knowledge of general health care, and although I had no children of my own, with the aid of an interpreter I was able to give helpful advice.[51]

In other words, despite a complete lack of qualifications, experience or even linguistic capability, Ward assumed that her gender – her innate caring role as a woman – and her societal position gave her authority. Beyond the Gold Coast, Dr Fraser, working in Nyasaland reforming hygienic practices of mothers, emphasised women's fear of new ideas. She said that 'fear and customary taboo were crippling to my work.' She gradually contested this until – the happy ending to this article – African women were able to laugh at how 'stupid' they had been.[52] Another British woman visitor to the Gold Coast was, on account of her gender, not her experience, sent to visit a Gold children's clinic. She describes the 'Mammies' as quite a 'nuisance' – '[t]hey would not sit down and wait their turn and, not unlike the English parent in *certain circles*, they had tremendous faith in a bottle of medicine.'[53] Certainly, in comparison to the doctors and assistants for whom the author is left 'full of admiration,' these 'mammies' appear very much in need of aid.[54] Whilst both of these women express sympathy for African mothers, their attitudes are condescending.

Jessie Griffith was a qualified midwife whose husband was employed by the colonial service. Her account of volunteering and running a mother and baby clinic in Savelegu shows how she differentiated between Gold Coast women and 'mammies.' Firstly, she noted that 'educated African wives gave up wearing the Mammy's cloth and wore European dress.' She socialised with these educated wives, 'the wives of teachers, lawyers, missionaries etc. with complete ease and happiness.' In contrast she describes 'watching' the Mammies from afar at the market. She noted their 'special dignity,' 'they worked hard ... [walking] as far as 12 miles and return again with a four gallon tin of brown infected water.'[55] The physical distance in her description reflects the wide disparity between herself and the 'mammies.' Her description is the epitome of the 'beast of burden' trope, Africans working hard in ignorance (note the dirty water) but with noble dignity.

Many scholars have commented on the subjectification of women through discourses of developmental humanitarianism. Women have frequently been framed as victims, especially of their own patriarchal societies.[56] Chandra Mohanty has argued that 'third world women' in contemporary development practice are depicted as constantly battling oppressive tradition, illiteracy, poverty, fanaticism, which 'freeze[s] third world women in time, space, and history.'[57] Her observation can certainly be applied to interwar colonisers in Africa. In the 1920s and 1930s they, and humanitarians, took an interest in women for the first time.[58] This led to the production of knowledge about and the formation of the subjective category of the 'African woman.' The construction of this figure as vulnerable, victimised and ignorant led to particular responses in terms of healthcare. Women were drawn into colonial governance and became simultaneously objects of gendered knowledge and compassion.

Colonial governments came under pressure regarding women's welfare. The Gold Coast government was obliged to answer questions from London about women's and girls' education and health.[59] For example, a circular was sent to colonial governments in Africa in 1930 to determine whether the circumcision of girls was practised, and if so, how governments were responding. The governor of the Gold Coast, G. C. du Boulay, replied that the practice did not exist in Ashanti or the Colony but was 'widely prevalent' in the Northern

Territories, causing 'intense suffering to the girl.'[60] Two years later, the matter arose again in the British Parliament.[61] Acting Governor Northcote informed Sir Philip Cunliffe-Lister, Secretary of State for the Colonies, that MOs in the North were carrying out a 'campaign of propaganda' against the practice but that its force was measured so as not to arouse 'suspicion and resentment.' Meanwhile, Catholic missionaries were making some progress by banning it amongst their members.[62] Unsatisfied by Sir Philip's response in Parliament, Colonel Wedgewood asked if he would put an end to 'ugly practices on African women,' by providing them with education.[63] Two interesting points arise here. Firstly, it reflects the growing notion that colonial governments ought to be providing welfare and education specifically for women. Secondly G.C. du Boulay's original reply to Lord Passfield in 1930 focused on circumcision primarily as a population issue. He addressed it in terms of its effect on women's 'fecundity' and reassured the Secretary that the colony's population was increasing. Furthermore, he pointed out the positive work being done by infant welfare clinics, suggesting that they were considered a panacea for harmful practices for African women.[64]

As explained previously, in the Gold Coast, colonial health services had first served working men. Dr Mary Blacklock, WMO, who worked to improve the conditions of women across the empire, pointed out the systematically gendered nature of medical services:

> the early activities in the development of most colonies were chiefly the concern of men … Men from the home countries generally originated these works and it was the male members of the local populations who assisted in developing them. As a result of this … hospitals were engaged chiefly in treating men patients.[65]

Meanwhile, women were held responsible for maternal and infant mortality as we saw in the previous chapter. Dr Blacklock wrote that 'when efforts were made to improve matters, surprising difficulties were often encountered. Difficulty sometimes arose from the timidity of local women and from their suspicion of strange foreign customs and institutions.'[66] This statement offers a logical explanation for women's reluctance but still manages to express surprise at it. African women were therefore trebly hindered – in the eyes of colonialists and humanitarians – because of their gender, their race and because of their ignorance. These three categories of identity intersected in the sense that African women's racial and social background was seen to hinder them more than their male counterparts.

Women were viewed as particularly vulnerable to a general lack of knowledge on hygiene amongst the population. Dr Selwyn-Clarke observed that:

> in many … primitive communities, where laws of hygiene are not carefully observed owing to ignorance or neglect, loss of life, particularly in children under one year and in mothers at childbirth – is very high.[67]

He saw the risk due to ignorance as particularly high in the Gold Coast, where 'a considerable amount of ill health among the women … is attributable to the filthy and sometimes violent methods practiced by native midwives.'[68] Women and very young children were almost always lumped together as one vulnerable group, which led to women's health being subsumed into a general provision of 'child' or 'infant' welfare, especially when services were first established.

Arturo Escobar describes the 'underdeveloped woman' depicted as 'oppressed by its own stubbornness, lack of initiative and traditions.'[69] This reflects entirely Blacklock's thoughts on the needs of colonised women in the 1930s. In fact, Blacklock's central point that women would fear entering medical institutions, chiefly because of the presence of men, homogenises women across the empire. She wasn't the only colonial official to misread women's 'traditional' practices. For example, colonial officials argued that African women did not attend hospitals to give birth because of their loyalty to the practice of giving birth in their 'kitchens.'[70] Gold Coast women rarely had kitchens as such, and although it is doubtless the case that women preferred home births, the reasons for this were varied. Indeed, both Blacklock and Escobar's evaluation of 'underdeveloped' women can be revised when we see, for example, the way in which they shaped services in the Gold Coast earlier in this chapter.

Save the Children

In 1931, Save the Children organised a conference on the 'African Child.' This conference examined the educational, occupational and health needs of African children, at a time when the definition of an African 'child' was contested under colonial rule.[71] It also gave much attention to the 'African Mother' in her own right. The conference was dominated by European missionaries.[72] There were only five Africans among representatives, including J. W. de Graft Johnson, a delegate from the Gold Coast. There were a number of Red Cross representatives and delegates from the Gold Coast, including missionaries, colonial officials, anthropologist R. S. Rattray and The Reverend A. G. Fraser, Principal of Achimota College. Delegates from the Gold Coast were all men, with the exception of Miss Sutherland from the Church of Scotland Mission. Three of their wives attended as 'associate members,' underlining women's roles in aiding women and children in the colonies but not necessarily as leaders.[73]

The conference was held in Geneva, home to the League of Nations. However, since the conference was directed by an independent, humanitarian organisation, critiques of imperialism ran through it. There was a tension between delegates' belief that development was necessary for Africans' well-being and the harm that this might do to Africa's children. The 'abuses of industrialisation' were listed as a matter to be 'taken up without delay.'[74] In the lead-up to the Conference in March 1931, Save the Children's periodical addressed the key contradiction of imperialism: was its purpose of keeping Africans subjugated or work towards their 'well-being and development' for the 'general welfare of mankind'?[75] Later in June 1931 a short article was published by the Secretary of State for the Colonies, Lord

Passfield, stating that the reduction of infant mortality would be of 'the greatest economic benefit' to Africa. This, he says, 'is not merely a humanitarian question.'[76] Save the Children emphasised children's potential long-term impact on the social and economic development of the continent. This attitude lies at the heart of developmental humanitarianism. Indeed, Emily Baughan has shown that any serious critique of imperialism at the conference, particularly from its black delegates, was shut down as 'political' and outside of the conference's remit. Overall, this was an endorsement of imperialism-as-trusteeship.[77]

Delegates stressed the significance of 'social maladies' and 'anti-moral, anti-hygienic and superstitious practices widespread in Africa' as causes for infant mortality, placing blame on African women.[78] However, African women became objects of compassion both by virtue of their poverty and their gender. Delegates there spoke of their 'burden,' living in 'wretched huts,' underfed and working long hours. They concluded that African women were 'more "beasts of burden" than human beings.'[79] 'The African woman' was an 'economic asset' with 'cash value,' chosen by husbands on the basis that 'she will be able to bear children,' according to Save the Children's magazine *The World's Children*.[80] Somewhat contradictorily, the 'tribe' or African social structures were said to be breaking down, leaving women and children vulnerable due to a lack of social services.

Birth was seen as a particularly dangerous time for women. One representative from South Africa, Dr Secherhaye, stated: 'I can testify myself to the ease with which a confinement becomes a drama in which the life of the mother and baby is at stake … Impossible to paint the moral and physical sufferings which are involved in a difficult birth among the heathen.'[81] Note here that this is not only a physical problem but also a moral one. This narrative, and the strength of the language it was expressed in, had a dehumanising effect. Arguably without much real understanding, humanitarians adopted narrative conventions that painted African women as victims of a patriarchal and barbaric society.[82]

Health was an important topic at the conference. Before it began, Save the Children made enquiries to colonial officials, missionaries and educators as to current regimes of healthcare in Africa.[83] Respondents, who were mainly missionaries, were asked to identify social factors in high rates of infant mortality and asked whether African women received any instruction in childcare or health. It also pushed respondents to describe 'superstitious or unhealthy practices of midwives that augment levels of infant mortality' or indeed any other 'customs or practices' doing the same.[84] The way these questions were constructed indicates that the causes of infant mortality were pre-decided: blame lay with women's social conditions and cultural practices. However, although discussion at the conference mainly reiterated problems such as the ignorance of mothers, not feeding babies properly and even infanticide, it was pointed out that labour patterns – particularly women working through pregnancies – resulted in infant mortality.[85] During the conference itself, the issue of forced labour was discussed, implicitly laying the blame for infant mortality on colonial governments as well as Africans.[86]

Save the Children's language highlights the paternalism that Michael Barnett amongst others identifies in humanitarian ideology.[87] Blame towards African mothers for their 'archaic beliefs' and 'ignorance of elementary hygiene' was mixed with expressions of sympathy for women who were 'beasts of burden,' a common metaphor for African women in this period.[88] Baughan has pointed out that Save the Children's interest in African children was to integrate them into the global economic order and to ensure that they benefitted from this.[89] Crucially, delegates relied above all on maternal solutions. It was principally through reforming motherhood that humanitarians saw the way forward for imperialism in the interwar period.

The Red Cross

When clinics closed in the Gold Coast, it was an international humanitarian organisation to whom the Dr Selwyn-Clarke turned. The Red Cross had been providing medical care internationally since its establishment in 1863. Its style was that of 'emergency humanitarianism,' responding to urgent needs, typically in war time.[90] However, it underwent significant changes following World War I as the International Committee for the Red Cross began reforming its peace-time role. Although many within the organisation defended the traditional role of the Red Cross, the head of the American Red Cross, Henry Davison, pushed for change. He worked to realise his vision of an organisation that looked to the health and welfare of needful beneficiaries in a new peace-time role.[91] Barnett identifies this move to a longer-term commitment to look at and tackle the *causes*, rather than the outcomes, of suffering, as the 'most revolutionary shift' in humanitarianism.[92]

A shift to a developmental role for the Red Cross allowed it to take on a more governmental one in the Gold Coast, as it provided health structures and challenged women's childbearing and rearing practices. Indeed, the British Red Cross (BRC), from which the new Gold Coast Branch derived, was part of imperial structures. In 1930, The British Empire Red Cross Conference was held in London. A report on the conference stated that the BRC aimed to fulfil a covenant of the League of Nations to 'encourage and promote in every country in the world the establishment of a duly organised voluntary national Red Cross organisation.'[93] Delegates concluded that branches should be opened in the colonies and should call to 'the attention of the Red Cross Societies within the British Empire the importance of social and economic conditions as factors in the health and welfare of the people.' Branches should 'investigate and consider the effect of these conditions upon public health.'[94] The aims of the Red Cross within the British Empire became developmental. As Lester and Skinner assert, humanitarianism not only *resembled* empire; the two were interdependent, as can be seen in this case.[95]

From within the colonial government, the fiercest protests against clinic closures came from Dr Selwyn-Clarke, Secretary of the GCLMCW. Arguably, the welfare activities that the League promoted had already made it difficult for the government to cancel them.

Dr Selwyn-Clarke claimed that without ante-natal care, pregnant women were left vulnerable to death in childbirth and that without preventative and educative work and well-baby checks, infants were vulnerable to disease and death.[96]

Archives leave no doubt that Selwyn-Clarke felt passionately about the health of women and children. However, he saw, like other colonial officials, links between this and economic development. In 1932, he prefaced his report on the GCRC with an economic overview of the colony. He emphasised the potential for exports of gold, diamonds, manganese and above all cocoa, noting that 'the resources of the colony absorb a considerable amount of unskilled labour and it is considered that the country could support at least three times its present population.'[97] We should remember that at this time, Selwyn-Clarke was attending LNHO conferences, which emphasised economic development as a prerequisite for health.[98] Humanitarian work was understood as part of economic development.

Whilst on leave in London in 1932, Selwyn-Clarke approached the Secretary General of the BRC. He requested permission for the Gold Coast League to become an affiliate organisation, and eventually to establish a Branch on the Gold Coast.[99] The governor of the Gold Coast at the time supported the transition and praised Selwyn-Clarke's efforts in making links with the BRC in the metropole.[100] GCRC was inaugurated in 1932 with the precise goal of providing for the welfare of mothers and babies after government retrenchments.[101] One of the first things Selwyn-Clarke organised was meetings with missions, Paramount Chiefs and the public. He suggested that interest in the new venture be stimulated throughout the Gold Coast. The Branch used posters and health films as well as lantern-illustrated health talks to spread health propaganda and interest.[102] Public meetings explained that GCRC's particular aim was to maintain and extend through voluntary work the 'medical and allied services for women and children.'[103] Indeed, GCRC's venture was dependent on voluntary work and funds from those in the Gold Coast, as well as the BRC. Its success is testimony to strengthening civil society. Various 'leading Africans' promised funds at the Branch's inception.[104]

Selwyn-Clarke envisaged that GCRC be run and funded by 'leading Africans but with a sprinkling of European members to assist from their knowledge of similar associations elsewhere.'[105] He wrote that 'it was now necessary to develop an organisation which would include chiefs, missionaries, merchants, Government officials, in fact all classes of society without distinction as to race or colour.'[106] Although he promised 'all classes of society,' in actual fact this became an activity for elite and professional classes. The Committee featured a range of prominent Gold Coasters, including Drs Nanka-Bruce and C. E. Reindorf, Ruby Quartey-Papafio, Mrs Kojo-Thompson and a number of chiefs including Nana Sir Ofori Atta, as well as other educators and religious leaders.[107] However, the idea that Europeans should be included because of their knowledge of how such associations ought to be run suggested that they should take leading roles. Indeed, the top GCRC positions were *all* taken by colonial officials, and none were women. The Patron was the Acting Governor, whilst the Branch's chairman was the Director of Medical and Sanitary Services.

Therefore, although the GCLMCW made up the nucleus of the organisation, its leadership was radically different. But those working on the front line were all women, including volunteers, Red Cross Sisters, the scattering of WMOs that remained, and midwives trained in Accra.[108] The first 'Sisters' who arrived from

Britain were Mrs Thompson and Mrs Browning. Whilst Mrs Thompson was a qualified nursing sister, Mrs Browning was not but had volunteered in the field when living on the Gold Coast alongside her husband.[109] There were worries from certain colonial officials that a 'jolly little scandal' may arise from the lack of oversight from MOs.[110] Nonetheless, these Sisters took over the first two Red Cross Clinics in Sekondi and Cape Coast in 1932. This was followed in 1934 by a third in Kumasi. As GCRC found its feet towards the mid-1930s, more clinics were held in rural villages – branching out from towns. In Accra, there were multiple weighing centres and welfare clinics. Their number grew throughout the 1930s. They were staffed predominantly by members of the GCLMCW. Thus, one organisation had merged almost entirely into another. [111]

Volunteers gave 'friendly' health talks to African women. Others continued house-to-house visits, entering women's homes and talking to them about their personal and domestic hygiene.[112] During these visits, volunteers were expected to 'point out faults in a friendly and helpful manner.'[113] Red Cross Annual Reports praised volunteers and gave them credit for making a success of clinics through their interpersonal work with mothers and babies.[114] Volunteers were advised by the Senior Nursing Sister at the Children's Hospital in Accra, to have 'intimate knowledge of the homes and lives of the mothers and children visited.'[115] Presumably, it would have been more difficult for a man to gain 'intimate knowledge' of Gold Coast women's lives. The organisation therefore continued to rely on women even after the higher echelons were taken over by male colonialists. As well as volunteers and midwives, clinics relied upon other labourers and health workers occupying roles such as dressers and dispensers. Crucially, dressers were often women and also held the role of 'interpretress.'[116] They were needed to translate both language and biomedical practice.[117] Sylvia Ward, a British woman who volunteered with domiciliary visits to mothers and babies, noted 'with the aid of an interpreter I was able to give helpful advice.'[118] Clinics' functions ranged from weighing babies to small maternity homes where women could give birth and children could be treated for minor illnesses. Staff ran ante-natal and post-natal clinics, and midwives delivered babies. They measured expectant mothers, carried out ante-natal tests and prescribed medication.

Education and Social Development

From its inception, GCRC work went beyond the medical. Writing to elicit support from the Secretary of Native Affairs in May 1932, Dr Selwyn-Clarke stressed that the organisation would 'provide means for the prosecution of other undertakings affecting the health of the community as a whole. The educational value of such an institution needs no emphasis.'[119] Indeed when the Red Cross began, they decided that 'educational and advisory methods [would] be their first aim.' Education started in terms of advice to mothers. Red Cross Sisters and volunteers gave mothers advice on pregnancy hygiene and on 'feeding, bathing and clothing their children, vaccination and birth registration.'[120] Volunteers at weighing clinics were advised to stop what they were doing for a few minutes to give short talks.

These could be on a range of topics from 'vaginal discharge' to '"Native" and European medicine' (presumably in favour of the latter) or even 'crying babies and what to do with them.'[121] Selwyn-Clarke saw Africans' (apparent) rejection of western medicine in favour of their own practices as a dangerous inconvenience to be surpassed. He wrote that medical staff 'must confront a long inheritance of tribal custom, traditions.' One of these was in childbirth when 'grandmothers or handy women ... took charge' and 'treatment in difficult or delayed deliveries sometimes included stuffing salt, leaves or grass into the vagina, at others placing a board across the abdomen and seating a heavy person on each end of it.'[122] Changing these perceived cultural norms was a crucial part of Red Cross work. Advice given in clinics generally steered women away from what officials saw as 'ignorant' and 'dangerous' methods at childbirth and for child-rearing. The alternative was encouraging women to attend clinics regularly for examination. The aim to educate members of African communities reflected colonial officials' attitude that the problem of high maternal and infant mortality could be explained through the ignorance of mothers and female birth attendants.

Another key space in which the Red Cross operated was schools. It was here that the importance of its relationship with the Christian missions became apparent.[123] In 1931, only 24 out of 336 schools in the colony were government run. A significant number were run by Christian missions: 180 by Presbyterians, 57 by Wesleyans and 48 by Roman Catholics, although all of these were assisted financially by the government.[124] In the 1930s, these schools began cooperating with the Red Cross, setting up Junior Red Cross Links, made up of students and teachers. Indeed, connections with these schools were invaluable as they raised, through subscriptions and fundraising events, £337.1.6, which made up around half of the Red Cross income.[125] In 1935, there were 33 Junior Red Cross Links across the colony, representing almost 10% of schools. Link members took part in health education, welfare work and first aid, as well as helping at weighing stations and delivering hygiene lessons to mothers.[126] Participants from the Wesleyan Girls' School in Accra frequently spent time at Princess Marie Louise Hospital, where they were described as 'most helpful as fresh, vigorous interested *interpreters*,' again emphasising the important role of building bridges between mothers and health work.[127] Most importantly, students in the Links acted as 'veritable missionaries for health,' as one Red Cross report described them.[128] Students regularly travelled back to their towns and villages where they encouraged their communities and chiefs to engage with Red Cross ideals on hygiene and health.[129] How seriously they were taken, we cannot know from Red Cross reports; however it obviously thought the work invaluable.

Humanitarian Governance

Scholarship on global health in the last 20 years has begun to account for networks and medical marketplaces. Hunt characterises global health as NGOs 'sitting alongside and within zones of instability, displacement, and warfare.'[130] Meanwhile, Gregory Mann points out that NGOs often step into the role of the state, calling this 'nongovernmentality.' He argues that there is a need to look 'beyond familiar political formations' in post-independence era Sahel, to 'communities of solidarity and aid, social science and activism.'[131] We see a precedent for these characteristics of global health as the Red Cross, as a non-governmental organisation (NGO), stepped in to provide health infrastructure that the colonial state could, or would, not. Work that had

> hitherto been carried out directly by the Medical Department should, in future be organised independently under the aegis of the Red Cross Society. A grant would be received from the society in England, and the interest of Government organisations, unofficial organisations etc. in the Colony would be secured by means of the central committee.[132]

This approach of treating the NGO as a governmental structure brings to light its relationship with and beyond the colonial government and, as Mann advocates, helps us to look beyond the colonial/post-colonial frame.[133] Red Cross clinics sat alongside an absence of colonial health services in the rest of the country.

Usually, clinic buildings or some of the equipment or staff would be provided by the government, whilst funds and organisation depended on the Red Cross.[134] The organisation was given tax exemption on imports as well as semi-official status as soon as it was inaugurated.[135] However, colonial officials specifically pointed to the importance of voluntary work and the importance of expanding that work in the face of government cutbacks.[136]

Furthermore, this non-governmental work was dependent on African civil society, located above all in the coastal towns of the Gold Coast and made up of merchants, professional classes, traditional leaders and those aligned with colonial political structures. The first Red Cross clinics were established in Sekondi and Cape Coast, funded by African-led Town Councils who took 'considerable interest in [the] matter.'[137] They took over the organisation, funding and staffing of clinics that had previously been run by the government or volunteers. In 1934 a clinic was established in Kumasi and a year later in Koforidua. This meant that by the mid-1930s, the Red Cross was operating in the five largest urban spaces on the Gold Coast. It was the children of this elite group, who attended, for example the Wesleyan Girls' School mentioned above, that took part in Red Cross Links. At Achimota school, the most progressive the colony had to offer, volunteer work in the form of social service was expected from students and staff alike.[138] This also followed a pattern of geographically restricted medical services

The notion of medical services dependent on donors and volunteers was something that the Gold Coast government encouraged. In 1932, the governor wrote that '<u>now</u> is the time to foster voluntary effort. If the Red Cross takes root <u>now</u> it will probably mean that when prosperity returns to the colony, heavy outlay might be avoided.'[139] It was not just GCRC and its volunteers who were expected to prop up medical services. Dr Selwyn-Clarke noted that chiefs in the Eastern Province should raise their own funds for a WMO and infant welfare clinic.[140] GCRC was dependent on fundraising, a role in which it became quite visible through Red

Cross 'Flag Day' and 'Flag Week,' when announcements were made in churches and events such as jumble sales and football matches were organised. Chiefs were also relied upon as sources of funding and encouraged to take ownership of certain projects, for instance, the extension of the Maternity Hospital that the Red Cross funded in 1934.[141] This expectation of funding for health projects, or contributions to humanitarian fundraising campaigns, coincided with the establishment of stool treasuries in the mid-1930s. These treasuries meant more rigorous account keeping for local authorities, overseen by colonial officials.[142]

Attendance at Red Cross Clinics

It cannot be argued by any stretch of the imagination that a majority of women were attending clinics. As Esi Yawaa from Mpaesem in Central Region reflected on her mother's childbearing years: 'in the past we were only born in the house … we didn't know about the hospital.'[143] A number of women born in the 1930s testified that their mothers relied solely on local herbs, healers and family members during their pregnancies. Knowledge about herbs, pregnancy and childbirth was common. Some women did go to the village herbalist and buy particular medicines during pregnancy 'to make the baby strong,' but many others got herbal remedies from family members: grandfathers and fathers as well as women. Infertility was one of the most frequent reasons that women attended herbalists or shrines. This was not a priority in either government or Red Cross clinics: there is no mention in reports of infertility or even frequent miscarriages being attended to in clinics. Although there might have been unofficial or occasional recourse to clinics for fertility matters, this left a gaping hole in medical provision for women and may explain, in part, women's practice of adhering to multiple medical systems and options in the course of their reproductive lives.

Sometimes, women did not choose to attend clinics at all. One Red Cross Sister reported in 1938 that the clinic she established in Moree, near Cape Coast, saw the small number of 16 patients dwindle and disappear altogether within three weeks.[144] Furthermore, not all chiefs were keen on providing support for Red Cross services. For example, one rural chief insisted that if Sister Grand wanted the clinic room cleaned, she would have to pay. After Sister Grand refused, she returned the next week to find the clinic room closed up and 'in a filthy condition.' She stopped visiting, complaining that she had 'understood that our efforts at these Bush Clinics were appreciated and that we would be given every assistance by the Chiefs.'[145]

However, in general, women, particularly those living in towns, appear to have been enthusiastic about attending Red Cross clinics for treatment for themselves and their children.[146] As has been noted above, the proposed closure of clinics in the early 1930s was met with considerable protest. Furthermore, numbers of attendances at GCRC clinics grew.[147] For example, attendances at the Sekondi clinic jumped from 7,476 attendances in 1933 to 9,735 the following year. In Cape Coast, the numbers were 6,608 in 1933 to 13,531 in the following year.[148] Dr Williams described the clinic in Kumasi as very popular in 1935, noting that 'patients may come from great distances.'[149] Indeed, in 1933, the Red Cross reported the 'keenness of the people of Kumasi, encouraged by Nana Prempeh II, ably supported by his Head Chiefs.'[150] The number of clinics slowly increased, with more being held outside of provincial capitals. And women appear to have travelled significant distances to attend clinics: a number of women born in the 1930s from villages up to 20 km away from Cape Coast remembered that their mothers attended 'Jubilee' in Cape Coast, which was the Red Cross Clinic.[151] In fact, by 1935, 3,500 women visited 'Jubilee' clinic for ante-natal and post-natal care alone, and 7,000 attendances were recorded for babies.[152] Although this figure is relatively low in proportion to the female population of Central Province, it represents a sizeable proportion of Cape Coast, whose population in 1931 was 136,044.[153] Domiciliary visits were also in their thousands in the town; in 1934, 6,500 visits were recorded.[154] Weighing centres in Accra saw tens of thousands of babies. For example, in 1935 alone, babies were weighed 29,000 times and 37,450 times in Kumasi. Even if we suppose that mothers attended monthly with babies, this accounts for around 3,100 individual babies in Kumasi, a town with a population of 172,196 in 1931. It pays to remember that even when infants' attendances were counted, it was mothers who were on the receiving end of advice and educational work. Reports made by the BRC in the 1930s give a picture of a steadily growing organisation, which was well patronised.[155] Clinics apart, the government reported that the public was 'rapidly learning the value' of trained midwives. So much so that it planned to reduce subsidies paid to government-trained midwives outside of clinics.[156]

Maternal and Child Welfare and Gold Coast Civil Society

The two unnamed 'African ladies' mentioned earlier in their roles keeping Sekondi maternal and child welfare clinic open were part of an elite class of women whose status was linked to these clinics. In the 1930s, Gold Coast civil society was increasing in size, dynamism and influence. This was cultivated in part through humanitarian work organised through the elite class and their organisations.[157] Although these particular women remained 'unnamed' in the colonial archive, it is their volunteer status in a humanitarian movement that means they are visible there at all. And it arguably gave them legitimate power and authority in Sekondi, perhaps the opportunity to direct other women and to display individual expertise. The power wielded by these unnamed women was undoubtedly linked to their class: a growing class of elite, urban Africans. These Sekondi women and others volunteering with the Red Cross, had access to the networks and economic resources of the elite.[158]

Leaders of the GCRC were members of nascent civil society, as the membership mentioned earlier in this chapter indicates. Despite its widening availability, maternal and child welfare was still associated with a higher class made up of professionals, 'traditional' leaders and those aligned with colonial power. It went some way to forming that group's identity. As mentioned, Governor Guggisberg expressed surprise and disappointment in 1923 at the fact that 'the more *enlightened citizens*, both African and European' had not founded child welfare associations.[159] This indicates that citizenship was connected to 'enlightened' status, as was maternal and child health. It places a moral expectation on this class to bring others to their level. In this period, status hierarchies were shifting. Education and progress began to be valued over traditional structures.[160] Civil society was growing, and urban Africans were performing citizenship in the colonial state.[161] In Britain, as Helen McCarthy has put it, voluntarism had been 'integral to the consolidation of middle-class identity and power since the eighteenth century.'[162] Arguably, a similar dynamic can be seen here as. Elite Africans – especially women – were able to claim citizenship through their roles in a humanitarian organisation. What is more, this status was solidified in its differentiation from the tropes of 'backward' women explored above.

Those attending clinics were on average better off, and perhaps better educated than the majority of women. This conclusion can be drawn from their location – as noted, clinics were held in towns with midwives and volunteers making brief forays into the 'bush.' Indeed, Dr Vane Percy mentioned that she saw no reason not to charge those attending clinics and that, indeed, those attending Princess Marie Louise Children's Hospital were all in a position to pay a private practitioner.[163] Dr M. C. Quin stated that when welfare centres were established, it was the wives and families of government employees who attended, whilst the men went to the hospital. He implies that there was something morally correct about this class of women avoiding the hospital, a place where men went, and that the centres had given them an option for healthcare that they did not have previously.[164] Clinics were evidently not envisaged to provide for the destitute or impoverished.

The fact that GCRC's financial statements were published in the *Gold Coast Independent* indicates a connection with the newspaper-reading public.[165] This is significant since, as civil society consolidated in the 1930s, newspapers became a very important site of social expression.[166] Meetings for the 'Gold Coast League for Maternal and Child Welfare, British Red Cross' were also advertised there, establishing the 'visibility as a social group,' as Stephanie Newell has phrased it.[167] Members met at the Government Girls' School, and talks were given by doctors. For example, in December 1934, Dr Nanka-Bruce spoke on 'Some Common Disorders Associated with pregnancy,'[168] and in September of that year, Dr Cummins spoke on, 'Some causes of ill health among children.'[169] Given that the Government Girls' School represented an exclusive space for educated people, these meetings were implicitly exclusionary. Newell has argued that literary networks grew alongside British colonialism on the Gold Coast, as a vital aspect of culture.[170] Although she focuses on literature of debate groups, newspapers and public talks were arguably just as important in forming mutual cultural resonance. Certainly, maternal and child welfare entered the sphere of 'public debate and the "ethical" agency of the reader.'[171] Those reading newspapers and taking part in public debates were putting their education on display in the public sphere and cultivating social groupings by doing so. For women, in particular, public intellectual and cultural events linked to maternal and child welfare were crucial for establishing themselves as 'progressive.'

One of the ways in which the GCRC was most visible was through fundraising. An advertisement for a fundraising event in 1933 appeared in the *Times of West Africa*. The title 'Now for the Red Cross' appeared on the front page, followed by the enticing subtitle 'A Maternity Ward We Can Call Our Own.' On 6 December, the great and the good gathered at this event, including Dr Nanka-Bruce. The appeal was publicly backed by the governor, and numerous influential people were scheduled to speak.[172] It is also noteworthy that GCRC was able to raise considerable amounts of money, quite quickly, from subscriptions. Within its first ten months, the Society had 31 life members, 104 Associate members and raised £664 from individual subscriptions and fundraising through schools.[173]

Women volunteers for the Gold Coast League, and later the Red Cross, played into a gendered division of labour that befitted this class. Women were encouraged to take on domestic roles, and girls' education began to reflect this. Housecraft and needlework were core parts of schools' syllabi, as was, by the 1930s, infant care. In general, education was linked to a stratification of Gold Coast women based on their mothering. Domestic science was introduced into the curriculum as a compulsory subject for female pupils. It included 'Laundry, Cookery, Child Welfare and Needlework.'[174] In 1934, Mrs Northcote, wife of the Acting Governor, published a book on cookery. Sales proceeds went to the Red Cross.[175] This event captures the mix of 'educated but domestic' that was supposed to characterise women of the organisation. In a society in which, as journalist Mabel Dove wrote, 'there is a feeling among the men folk of this country that we women are not capable of really doing anything,' maternal and child welfare organisation arguably provided an opportunity for women to prove them wrong.[176]

The drive for a certain mode of domesticity was linked to the work of Christian missions. The period saw the emergence of what Apter terms, 'mission school gentry.'[177] Both the Scottish Mission and the Wesleyan Mission had 'Women's Work' sections, run by women missionaries or missionary wives. Missionaries aimed to provide the foundations upon which Christian families could be built. The Wesleyan mission saw West African girls as integral for encouraging Christian homes. They argued that in West Africa, the future,

> as in every land is largely in the hands of mothers and home makers. In a country where there is no ideal of home, as we know it in Christian countries, and where the moral standard is often appallingly low, there is much that only women can do.[178]

Clearly, domesticity and motherhood were portrayed as crucial for the reproduction of 'moral' Africans.

The fact that the GCLMCW was made up of both African and European women was something about which Selwyn-Clarke was particularly proud. He stated that the League was to 'assist in breaking down the racial barriers which are a bar to progress by the association of European and African women in social service.'[179] Women's gendered identities: their propensity for caring and understanding other women's needs were expected to override racial divisions. Women who joined the

League were often the female relatives of high-profile men, whilst those women who attended clinics were encouraged to join as volunteers. Women were not only passive recipients in maternal and child welfare but played a role as 'middle figures' as Hunt labelled those translating biomedical systems to African populations at large.[180] Encounters between elite women and the Gold Coast mothers were not framed as dictatorial. Rather, the idea was to 'engage the women-folk in friendly discussion.'[181] However, the organisation aimed to 'dispel the suspicion with which the welfare centres were regarded by the less informed and poorer section of the population.'[182] Again, those more socially advanced were responsible for their less fortunate counterparts. Selwyn-Clarke wrote 'that the well-educated section of the community approves of Child Welfare is shown by the fact that many African ladies give valuable assistance work by giving up their services voluntarily for that purpose.'[183] In other words, women's social status was based on their attitude to child welfare. The less- or uneducated population was lumped together and their assumed 'suspicion' of welfare centres placed in opposition to those women who knew better. Therefore, whilst racial divisions were supposed to be overcome, racialised socio-economic divisions were emphasised.

Despite being on the 'right' side of the divide regarding their attitude to child welfare, Gold Coast women volunteers were still characterised by their Africanness. African and European ladies were expected to act as 'a partnership that combined a knowledge of local ways and languages with that of biology, hygiene and infant care.'[184] The word 'partnership' is interesting here as it suggests equal terms. However, there is a clear division of knowledge envisaged between 'local ways' and knowledge of 'biology, hygiene and infant care,' which is the remit of European women. The gloss of science remained something that Europeans supplied, at least in the eyes of the League's secretary Selwyn-Clarke. However, in 1937, the first African was selected as Secretary Manager of the Red Cross. The report for that year noted that 'the appointment is a very popular one,' presumably amongst the Society's members. They noted, '[h]e has a long association with the Health Branch of the Medical Department and is thoroughly conversant with the health problems affecting the community,' as if to reassure British readers doubting his capabilities.[185] Nonetheless, his appointment arguably represents a shift in the organisation of the Society to make good on the rhetoric of racial equality.

Conclusion

Developmental humanitarianism became a crucial factor in establishing maternal and infant health in the 1930s. The colonial government embraced the Red Cross as a humanitarian organisation that could take responsibility for maternal and infant welfare. As a result, the Red Cross tapped into an emerging elite and fostered volunteerism and the beginnings of 'self-help,' a concept that will be explored further in the next chapter as we move into the 1940s. Whilst there is no doubt that visiting a GCRC clinic would have been one recourse for healing among many women on the Gold Coast, it was an option that was increasingly taken.

Humanitarian intervention was based on compassion for 'the African woman,' which influenced health services as female-only spaces and a focus on reproductive health dominated. Despite obstacles supposedly linked to the perseverance of 'tradition,' medicalisation of pregnancy and child-rearing was, by the end of the 1930s, becoming normalised. However, development discourses constructed two strata of African women on the Gold Coast. One framed women as timid victims, ignorant and overly attached to tradition. The second saw Gold Coast women buying in to colonial tropes and practices regarding maternal and infant welfare in order to consolidate their elite status and position themselves as progressive, in contrast with their 'less fortunate' sisters.

Notes

1 Michael N. Barnett, *Empire of Humanity: A History of Humanitarianism* (Ithaca, NY: Cornell University Press, 2011), 52; Rob Skinner and Alan Lester, 'Humanitarianism and Empire: New Research Agendas', *The Journal of Imperial and Commonwealth History* 40, no. 5 (1 December 2012): 731.

2 Lara Putnam, 'Global Child-Saving, Transatlantic Maternalism, and the Pathologization of Caribbean Childhood, 1930s–1940s', *Atlantic Studies* 11, no. 4 (2 October 2014): 492.

3 Susan Pedersen, 'The Maternalist Moment in British Colonial Policy: The Controversy over "Child Slavery" in Hong Kong 1917–1941', *Past & Present* 171 (2001): 164.

4 NA, CO 96/702/1: Dr Duff, Director of Medical Services, 'Memorandum: The Medical Department – Gold Coast 1910–1932. A Balanced Service', 23 June 1932, 11.

5 The following histories touch on the role of the Red Cross: Stephen Addae, *The History of Western Medicine in Ghana 1880–1960* (Edinburgh: The Pentland Press, 1997); Jean Allman and Victoria B. Tashjian, *I Will Not Eat Stone: A Women's History of Colonial Asante* (Portsmouth, NH: Heinemann, 2000); K. David Patterson, *Health in Colonial Ghana: Disease, Medicine, and Socio-Economic Change, 1900–1955* (Waltham, MA: Crossroads Press, 1981). Anne Hugon goes into more detail about it: Anne Hugon, *Être mère en situation coloniale: Gold Coast, 1910–1950*, Histoire contemporaine 28 (Paris: Éditions de la Sorbonne, 2020), 104–9.

6 Hugon, *Être mère en situation coloniale*, 106.

7 Megan Vaughan, *Curing Their Ills: Colonial Power and African Illness* (Cambridge: Polity, 1991).

8 PRAAD, Cape Coast, ADM 23/1/441: 'Letter from Central Province Commissioner', 30 September 1930.

9 See Introduction for details of interviews carried out between October 2017 and July 2019.

10 NA, CO 96/702/1: Memorandum, Dr Selwyn-Clarke, n.d., but July 1932, 8.

11 NA, CO 96/702/1: Letter from Acting Governor to Lord Passfield, Secretary of State for the Colonies, 23 July 1930, 3.

12 NA, CO 96/702/1: Letter from Dr Duff, Director of Medical Services, to Mrs Vane Percy and Mrs Hendrie, 20 May 1932, 1.

13 NA, CO 96/702/1: Dr Duff, Director of Medical Services, 'Memorandum: The Medical Department – Gold Coast 1910–1932. A Balanced Service', 23 June 1932, 2–11.

14 NA, CO 96/702/1: 'Memorandum, Dr Selwyn Clarke', n.d. but July 1932, 10 and Memorandum, M. C. Quin, 8 October 1931, 1.

15 NA, CO 96/702/1: Memorandum, J. M. Mackay, 22 February 1932, 2.

16 NA, CO 96/702/1: Letter from Nora Vane Percy to Dr Duff, 13 June 1932, 1.
17 NA, CO 96/702/1: Memorandum, C. D. Williams, 3 March 1931, 1.
18 NA, CO 96/702/1: Memorandum, Dr Selwyn-Clarke, n.d., but July 1932, 10.
19 Ibid., 12.
20 NA, CO 96/705/10: Letter to Dr Stanton from Dr Alice Piegrome, 16 January 1932, 2.
21 PRAAD, Accra, CSO 11/1/209: 'Letter from Governor Northcote to Lord Passfield, Secretary of State for the Colonies', 30 January 1931.
22 NA, CO 96/702/1: 'Letter to Mrs Vane Percy and Mrs Hendrie from Dr Duff', 20 May 1932, 2.
23 BDL, MSS.Afr.s.1872/154, Box 43: C. D. Williams 'Maternal and Child Health Services in Developing Countries', reprinted from *The Lancet* 15 February 1964, 345–48.
24 NA CO 96/705/10: Letter from Dr Selwyn-Clarke to The Colonial Secretary, Accra, 28 June 1932, 3.
25 NA, CO 96/702/1: Memorandum, Dr Selwyn-Clarke, n.d., but July 1932, 8.
26 Thomas Spear, 'Neo-Traditionalism and the Limits of Invention in British Colonial Africa', *The Journal of African History* 44, no. 1 (March 2003): 26–27.
27 BDL, MSS. Brit.Emp.s.470, Box 10: *Second Annual Report of the Gold Coast (Central) Branch, British Red Cross Society for the Year 1934*, Government Printer, Accra, 1935, 1.
28 PRAAD, Accra, CSO 11/6/9: 'Letter from Kumasihene"s Office to Sir Alexander Ransford, Governor of the Gold Coast', 22 March 1932, 1–3.
29 PRAAD, Cape Coast, ADM 23/1/976: Petition to the Commissioner of Central Province from the Town Council of Cape Coast, 10 February 1932, 1–2.
30 PRAAD, Accra, CSO 11/6/4: 'Infant Welfare', 22 July 1932, 1.
31 PRAAD, Accra, CSO 11/6/1: 'Infant Welfare Clinic at Dsoje', 1930–1932, 1.
32 PRAAD, Cape Coast, ADM 23/1/976: 'Letter to the Chairman of the Red Cross Society, Cape Coast, from Omanhene of Asebu', 13 June 1933, 1.
33 NA, CO 96/705/10: Letter to Dr Stanton from Dr Alice Piegrome, 6 January1932, 3.
34 PRAAD, Accra, CSO 11/6/8: Letter to Deputy Director of Health Services from Medical Officer of Health, Sekondi, 14 May 1932, 1–3.
35 PRAAD, Accra, CSO 11/6/8: Letter from Dr Duff, Director of Medical and Sanitary Services, 18th March, 1932, 2. Dr Piegrome had worked for the colonial service before her contract was terminated upon her marriage in 1930. In 1932, she contacted the colonial office asking to take over the Sekondi clinic where her husband was stationed. She was eventually appointed on a salary that was less than a third of what she had been paid previously.
36 NA, CO 96/705/10: Letter to Dr Stanton from Dr Alice Piegrome, 6 January 1932, 4.
37 Iris Borowy, *Coming to Terms with World Health: The League of Nations Health Organisation 1921–1946* (Frankfurt am Main: Lang, 2009), 184.
38 Ingrid Sharp and Matthew Stibbe, 'Women's International Activism during the Inter-War Period, 1919–1939', *Women's History Review* 26, no. 2 (4 March 2017): 167.
39 Allman and Tashjian, *I Will Not Eat Stone*, 33.
40 Ibid., 18–25.
41 Nancy Rose Hunt, '"Le Bébé En Brousse": European Women, African Birth Spacing, and Colonial Intervention in Breast Feeding in the Belgian Congo', in *Tensions of Empire: Colonial Cultures in a Bourgeois World*, ed. Frederick Cooper and Ann Laura Stoler (London: University of California Press, 1997), 288.
42 Annemieke van Drenth and Francisca de Haan, *The Rise of Caring Power: Elizabeth Fry and Josephine Butler in Britain and the Netherlands* (Amsterdam: Amsterdam University Press, 1999), 12.
43 Eliza Riedi, 'Options for an Imperialist Woman: The Case of Violet Markham, 1899–1914', *Albion: A Quarterly Journal Concerned with British Studies* 32, no. 1 (2000): 60.

44 PRAAD, Accra, CSO 11/6/4: Memorandum in file "Infant Welfare Centres", 31 March 1932, n.d. but August, 1932.
45 NA, CO 96/702/1: 'Memorandum from Dr M C Quin', 8 October 1931, 2.
46 NA, CO 96/705/10: 'British Red Cross Society. Gold Coast Branch', 28 June 1932, 2.
47 Helen McCarthy, 'Service Clubs, Citizenship and Equality: Gender Relations and Middle-Class Associations in Britain between the Wars', *Historical Research* 81, no. 213 (2008), 534.
48 Ulrike Lindner, 'The Transfer of European Social Policy Concepts to Tropical Africa, 1900–50: The Example of Maternal and Child Welfare', *Journal of Global History* 9, no. 2 (July 2014): 213.
49 Putnam, 'Global Child-Saving', 493.
50 Lidner, 'The Transfer of European Social Policy', 214.
51 BDL, MSS.Afr.s.1985, Gold Coast Wives: Mrs Sylvia Ward, 1985, 9.
52 'Mothercraft in East Africa', *The World's Children*, vol. XI, no. 8, May 1931, 151–53.
53 Ibid., 152. My italics.
54 Ibid., 153.
55 BDL, MSS.Afr.s.1985, Gold Coast Wives: Mrs Jessie Griffith, 1985, 13–14.
56 Lila Abu-Lughod, 'Do Muslim Women Really Need Saving? Anthropological Reflections on Cultural Relativism and Its Others', *American Anthropologist* 104, no. 3 (2002): 783–90.
57 Chandra Talpade Mohanty, 'Introduction', in *Third World Women and the Politics of Feminism*, ed. Chandra Talpade Mohanty, Ann Russo, and Lourdes Torres (Bloomington, IN: Indiana University Press, 1991), 5.
58 I refer to 'humanitarians' here as opposed to Christian missions which had been working with women and on issues relating to family life for a lot longer.
59 Jessica Cammaert, *Undesirable Practices: Women, Children, and the Politics of the Body in Northern Ghana, 1930–1972* (Lincoln, NE: University of Nebraska Press, 2016), 7–8.
60 NA, CO 323/1067/5: Letter to Lord Passfield, Secretary of State for the Colonies, from Gold Coast Governor, 23 July 1930, 1.
61 PRAAD, Accra, CSO 21/10/24: Copied from file 1207/20, Downing Street, 3 May 1932.
62 PRAAD, Accra, CSO 21/10/24: Letter from Northcote to Sir Philip Cunliffe-Lister, 26 October 1932, 1.
63 PRAAD, Accra, CSO 21/10/24: Extract from Official Report of 13 April 1932.
64 CO 323/1067/5: Letter to Lord Passfield, Secretary of State for the Colonies, from Gold Coast Governor, 23 July 1930.
65 PRAAD, Accra, CSO 11/1/413: 'Certain Aspects of the Welfare of Women and Children in the Colonies' by Dr Mary G. Blacklock, reprinted for the Colonial Office from the *Annals of Tropical Medicine and* Pathology, 223.
66 Ibid., 228.
67 BDL, MSS.Brit.emp.s.470, Box 9: 'A Red Cross Branch on the Gold Coast', n.d., 2.
68 NA, CO 323/1067/5: 'Letter to Lord Passfield, Secretary of State for the Colonies, from Gold Coast Governor', 23 July 1930, 1.
69 Escobar, *Encountering Development*, 8.
70 PRAAD, Accra, CSO 11/4/9: 'Synopsis of the Maternity and Infant Welfare Movement in Accra' Enclosed in Letter to Acting Director of Medical and Sanitary Service, 13 January 1933, 1933.
71 Sarah Walters, '"Child! Now You Are": Identity Registration, Labor, and the Definition of Childhood in Colonial Tanganyika, 1910–1950', *The Journal of the History of Childhood and Youth* 9, no. 1 (1 March 2016): 66.
72 Dominique Marshall, 'Children's Rights in Imperial Political Cultures: Missionary and Humanitarian Contributions to the Conference on the African Child of 1931', *The International Journal of Children's Rights* 12, no. 3 (1 September 2004): 273.

73 Evelyn Sharp, *The African Child: An Account of the International Conference on African Children, Geneva* (London: Weardale Press, 1931), 104–9.
74 Sharp, *The African Child*, 112.
75 'The Outlook', *The World's Children*, vol. XI, no. 6, March, 1931, 106.
76 'Health Factor in Africa's Prosperity', *The World's Children*, vol. XI, no. 9, June 1931, 163.
77 Emily Baughan, *Saving the Children: Humanitarianism, Internationalism, and Empire*, Berkeley Series in British Studies 19 (Oakland, CA: University of California Press, 2022), 91–96.
78 Sharp, *The African Child*, 112.
79 Ibid., 37.
80 'Glimpses of African Child Life', *The World's Children*, vol. XII, no. 10, July, 1932.
81 Ibid., 36.
82 Samuel Martínez and Kathryn Libal, 'Introduction: The Gender of Humanitarian Narrative', *Humanity: An International Journal of Human Rights, Humanitarianism, and Development* 2, no. 2 (8 September 2011): 162.
83 LN, 8F/124/67/321: 'Commission d"etudes des questions concernant l"enfance non-europeenne', 8th September, 1930, 1.
84 Ibid., 2.
85 Ibid.
86 Sharp, *The African Child*, 30.
87 Barnett, *Empire of Humanity*, 60.
88 Sharp, *The African Child*, 37, 41.
89 Baughan, *Saving the Children*, 79.
90 Skinner and Lester, 'Humanitarianism and Empire', 730–31.
91 John F. Hutchinson, *Champions of Charity: War and the Rise of the Red Cross* (Boulder, CO: Westview Press, 1996), 279–344.
92 Barnett, *Empire of Humanity*, 52.
93 'British Empire Red Cross Conference', *The Lancet* 1, no. 5568 (17 May 1930): 1083.
94 'British Empire Red Cross Conference', *British Medical Journal* 1, no. 3620 (24 May 1930): 968.
95 Skinner and Lester, 'Humanitarianism and Empire.'
96 NA, CO 96/702/1: Memorandum, Dr Selwyn-Clarke, n.d. but July 1932.
97 PRAAD, Accra, CSO 11/1/274: Letter to Colonial Secretary from Dr Selwyn-Clarke: 'British Red Cross Society Gold Coast Branch', 28 June 1932.
98 See chapter 1.
99 NA, CO 96/702/1: Memorandum, Dr Selwyn-Clarke, n.d. but July, 1932, 16.
100 NA, CO 96/705/10: Letter from Governor Northcote to Sir Phillip Cunlife-Lister, Colonial Office, 5th August, 1932, 4.
101 BDL, MSS.Brit.Emp.s.470, Box 9: 'The British Red Cross Society on the Gold Coast' by Dr P. S. Selwyn-Clarke reprinted from *The West African Medical Journal*, January, 1934, 1–2.
102 BDL, MSS. Brit.Emp.s.470, Box 9: *Second Annual Report of the Gold Coast (Central) Branch, British Red Cross Society for the Year 1934*, Government Printer, Accra, 1935, 12.
103 BDL, MSS.Brit.Emp.s.470, Box 9: 'A Red Cross Branch on the Gold Coast', 2.
104 NA, CO 96/702/1: Memorandum, Dr Selwyn-Clarke, n.d. but 1932, 16.
105 Ibid.
106 BDL, MSS.Brit.Emp.s.470, Box 9: 'The British Red Cross Society on the Gold Coast' by Dr P. S. Selwyn-Clarke reprinted from *The West African Medical Journal*, January, 1934, 1.
107 PRAAD, Accra, CSO 11/1/274: 'British Red Cross Society Gold Coast Branch', n.d. but 1932.

108 PRAAD, Accra, CSO 11/1/274: 'Resume in Brief of the Activities of the Gold Coast Branch of the Red Cross Society', n.d., 2.
109 NA, CO 96/705/10: Note in file: Maternity and Child Welfare, 7 September 1932.
110 N A, CO 96/705/10: Note in file: Maternity and Child Welfare, 2 September 1932.
111 BDL, MSS.Brit.Emp.s.470, Box 9: 'The British Red Cross Society on the Gold Coast' by Dr P. S. Selwyn-Clarke reprinted from *The West African Medical Journal*, January, 1934, 1.
112 BDL, MSS.Brit.Emp.s.470, Box 10: *First Annual Report of the Gold Coast (Central Council) Branch, British Red Cross Society for the Year 1933*, Government Printer, Accra, 1934, 4.
113 BDL, MSS.Afr.s.1872/154, Box 43: 'Gold Coast Handbook of Nursing. Children's Section. Accra' by H. M. Barr, 1937, 14.
114 BDL, MSS.Brit.Emp.s.470, Box 10: *Sixth Annual Report of the Gold Coast (Central Council) Branch, British Red Cross Society for the Year 1938*, Government Printer, Accra, 1939, 13.
115 BDL, MSS.Afr.s.1872/154, Box 43: 'Gold Coast Handbook of Nursing. Children's Section. Accra' by H. M. Barr, 1937, 14.
116 See for example: PRAAD, Accra, CSO 11/6/2: 'Memorandum to the Director of Medical and Sanitary Services', 2nd December, 1930, 2; and CSO 11/6/8: 'Sekondi Clinic', 1932. A 'Dresser Interpreter' is also included in the starting costs of the Red Cross clinics: CO 96/705/10: Enclosure 2: Cape Coast Clinic, 5 August 1932, 1.
117 Nancy Rose Hunt, *A Colonial Lexicon: Of Birth Ritual, Medicalization, and Mobility in the Congo* (Durham, NC: Duke University Press, 1999), 7–8.
118 BDL, MSS.Afr.s.1985, Gold Coast Wives: Mrs Sylvia Grace Ward, 1985, 9.
119 PRAAD, Accra, CSO 11/1/272: Letter from Dr Selwyn-Clarke to the Secretary for Native Affairs, 15th May, 1932, 1.
120 PRAAD, Accra, CSO 11/6/8: 'Further Notes by the Deputy Director of Health Services', 4 August 1932, 1.
121 BDL, MSS.Afr.s.1872/154, Box 43: 'Gold Coast Handbook of Nursing. Children's Section. Accra' by H. M. Barr, 1937, 15.
122 BDL, MSS.Brit.Emp.s.470, Box 5: *Draft Footprints, the Memoirs of Selwyn Selwyn-Clarke*, Sir Percy Selwyn Selwyn-Clarke, 1972, 59.
123 For more detail on this relationship see: Holly Ashford, 'The Red Cross and the Establishment of Maternal and Infant Welfare in the 1930s Gold Coast', *The Journal of Imperial and Commonwealth History* 47, no. 3 (2019): 528–30.
124 A. W. Cardinall, *The Gold Coast, 1931* (Accra: Government Printer, 1933), 192.
125 NA, CO 96/705/10: British Red Cross Society Gold Coast Branch: Statement of Accounts, 1933, 1.
126 BRC, RCC/1/29/11: *Report of the British Red Cross Society for the Year 1934*, London, 1935, 51.
127 NA, CO 96/702/1: "Princess Marie Louise Hospital", 24 March 1932, 2. My italics.
128 BRC, RCC/1/29/9: *Report of the British Red Cross Society for the Year 1932*, London, 1933, 39.
129 BRC, RCC/1/29/11: *Report of the British Red Cross Society for the Year 1934*, London, 51.
130 Nancy Rose Hunt, 'Health and Healing', in *The Oxford Handbook of Modern African History*, ed. John Parker and Richard Reid (Oxford: Oxford University Press, 2013), 387–88.
131 Gregory Mann, *From Empires to NGOs in the West African Sahel: The Road to Nongovernmentality* (Cambridge: Cambridge University Press, 2014), 2.
132 NA, CO 96/705/10: Note in file: Maternity and Child Welfare, 6 July 1932.
133 Mann, 3.
134 PRAAD, Accra, CSO 11/6/8: 'Inter-Office Memorandum no. 26', 22 July 1932.

135 PRAAD, Accra, ADM 14/2/18: *Legislative Council Debates 1932–1933*, Government Printer, Accra, col. 269.
136 NA, CO 96/705/10: Minutes of the 1st Meeting of The Central Committee of the Gold Coast Branch, Red Cross Society, Accra, 11 June 1932, 2.
137 NA, CO 96/705/10: Note in file: Maternal and Child Welfare Centres, 1932.
138 BDL, MSS.Afr.s.1985 Gold Coast Wives: Mrs Sylvia Ward, 1985, 9 Mrs Jessie Griffith, 1985.
139 PRAAD, Accra, CSO 11/6/8: 'Letter to the Colonial Secretary, Accra', 5 August 1932.
140 PRAAD, Accra, CSO 11/6/7: 'Resolution by the Eastern Province Council', 3. Of course, I should make clear here that I am stressing the absence of the *colonial* state, not Chieftaincies.
141 PRAAD, Accra, CSO 11/1/288: 'Red Cross Society (G. C. Branch) - Proposal to Appeal for Funds for Enlarging Accra Maternity Hospital', August 1933.
142 Sara Berry, 'Unsettled Accounts: Stool Debts, Chieftaincy Disputes and the Question of Asante Constitutionalism', *Journal of African History* 39, no. 1 (1998): 60.
143 Interview with Esi Yawaa. Koforidua, Central Region, 27 November 2017.
144 PRAAD, Cape Coast, ADM 23/1/976: 'Letter from Commissioner Central Province to District Commissioner, Cape Coast', 15 November 1939.
145 PRAAD, Cape Coast, ADM 23/1/976: Letter E. Grand, Health Sister, to the Chairman of the Cape Coast Branch of the Red Cross Society, 4 August 1939.
146 NA, CO 96/702/1: "Letter from Acting Governor to Lord Passfield, Secretary of State for the Colonies', 23 July 1930.
147 Red Cross reports count attendances in different ways from year to year. However, figures suggest considerable growth every year, in every region. Figures are taken from BDL, Mss.Brit.Emp.s.470, Box 10, Red Cross Gold Coast Branch Annual Reports. Medical reports do not differentiate between those attending Red Cross clinics, mission clinics or government clinics until 1935.
148 Report on the Medical Department for the year 1933–1934 Gold Coast, Accra, 1934, 41.
149 Wellcome, PP/CDW/B.1/1: C. D. Williams, 'Maternal and Child Health in Kumasi in 1935', later published in *Journal of Tropical Pediatrics* (1956): 8–9.
150 BRC, RCC/1/29/10: *Report of the British Red Cross Society for the Year 1933*, London, 1934, 51.
151 Jubilee School sits opposite the clinic and is one of the oldest schools in the town, hence the popular naming of the clinic. Interview with Cecilia Fynn Essien, Cape Coast, Central Region, 28th November, 2017. Interview with Aba Efrim, Nkanfoa, Central Region, 13 February, 2018. Interview with Ama Yemaba, Nkanfoa, Central Region, 13 February, 2018. Other women mentioned attending this clinic later, and it still functions as a maternal and child health clinic today. Interviewees also referred to it as 'health insurance' since that is where women in the National Health Insurance scheme can go.
152 BRC, RCC/1/29/10: *Report of the British Red Cross Society for the Year 1935*, London, 1936, 51.
153 Cardinall, *The Gold Coast, 1931*, 145.
154 BRC, RCC/1/29/10: *Report of the British Red Cross Society for the Year 1934*, London, 1935, 53.
155 BRC, RCC/1/29/9-14: Reports of the British Red Cross Society, 1932–1927.
156 PRAAD, Accra, CSO 11/1/343: 'Letter from Dr Duff, Director Medical and Sanitary Services, to Colonial Secretary', 23 November 1933, 1.
157 For example, a crucial aspect of the culture at Achimota School was its voluntary social service work in the area. BL: MSS.Afr.s.1985: Gold Coast Wives: Sylvia Grace Ward, 1985.

158 Diana Elizabeth Kendall, *The Power of Good Deeds: Privileged Women and the Social Reproduction of the Upper Class* (Oxford: Rowman & Littlefield, 2002), 4–5.
159 SOAS, CBMS/IMC, Box 264: 'The Post-War Gold Coast. A Review of the Events of 1923' by Sir Gordon Guggisberg, Governor, 1924, 87. My italics.
160 David E. Apter, *Ghana in Transition* (New York: Atheneum, 1963), 150–57.
161 Jeff Grischow and Glenn H. McKnight, 'Rhyming Development: Practising Post-Development in Colonial Ghana and Uganda', *Journal of Historical Sociology* 16, no. 4 (1 December 2003): 519.
162 Helen McCarthy, 'Service Clubs, Citizenship and Equality', 532.
163 NA, CO 96/702/1: Letter from Nora Vane Percy to Dr Duff, 13 June 1932, 3.
164 NA, CO 96/702/1: 'Memorandum from Dr M C Quin', 8th October, 1931.
165 'Accra (Eastern Province) Division of Central Council Branch, British Red Cross Society. Statement of Accounts as For The First Half Year 1934', *Gold Coast Independent*, 18 August 1934, 775.
166 Stephanie Newell and Audrey Gadzekpo, eds., *Selected Writings of a Pioneer West African Feminist* (Nottingham: Trent Editions, 2004), xi.
167 Stephanie Newell, *Literary Culture in Colonial Ghana: "How to Play the Game of Life"* (Manchester: Manchester University Press, 2002), 31.
168 'Gold Coast League for Maternal and Child Welfare', *Gold Coast Independent*, 8 December 1934, 1163.
169 'Gold Coast League for Maternal and Child Welfare', *Gold Coast Independent*, 29 September 1934, 923.
170 Newell, *Literary Culture*, 3.
171 Ibid., 5–6.
172 'Now for the Red Cross', *The Times of West Africa*, 23 November 1933, 1.
173 BRC, RCC/1/29/10: *Report of the British Red Cross Society for the Year 1932*, London, 1933, 39.
174 Cardinall, *The Gold Coast, 1931*, 190.
175 'Red Cross Honours His Excellency', *The Gold Coast Independent*, 20th October, 1934, 995.
176 Newell and Gadzekpo, *Selected Writings*, 14.
177 Apter, *Ghana in Transition*, 152.
178 SOAS, WMMS: *The Glory of the Garden 1928: The Seventieth Annual Report of the Woman's Department*, 1929, 62.
179 BDL, MSS. Brit.Emp.s.470, Box 10: *Second Annual Report of the Gold Coast (Central) Branch, British Red Cross Society for the Year 1934*, Government Printer, Accra, 1935, 1.
180 Hunt, *A Colonial Lexicon*, 160.
181 Ibid.
182 PRAAD, Accra, CSO 11/1/274: Letter to Colonial Secretary from Dr Selwyn-Clarke: 'British Red Cross Society Gold Coast Branch', 28 June 1932, 1.
183 BDL, MSS. Brit.Emp.s.470, Box 10: *Second Annual Report of the Gold Coast (Central) Branch, British Red Cross Society for the Year 1934*, Government Printer, Accra, 1935, 1.
184 BDL, MSS.Brit.Emp.s.470, Box 5: Draft *Footprints, the Memoirs of Selwyn Selwyn-Clarke*, Sir Percy Selwyn Selwyn-Clarke, 1972, 60.
185 BRC, RCC/1/29/14: 'Report of the British Red Cross Society 1937', 78.

3 Social Development and Medicalising Reproduction, 1940–1956

Antenatal care was increasingly common in the 1950s: 'when the hospital came, everybody was going there,' testified Esi Yawa. Indeed, we see a significant increase in women attending clinics and hospitals through the 1940s and 1950s so that the medicalisation of pregnancy became standard. Delivering in hospital, though, remained rare, especially for rural women, Esi remembered: 'during the time I was in labour there was no car but there was a woman who was a birth attendant, so they went to call her.'[1] In the 1940s, biomedicine increasingly became an option available to Gold Coast women. The motives behind women's choice to seek biomedical intervention expose a complex web of power, health and body politics.[2] As the discourses around health and development shifted to widen women's options, new choices had to be made. A push for 'modernisation' both through large-scale projects and the community development projects described in this chapter changed what was expected of women. However, medicalisation was not imposed on a passive population. Rather, it shifted the framework in which women made health-related choices. Women entered a marketplace of options. Women – and families – made choices about their healthcare based on a combination of pragmatism and social obligation. This chapter outlines changes in medical services. It shows that whilst medical and scientific knowledge was increasingly disseminated through hospitals and Mass Education, other knowledge systems surrounded women's pregnancies, deliveries and reproductive careers.

Following World War II, the discourse and practice of development flourished. The world saw an ideological shift as development became ubiquitous.[3] What emerged was a global 'moral community' as Frederick Cooper and Randall Packard have characterised it. The relationships between colonial governments and the international community explored in Chapter 1 were expanded in the post-war era as governments of both independent and colonised 'underdeveloped' nations worked with global structures of international aid.[4] Describing post-war global development in terms of its morality goes straight to the heart of the issue: so-called underdeveloped people were being directed to industrialise, strive for economic growth, to reform their social practices to comply with certain codes of behaviour. Women in Ghana were directed to reproduce in different ways, both to emulate progress in the new generation and to embrace biomedicine as a symbol

DOI: 10.4324/9781003274162-4

of modernity. Moral codes were moulded by health programmes, colonists' ideals of biological and social reproduction, and discourses of progress, modernity and development. These codes impacted women's sexual and reproductive lives.[5]

Indeed, whilst Cooper and Packard are not mistaken when they claim that development appealed to leaders in so-called underdeveloped places, I challenge their claim that this era of development practice differed greatly from the 'inherent superiority' of the earlier European civilising mission.[6] In fact, discourses that were explored in the previous chapter, characterising African women as helpless 'beasts of burden' or that focused on women's moral failings in childbearing and rearing, continued into the 1940s and 1950s. Although World War II *was* a trigger for development planning, it will become clear through looking at social development policies that many had their roots in late-1930s plans.[7] Through an analysis of medicalisation, community development and women's education we see that development in late colonial Ghana was not only 'bureaucratic' but also moralising.[8]

The evolution of colonial medical services in Ghana has been well documented. Existing accounts show that colonial officials reacted to shifting patterns of disease and therefore highlight curative services detached from Africans' social networks.[9] The introduction of biomedicine in Africa through colonialism arguably alienated women from their social contexts.[10] In some cases, women's reluctance to enter hospitals bears witness to this. However, more often colonial medicine became *part of* Africans' social context. 'Therapeutic pluralism' emphasises the multiplicity of options open to Africans in relation to their health and places these options into their social context.[11] I demonstrate here that social development, including the medicalisation of pregnancy, meant that the social context of women's health was shifting. Therapeutic pluralism and its evolution should be linked to gendered histories of development.

In the 1940s, social development was delivered in two tiers. New hospitals in urban centres were modernisation projects. On the other hand, the government pushed 'community development' and 'self-help' through local government. At the community level, MCH and women's education were stressed. Social development – on both levels described above – encouraged interaction with biomedicine.

Social Development Planning

The 1940s and 1950s featured significant change and challenges both to colonial and traditional authorities.[12] Dennis Austin credits the power of education for this, which engendered resistance against traditional forms of authority as well as the colonial government.[13] Furthermore, World War II disrupted the lives of colonial subjects; conceptions of 'colonial development' once again shifted. Production of resources needed in war time, for example rubber, changed the Gold Coast economy.[14] After the war, living conditions for Gold Coasters worsened as the economy went into decline and then stagnation, linked particularly to the purchasing power of cocoa.[15] This meant shortages, difficulties with transport and malnutrition. In the Gold Coast, widespread strikes both of mine and railway workers, and in the form of cocoa 'hold-ups,' prompted a response from the government.[16] The need for tutelage, which occupied the discourse of the interwar international world, gave way to the need to impart stability, welfare and – increasingly – political rights to colonial subjects. Ultimately, unrest in colonies meant that governments were 'forced' to prioritise social and economic development.[17]

Social development was a crucial part of post-war colonial development; the British government saw it as a way to safeguard the future of the empire.[18] It therefore stressed social security and economic development as positives of colonial rule and necessities for global security.[19] 'Mass Education and Community Development' drove colonial officials' policy, especially when it came to social reproduction.

This environment resulted in the 1940 Colonial Development and Welfare Act (CDWA). Spending on social areas, like health and education, was intended to improve production and create wealth, meaning that social and economic development were integrated.[20] Cooper argues that colonialist bureaucrats looked for 'rational solutions' to impose modernisation, an inevitable process that could be driven by technical expertise.[21] However, social development took on a moral character beyond economics, inherited from missionary and humanitarian practices. This moral sphere goes beyond the 'bureaucratic' nature of development. The colonial government's plans in Ghana were designed to be revolutionary. As penologist Alexander Paterson put it in a report to the governor of the Gold Coast, 'so will the young man free himself from the dead hand of the live grandfather.'[22] In other words, development programmes were designed to manage social change and ensure positive progress. Focusing on women's health provides a clear view of how development was domesticated and linked to issues such as nutrition, reproduction and gendered relationships.

A new Central Planning Committee would 'coordinate plans for the development of the economic resources of the country and for the development of social services of an adequate scale.'[23] Social services were, according to Governor Sir Alan Burns, 'of primary importance to the welfare and happiness of the people.' They comprised an amalgamation of categories, according to his 1944 memorandum on development planning. This included medical, education, labour, housing, prisons, and general infrastructure.[24] A Central Welfare Committee oversaw the heads of departments involved in social services from the mid-1940s.[25] The proposed Ten Year Development Plan written in 1946 allocated 11.18% of spending to medical services and 35% for social services. However, a larger sum was allocated to 'revenue-producing' activities.[26] Furthermore, the provision of social services should only grow as much as the colony's economy permitted. This was despite ostensible commitment of metropolitan funds. Sir Alan stated that 'it is essential that the economic development of the country should be a principal consideration in any scheme of development and I make no apology for considering it first.'[27] He further noted that the future income of the colony was unpredictable, making the allocation of budgets difficult.[28] As Robert Tignor demonstrates that late colonial development plans were 'primitive,' created neither by development economists nor long-term planners. He describes these colonial development plans as 'primitive.'[29]

In the late 1940s, the Gold Coast's social services were 'magnified a hundred times into a giant scheme of post war reconstruction,' according to an impressed Alexander Paterson. This included hospitals and 'educational and social programmes for the fit and unfit.'[30] A separate department for social services was established in the early 1940s, although it was not fully operational for some years.[31] This revolution in colonial welfare reflected that in the metropole. Paterson described this moment as 'the first chapter of the Book of Genesis ... with the Beveridge Report as an Appendix.'[32] This echoes Joanna Lewis's point that there was an intimacy between social engineering in the metropole and how the empire was administered following World War II.[33]

The provision of welfare across Africa was linked to the apparent challenge of detribalisation, attempts at stabilising the workforce and the provision of a 'better life' for Africans, which would stimulate economic production. The Colonial Office feared that although 'tribal societies' provided social security within families, this was disintegrating in the face of colonial modernity, thus necessitating government assistance. Social services, it argued, would evolve together with growing political and economic development.[34] Women were seen at once as crucial for maintaining stable domesticity and morality and as a threat to it. Growing numbers of women in towns were perceived as a necessity to counter the phenomenon of lone, urban men but also as a sign of deteriorating social fabric. Colonial officials feared that maladjustment to a rapid transition from rural to urban life would lead to increased prostitution, lack of social standards, and the spread of venereal disease from the 'asymptomatic female.'[35] Increased prostitution in coastal towns, particularly Takoradi, and the new phenomenon of 'pilot boys' sparked concerns in the Gold Coast.[36] In sum, the Sub-Committee on Women and Girls in Africa, sitting in 1943, noted that 'the African woman is facing a revolution in her morals' due to 'dying tribal customs.'[37] In other words, at the Colonial Office, development was governed by fears over morality and gender norms that were in the process of being realigned.

Social 'welfare' applied particularly to women and children, where other areas of development planning did not. Arturo Escobar has characterised it as a 'domain of knowledge and intervention', which involved gathering information about the population and venturing into the realms of education, employment and health.[38] Indeed, the Gold Coast government planned for social services on a much wider scale.[39] When Dr Turner, the Director of Medical Services, formulated a plan for his department in 1946, he pushed for a census as soon as possible and encouraged record-keeping.[40] Turner saw the accumulation of data and knowledge of the population as crucial in providing medical services: he envisaged the extension of the colonial state's reach. Late colonial governments intervened in Africans' lives more than ever before when the arrival of numerous 'experts' to the continent increased government oversight.[41]

Medicalisation and Modernisation

Governor Alan Burns emphasised that new hospitals needed to be established and those already in existence improved. This was to prove to 'primitive tribes' the efficacy of 'European medicine' and the government's awareness of its 'responsibilities to the sick.'[42] In the short term, curative methods also cost much less than preventative, not least because they reached a smaller proportion of the population. Large hospitals stood as symbols of development and modernity. Modernisation was a 'spectacle' which was played out in 'brick and mortar' constructions and equally in encouraging Africans 'to emerge as self-respecting and responsible citizens [and] to escape the unholy trinity of ignorance, poverty and disease.'[43] In other words, modernity became a prerequisite to citizenship in the post-war period in the same way that progressiveness had in the interwar period. In the late colonial period, urbanity was seen as proof of Africans' modernity.[44] The 1946 plan for the medical services was conservative in proposing four main hospitals situated at Accra, Kumasi, Sekondi and Tamale, in line with existing services, heavily weighted towards urban, curative provision.[45] It reflected an emphasis on centralisation and reliance on medical technologies characteristic of post-war modernisation projects. There was also a planned increase in ante- and postnatal services and in numbers of midwives and health visitors, meaning the midwifery school in Accra was to double its annual cohort of trainees.[46] Dr Turner proposed two hospitals for malnourished children located in Accra and Kumasi, noting that they would 'serve a very great need in educating mothers in correct methods.'[47] In general, it was envisaged that hospitals for children would not move outside urban centres, and welfare work would continue to be provided by volunteers.[48] We should perhaps not be surprised that the health service in Ghana, overseen by the British, favoured a curative approach with volunteers providing preventative services. This was the same trajectory followed by the newly established British National Health Service.[49]

In 1951 Kwame Nkrumah became Prime Minister, ruling alongside the British Colonial government. At this point, there were 1486 'non-paying' hospital beds available in the country and 96 further 'paying' beds.[50] The Convention People's Party (CPP) revised development plans, creating the First Development Plan, a compressed version of the Ten-Year Development Plan.[51] The budget for the new development plan was £120m, in a period of unique prosperity for the Gold Coast.[52] The CPP and the British government were in agreement about the need for economic and social development.[53] The construction of new hospitals commenced as well as extensions to current hospitals and clinics. A polyclinic was constructed in Accra and the Central Hospital in Kumasi expanded. Construction began on five new hospitals, in the Northern Territories, which had been sorely neglected.[54] In 1953 a working group discussed plans to update the Accra group of hospitals. This included the reconstruction of the Maternity Hospital and building a new children's unit. The working group considered that 'implementations of these recommendations would … provide at Korle Bu a proper medical unit, streamlined to meet modern requirements and to provide a prompt service to the public.'[55] 'The public' is framed as a consumer of this service, which is articulated in developmentalist language as 'streamlined' and 'modern.' At the launch of the Second Five-Year Development Plan in 1959, Nkrumah stated: 'you have all seen many changes in our capital and the many fine new buildings ... everyone can see very large numbers of schools, hospitals.'[56] There is an emphasis on large projects and visible proof of development. However, there was ambiguity between the aim of modernisation and the wish to provide local healthcare. Although Nkrumahist rhetoric often espoused the benefits of centralisation, industrialisation, standardisation and other markers of modernisation, there was also value attached to localised health and development programmes. As Daniel Immerwahr has argued in the context of US development practice, in the face of the strength of modernisation as a historical force, the local or community level aspects of development are often forgotten.[57]

Women Attending Hospitals

Interest in women's pregnancies meant that they came into contact with curative services for a range of reasons. By the late 1930s, Medical Officers perceived changes at Accra Maternity Hospital. It now catered more to women suffering from diseases unrelated to their pregnancies. Because of the increase in district midwives in Accra, more women were advised that if they were ill, they should go to the Maternity Hospital for delivery. Births themselves were therefore 'normal,' but the women giving birth needed medical care.[58] In fact, the overall effect of district work in Accra was to heighten the number of inpatients but lessen pressure on the hospital to provide outpatient services, as these were provided closer to women's homes.[59]

Rising numbers of midwives meant that this phenomenon went beyond Accra. With the midwives' hostel expanded in 1938,[60] by 1941, there were 40 midwives-in-training at the Maternity Hospital, and 10 graduated that year.[61] Ten years later, the number of trainees had jumped to 104; 40 of these attended a new school in Kumasi, opened in 1949.[62] Forty-three women qualified as midwives in 1952.[63] A third midwifery school opened in 1953: Mampong Midwifery Training School, for which Nkrumah laid the foundation stone. It had begun as an antenatal clinic five years previously, run by Anglican Sister Miriam.[64] The mission envisaged that the school would run courses for midwives with a 'rural bias,' making it unique since the Kumasi and Accra Schools trained midwives in urban hospitals.[65] By 1956, the school employed one MO, two Anglican Sisters and four 'African midwives.' Under their charge were 11 pupil midwives, around 230 outpatients and up to 29 inpatients.[66]

As more midwives opened private clinics or were employed by Local Councils, provision spread. For example, in 1953, private midwife Francisca de Medieros established a clinic in Aburi, supported by the Local Council.[67] That year she supervised 10 deliveries and saw 35 antenatal cases in the small town. By 1954, the Red Cross, which had been running a weekly mobile clinic at the market, decided that de Medeiros's presence obviated theirs. They transferred their mobile clinic to an area 'not lucky enough to have a midwife.'[68] Maternity services spread during this period, increasingly to more rural areas.

In general, there was a massive increase in those attending hospitals, dispensaries and dressing stations. People were attracted to the medical service because of the 'striking success' it had with diseases such as yaws, sleeping sickness and venereal diseases. In fact, between the mid- and late 1940s, the number of outpatients increased by more than 300,000, jumping from 475,571 to 777,949. Inpatients saw a similar increase from 38,128 to 59,042.[69] Furthermore, whereas male patients had previously far outweighed females, in 1953, the Ministry of Health (MH) noted widespread redistribution of beds to allow for an 'increasing number of women attending hospitals for obstetric and other reasons.' In fact, at the Gold Coast Hospital, female beds now outnumbered male beds because of the inclusion of the Maternity Hospital in this figure.[70] In Kumasi, a Maternity Hospital was opened in 1949 because of pressures on the welfare centre as growing numbers of women attended delivery.[71] Evidently, it became more likely that women would attend hospital during their lifetimes and more women were likely to do so when in labour. Inpatient admissions for reproductive health increased dramatically in the 15 years between 1937 and 1952 (Figure 3.1). Furthermore, although inconsistent, there was a general downward trend in death rates from these admissions (Figure 3.2).

However, the growing popularity of services stretched them. The 1952 Medical Report recorded 'embarrassment,' as the department could not keep up with demand.[72] Hospital reports convey results of systematic staffing problems. Accra Maternity Hospital faced 'difficulties' providing trained midwives for teaching

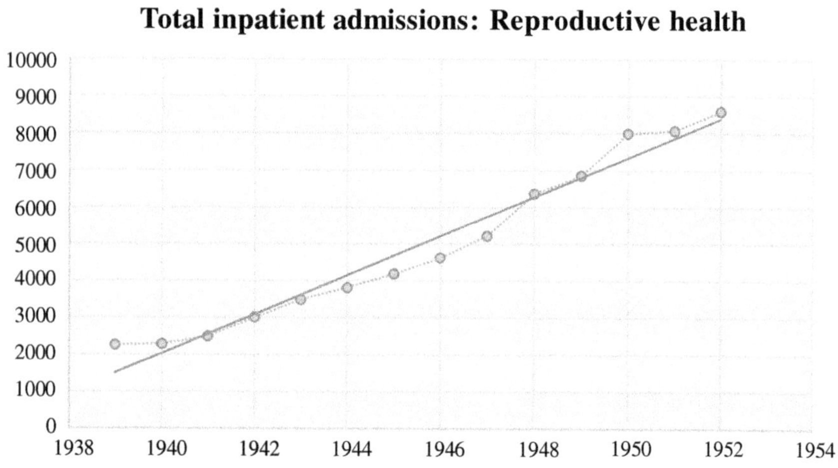

Figure 3.1 Inpatient admissions to hospitals for reproductive health.

Note: Reports of the Medical Department and Ministry of Health between 1939 and 1952. After 1952, the way that admissions were recorded in these reports changed.

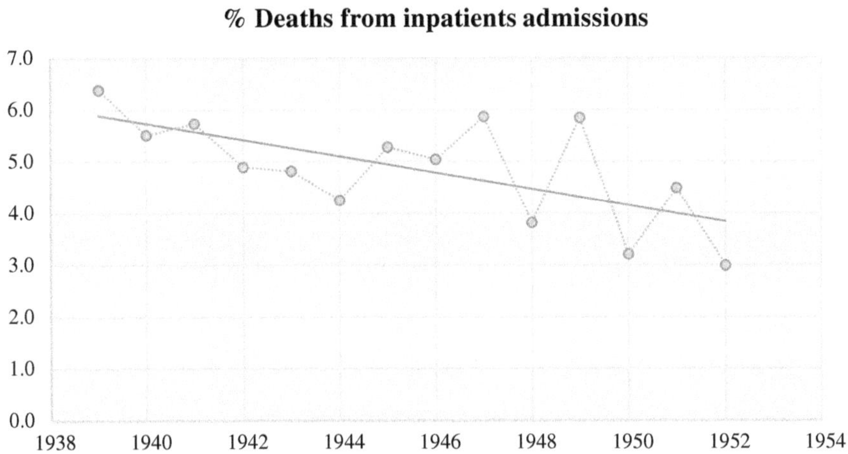

Figure 3.2 Deaths from inpatient admissions for reproductive health.

Note: Reports of the Medical Department and Ministry of Health between 1939 and 1952. The downward trend in death rates after 1948 may be linked to antibiotic use in the colony but as we can see, the trend pre-dates their introduction.

purposes.[73] In 1944 in Oda, one of two large towns in Birim Administrative District, 'large crowds' descended daily on the hospital. In the neighbouring Cape Coast District, the main maternity ward was 'lying empty' because of staffing issues.[74] In 1952, the Board of Visitors to Winneba Hospital reported overcrowding and extensions were needed to deal with pressure from maternity cases. Unfortunately, the shortage of female medical staff throughout the country meant that no extension was made.[75] The situation in Central Region in the 1940s meant that at times there were no accessible and functioning maternity services. In Western Region, the lone female nurse in the small town of Dunkwa in Western Province abandoned it in 1942,[76] whilst in nearby Tarkwa, the removal of the only female nurse met with extensive complaints.[77] Arguably, even if women could travel the distance to reach these hospitals, it did not make sense to do so unless there was an emergency since there were no specific services for obstetrics or gynaecology. In contrast, healthcare in the community was always available, 'when you get pregnant … they just pluck some leaves to prepare medication for you,' remembered Efua Ata.[78]

Whilst Governor Burns expressed a wish in the Ten Year Development Plans that the schedule for building hospitals should be sped up in line with staffing availability, he admitted a 'serious shortage' across all areas.[79] What probably did not help this situation was a decrease in proportional spending on health (Figure 3.3). The 1952 report on the *Health Needs of the Gold Coast* stated that: 'the service has not kept pace with the country's growing wealth and general

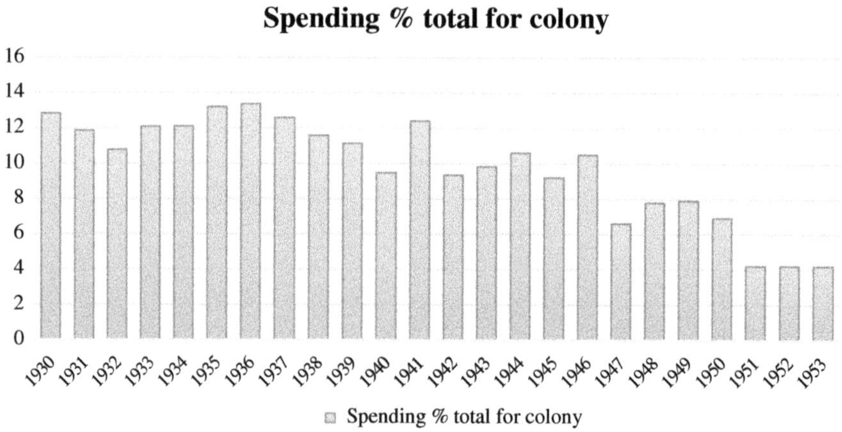

Figure 3.3 Medical spending as a proportion of total government spending 1930–1953.

Note: Statistics for Figure 3.3 are taken from Reports of the Medical Department and Ministry of Health between 1937 and 1952. As the graph indicates, figures were not available from every annual report.

development.'[80] By 1955, spending had risen again to 7.3% of total government expenditure.[81]

Because of the lack of hospitals or their distance from rural inhabitants, women often had to travel long distances to receive the medical care they needed in the 1940s and 1950s. In 1956, there were just 300 midwives in government employment and 295 in private practice, including those employed by local administrations or missions. Dr Poulton, WHO's MCH consultant for Africa, visited in 1957. He calculated that a minimum of 1,000 midwives were needed to meet the population's needs.[82] Looking back on a short period living in Accra in the 1950s and 1960s, Adjoa Ewusiwa attested, 'it was easier in Accra to have access to hospital.' In Central Region, in the 1950s, most women said that the closest hospital was in Cape Coast and that they also travelled to that town for antenatal care.[83] Esi Yawa, who lived in a village close to the town, went to the hospital throughout her first pregnancy but did not deliver there. It was too far and transport was unreliable.[84] Similarly, Aba Efrim, living in a nearby village, said, 'whenever you were in labour going to the hospital was difficult.'[85] For those living further away from Cape Coast, a clinic in Jukwa was intermittently staffed by a nurse. However, there was no transport between Abrafo and Jukwa, women living there reported having to walk 14 kilometres, even whilst heavily pregnant.[86]

Other women expressed fear of entering hospitals.[87] Gynaecologists and obstetricians ultimately held more power than their female patients. Women experienced a literal 'invasion' of their bodies, and, in the 1940s and 1950s Gold Coast, doctors were usually men.[88] Furthermore, they were likely to be European, unable to speak their patients' language, and to hold condescending views on women's own ideas about childbirth and rearing. This dynamic began to change. More staff employed in hospitals were Africans. Certainly, the face of the Red Cross centres changed. However, clinics remained alien to many women. Aba Efrim reflected on why women didn't go to the nearby Cape Coast hospital during labour. She commented: 'what I have noticed was most of them who went there did not come back.'[89] This speaks to a fear of entering hospitals. This was related to the idea that at hospitals, women would be 'cut,' in other words, be forced into surgery. In Nana Efua Ateifi's opinion, the problem was that:

> When you want to give birth at the hospital, every little thing they want to cut you. But for the traditional attendants, they don't cut ... you have the chance of having your family around to encourage you. Your mother will urge you on until you deliver.[90]

Here, the violence of the hospital is juxtaposed with the support of family members, particularly the mother. It also reminds us that avoiding hospital was not always a negative choice or a lack of choice, but a positive one.

The result of hospitals being located long distances from some women meant high death rates when they did make it to the hospital. For example, in 1953 almost half of the women presenting at Accra Maternity Hospital with postpartum haemorrhages did not survive. This was the most common cause of death linked to pregnancy.[91] In the same year, postnatal asphyxia and atelectasis was the ninth most common cause of death in hospital across the whole country.[92] Women presented at the hospital with pregnancy-related conditions but too late. Dr Poulton thought that maternal mortality was under-reported. He reported: 'no-one could estimate the number of maternal deaths in isolated communities with no qualified midwife available.' He had anecdotal evidence that figures would be high given 'repeated reports of patients dying through failure to reach hospital in time.'[93]

Attendance at colonial medical institutions, or even private maternity homes, was far from universal. 'The hospitals were far far far like Accra, Kumasi and the rest,' reported Effua Akyenoba of Aboadze in the Central Region. Although by the time she fell pregnant for the first time in the early 1950s, there were large hospitals situated in Sekondi and Takoradi, around 10 to 15 kilometres away, Effua apparently associated these medical facilities with urban life, out of her reach.[94] This suggests that as well as practicalities obstructing women from hospitals, a socio-economic divide was reinforced and governed women's choices.

In other cases, social obligation affected women's experiences of pregnancy and childbirth. Martha Boanno and Mary Abena remembered that each household had a particular healer who looked after their needs.[95] Others were in the care of family elders, be they professional herbalists or birth attendants or not. Mothers were often the first to be involved in daughters' pregnancies. Esi Atta said, 'when I was with [my mother] I would spit and vomit. My mother then looks at me and tells me I am pregnant.'[96] Many women travelled to stay with their mother's family whilst pregnant, at least the first time. Sometimes, this meant a significant change in the situation. For example, Aunty Angela lived between Abakrampa, where her husband was based, and Tema, where her mother lived. In her case, this meant that she attended hospital whilst staying with her mother in Tema, which she might otherwise not have done.[97] Esi Atta reported that when she went into labour, she told her mother who went to fetch the birth attendant.[98] Although this might seem like a benign event, it reminds us that the people around women had circumstantial decision-making power over how, when and with what aid they gave birth. Furthermore, women were often under obligation to give birth to their families. For example, Esi Koffuah explained: 'my Uncle didn't have children but me and my sister. So my parents and family wanted me to give birth to more children. We [Esi and her husband] could not plan anything.'[99] Although these social networks of reproduction and health were doubtless impacted by the introduction of biomedicine, it seems unlikely that they could be ignored.

The nuances of women's decision to seek other forms of care were rarely considered by medical officers. In 1945 one such Medical Officer pointed to the 'darker side of the picture':

> it is surprising and a little disappointing to find that, in this centre of so much education and enlightenment, there exists still a desire among Africans to take their sickness to the local fetish or herbalist while right here in town there exists a fine modern hospital.[100]

Here we see the imagery of darkness contrasted with the 'enlightenment' of urban spaces and the modern health infrastructure they offer. Through the lens of the colonial medical service, then, not accessing medical care continued to be framed as a moral failing and the antithesis of the modernity that was on offer.

Maternal and Infant Mortality

In 1953, Dr Cheverton, Director of Medical Services, stated that provision for female patients and hospital-based maternity work remained unsatisfactory: there was 'no evidence of improvement' in maternal mortality rates.[101] In fact, they appear to have risen (Figure 3.4). The data for maternal mortality were taken from registration areas and adjusted to apply to the wider population. Rising maternal mortality could be explained by data biases as maternal deaths were reported more consistently. Ironically, the fact that the 1940s saw the first widespread use of treatments that might be effective against maternal mortality – namely sulphonamides and antibiotics – may have driven more women to hospitals where their deaths would be registered, skewing the data.[102] It could also have to do with a dip in living conditions caused by the war and swollen shoot disease, which was having devastating effects on cocoa production by the mid-1940s.[103] Deaths from malaria also rose during this period. Since malaria can cause the death of a foetus in utero, it is possible that this was a cause.[104] More likely though, the expertise and the technologies needed to save the lives of women in childbirth were not yet

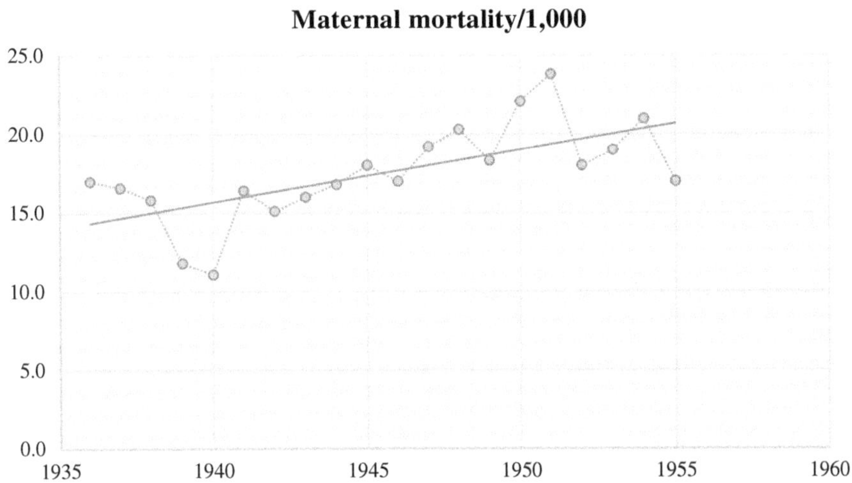

Figure 3.4 Maternal mortality rates 1935–1955. Reports of the Medical Department and Ministry of Health between 1935 and 1955.

widely available. Furthermore, most women were not attended to during childbirth by government-trained midwives which would have improved the outcomes as the most likely cause of death was obstructed labour or postnatal haemorrhaging.[105] Meanwhile, infant mortality appeared roughly consistent, despite medical campaigns against childhood diseases and increases in maternal and infant welfare services (Figure 3.5). This was probably the result of widening registration areas to places where the mortality rate was higher.

Women sought medical supervision during their pregnancies, but not for deliveries.[106] The sister in charge of Mampong Maternity Hospital wrote, 'I think many of the women who now deliver without a midwife would be willing to have a midwife, if she could attend them in their own compounds.'[107] In reality, there were not enough midwives to make this feasible, especially as midwives preferred to work in towns. In Nigeria, in the 1940s, two grades of midwives were introduced. The first resembled those in the Gold Coast: educated women who underwent three years of training. The second undertook six months of training, were 'illiterate' and had usually acted as the 'village midwife' previously.[108] However, in the Gold Coast this idea was rejected as 'fundamentally unsound' by the Advisory Committee on Education, despite agreeing that there were not enough medical staff. They believed that only supervision by 'educated' women was appropriate. They did, however, recommend that midwives maintain good relations with '"traditional" midwives', who could act as advocates for their work.[109] The Midwives Board opposed training local birth attendants because it was not in their interest to build up the professional competition.[110]

Although the dangers of the 'native midwife' by no means dissipated in the minds of colonial officials, by the 1950s the Social Welfare Department looked to

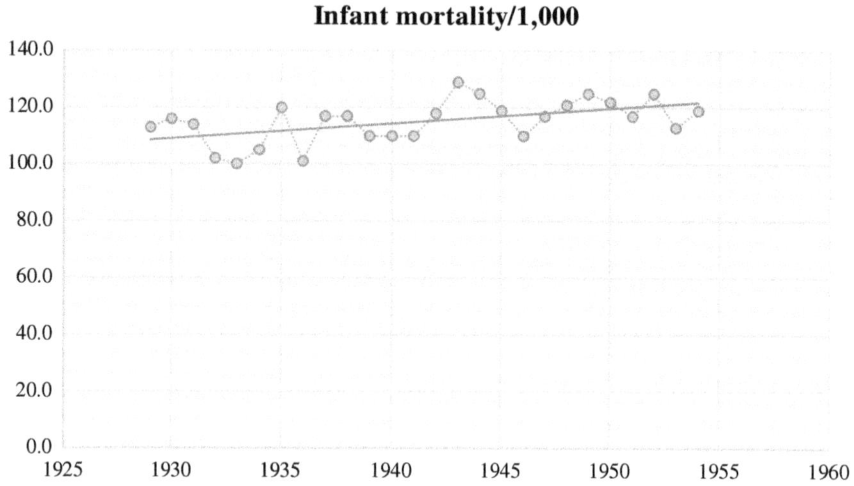

Figure 3.5 Infant mortality rates 1929–1954.

Note: Reports of the Medical Department and Ministry of Health between 1935 and 1955. Statistics for infant mortality were based on those deaths registered, usually in urban areas. This means that data is skewed. For example, the Annual Report on the Social and Economic Progress of the People of the Gold Coast, 1935–1936, Accra, 1936, 9, notes that infant mortality for that year was particularly high in comparison to the previous year due to the 'increased prosperity in rural areas' which allowed sick children to 'be brought in to the centres for treatment' so that their deaths would be recorded. The slight rise in infant mortality in 1950 likely has more to do with this than an actual increase in mortality.

decentralise and pass responsibility to local government. As such, they planned to train teams of men and women to 'provide the leadership necessary to implement Local Administration plan for the development of the area.' The Department decided that this team should comprise illiterate as well as literate people. Specifically,

> our experiment in the training of illiterate women leaders in child care and nutrition as Kpetoe in Togoland under British Trusteeship has proved that there is a vast reservoir of leadership amongst the ranks of the illiterate that can be tapped for community development work.[111]

The 'experiment' referred to here, in Togoland, invited 'traditional midwives' to receive classes on childcare and nutrition. This was an attempt to 'break down the practices and traditions' of the community's women through influential, older women.[112] Similarly, in Anomabu in Central Region in 1951, government-trained midwives shared ideas among one another to improve provision locally. They formed discussion groups with mothers and pregnant women. The activity was so successful that the Social Development Officer at Winneba suggested a similar programme for 'uncertified midwives' as 'in very many cases these women appear to be those to whom the others turn for leadership.'[113] This idea was not taken up by the District Commissioner, but its suggestion indicates a shift in attitude among certain officials towards birth attendants.

Welfare Centres

As well as providing curative centres, Governor Burns stressed that prevention, 'through education and propaganda' was of primary importance.[114] In other words, addressing – and reforming – Africans' wider approach to health. Attending ante-natal clinics became a normal part of women's pregnancies (Figure 3.6). The 1948 Medical Report stated:

> [t]here is a growing tendency for women to regard the routine visit to the ante-natal clinic as a pleasant social event, and with mounting attendances, the work at some of these centres became very heavy.[115]

Arguably, this was due in part to other women's advice to attend clinics. Cecilia Fynn Essien lived near Cape Coast, except for a period after she was married in the 1940s, when she travelled with her husband, a building contractor. Before giving birth to her ten children, she returned home. Her mother had attended the Red Cross clinic in Cape Coast, so when she suspected Cecilia might be pregnant, she sought confirmation there. Cecilia remembers being seen by a nurse and given medicines. There was family loyalty to this clinic: 'we all gave birth there' she remembers. Throughout her pregnancy, Cecilia attended clinic every Tuesday,

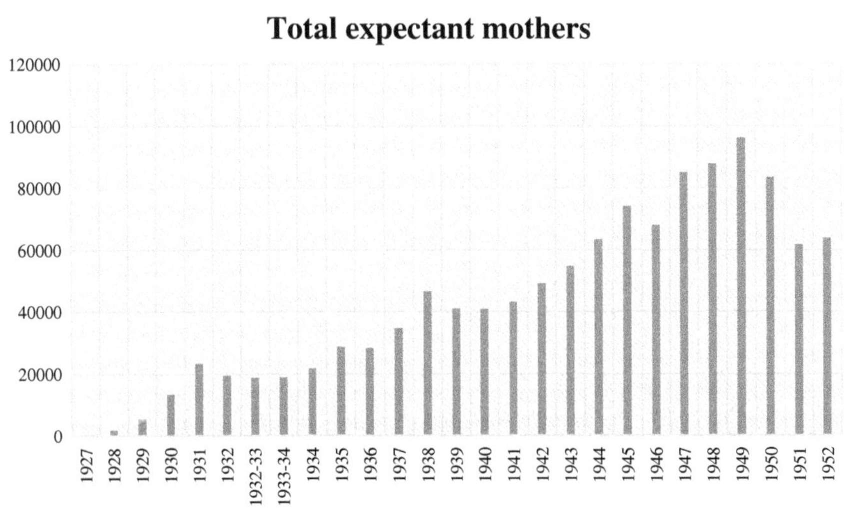

Figure 3.6 Expectant mothers attending clinics 1935–1951. Reports on the Medical Department and the Ministry of Health for the years 1935–1952.

where midwives examined her and tested her blood for sugar levels, as well as her urine and stool. Midwives advised her to take care of herself and eat nutritious foods. She remembers being 'treated well'; it cost little, the place was tidy, and women were seen privately. In short, 'they did a very good job there.'[116]

Cecilia described her first labour: 'from the beginning I was told that there was a problem, and that the child could not come out well. The leg was showing rather than the head.' However, 'the midwife did a great job by examining the stomach to ensure that the head rather comes first.' She said she 'was not scared, I knew whatever happened the child will come well.'[117] This memory of a first, and presumably difficult, birth is based on positive experiences of pregnancies and deliveries at this clinic, rather than necessarily this level of faith at the time in the midwife. Cecilia's memory of confidence in the clinic and medical procedure demonstrates the impact of belonging to the second generation of women attending clinics.

Historically, welfare centres had focused on reducing infant mortality rates; from the 1940s, the proportion of care shifted to expectant mothers (Figure 3.7). The exception to this was mainly the Catholic mission centres, where attendances for children reached around 90,000 annually by the late 1940s, whereas only around 4,000–5,000 mothers were treated at these clinics.[118] In government and Red Cross centres though, there was more demand for antenatal care and delivery services. Whereas in the mid-1930s, expectant mothers made up around 20% of attendances, this figure had almost doubled to 37% by 1950.

The clinics therefore became important for pregnant women. This was especially true of Red Cross clinics which, from 1948 onwards, recorded more

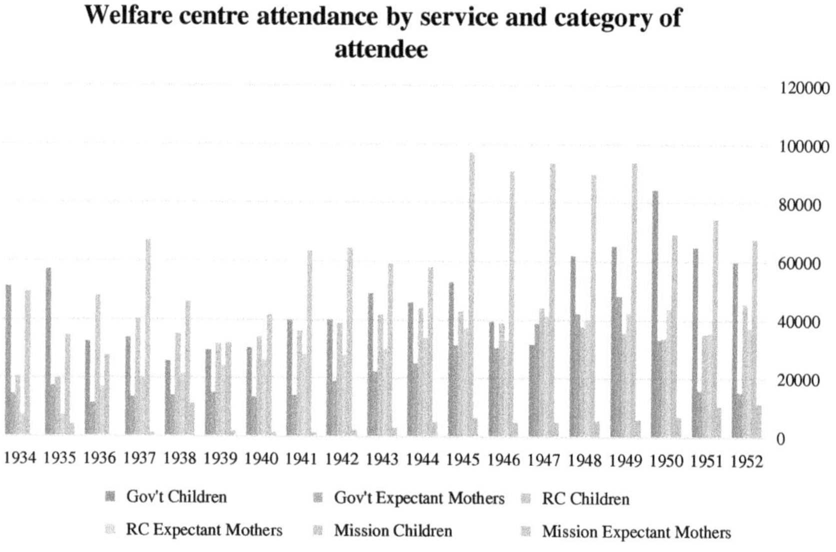

Figure 3.7 Attendances at welfare clinics. Statistics for Figure 3.7 are taken from Reports of the Medical Department and Ministry of Health between 1935 and 1951.

attendances for expectant mothers than children. Clearly, a significant proportion of reproductive health services were still delivered by non-government agencies, especially the Red Cross. In fact, the medical department's policy was to 'encourage outside agencies, especially voluntary agencies, such as Missions to erect and run hospitals.'[119] In other words, the tradition of voluntary work remained strong despite increased state provision. Attendances at government clinics accounted for around a quarter to a third of the total from 1935 onwards. This rose to about 40% after 1948. This was probably due to the government takeover of the Red Cross clinic in Kumasi and suggests increased governmental responsibility for MCH.

The Red Cross recorded attendance at its clinics at 130,000 by 1949, which was higher than Medical Reports suggested.[120] By 1954, the Red Cross oversaw three clinics at Cape Coast, Koforidua and Sekondi. There was an ambulance attached to each, which midwives took to clinics in neighbouring villages. In addition, in Accra, Ho and Ashanti there were three mobile clinics, reduced from five in 1949.[121] They also provided mobile clinics to mission societies.[122] Clinics were run by a combination of volunteers and medical staff.

When Lady Limerick, British Red Cross leader, visited the Gold Coast Branch in 1954, she noted that membership was 'mostly African,' suggesting that leadership of the Society had continued to move away from being dominated by Europeans, as it was in its early years.[123] By 1954, the Koforidua Red Cross clinic was run by an African midwife, Mrs Buckman. It employed ten staff and opened daily from 8 am. The midwife saw around 60 antenatal cases and 45 babies each morning.[124] The Western Region Matron described the Red Cross clinic at Takoradi as 'the largest and best run maternity and child welfare centre in the Gold Coast.' In 1954 Miss Vanderpuye, an African who had trained in the UK had been running the clinic for 16 years.[125] She was an 'outstanding and much respected personality.' In 1952, the clinic saw 9,000 children and 10,000 antenatal cases. Mothers were charged small amounts, which included any medicine they required; weighing sessions were free.[126] The Cape Coast clinic opened twice weekly. The remaining days the midwife, Mrs Coker, travelled to neighbouring villages with the mobile clinic. Two private midwives also saw their own patients at the Red Cross clinic.[127] In Ashanti, midwife Miss Mills ran the mobile clinic, another UK-trained African woman. The clinic visited a different village each week. The British Red Cross reported that though 'there is still a tendency to cling on to old beliefs and native medicines in certain areas, the services provided by the clinics are, on the whole, very much appreciated.'[128] Lady Limerick noted that the work of mobile clinics 'served its purpose in make the people more "midwife-minded,"' reminding us of the propaganda function of clinics.[129] The Red Cross contributed considerably to medicalisation of pregnancy and childbirth.

Schools' Junior Links' public work grew, promoting Red Cross healing practices. Lady Limerick reported that in the villages surrounding Cape Coast, pupils at girls' schools had 'done wonders,' washing and applying ointments to babies with 'the most horrible-looking sores, ulcers and bad burns cases.' She mentions 'an elderly woman sitting there, listening to every word of a lecture delivered by a 17-year old girl on food value, telling them what they should eat and how they should cook it!'[130] Lady Limerick's perception was doubtless skewed. This woman's respectful adherence to lessons taught by a young girl who was not a mother herself seems unlikely. Regardless, Links were important for the visibility of biomedical healing methods in the wider community.

However, the government was taking on more of the case load in its clinics and was establishing new maternity hospitals and midwifery training schools. In 1954, Lady Limerick, in consultation with Dr Cicely Williams, told the government that it was time for them to take over the 'pioneer service' the Red Cross had provided. It was no longer practical, they argued, for the Red Cross to take responsibility for Maternal and Child Health (MCH), especially given that 'the greatest mortality rates in the country' were among this demographic.[131] This is indicative of a shift in perception in which healthcare became the state's responsibility under the expansive plans for social development explored earlier in this chapter. But the government did not actually take over Red Cross maternal health provision until the early 1960s, demonstrating the ongoing importance of non-governmental and voluntary provision. However, as this examination of the Red Cross in the 1940s and 1950s has demonstrated, this was increasingly Africanised and came under the mantra of community 'self-help.'

Marketplace of Health

Furthermore, clinics were not the only option for women. One example of a 'marketplace' mentality to health is the demand from women attending clinics that they be given medicine to take away with them.[132] For example, in the early 1950s in Sekondi, Red Cross clinic attendance cost women 1/- regardless of whether they needed medicine or not. The midwife in charge, Miss Vanderpuye, reported that if women were not given medicine, they returned the next day demanding it. Interestingly, they said that it was their husbands who insisted on this. Perhaps men, who did not attend clinics, felt reassured by tangible evidence of their wives' medical care and the money spent there. Esi Koffuah reported that she went to the clinic every Thursday during her pregnancies, which her husband paid for. If she did not go, she said, he became quite annoyed.[133] The mention of money again suggests that husbands expected to see the return on their investment. Miss Vanderpuye began to give women 'some innocuous medicines' so that 'honour is satisfied all around!'[134]

This highlights the importance of commodities as proof of the value of clinics and indicates that men had a role in choosing healthcare for their pregnant partners. Indeed, Margaret Field states that in Ga society, it was men who approached the Gods when their partners became pregnant.[135] Most women I interviewed reported that their husband was the first person they reported pregnancies to; otherwise, it was their mother. Efua Ata said that it was her husband who chose which herbalist she went to during her pregnancy.[136] Interestingly, Kyei states that if a woman had fertility issues, it was her husband's responsibility to do all he could to help her conceive, including sending her to the hospital.[137] It is possible that men became more invested in their families' healthcare as the trend towards nuclear families and fathers' responsibility grew.[138] In any case, it seems pertinent to note that decisions over women's health were often made by their male partner.

Exemplifying a literal marketplace for health, Lady Limerick described the 'awful "medicine man"' in Kumasi. He had 'the most repellent looking bones, claws, crocodile's skulls, skins, tufts of hair, bat wings,' displayed outside his booth right beside the Red Cross clinic. Evidently, women attending the clinic to see the government-trained midwives could also take the opportunity to visit this healer.[139] What is more, healers operated as part of a diverse economy. Attending births or selling herbs was rarely a sole source of income. In Aboadze, for example, in the early 1950s, Effua Akyenoba's father was known and respected in the community as a medicine-man. He cured broken bones and attended to women during pregnancy and childbirth. He, like all of Effua's family, also worked as a fisherman.[140]

Spiritual healing was another option. Ekuah Nkrumah did not conceive a child in the first five years of marriage and chose an Imam to help with this problem. He carried out certain rituals including chanting and drawing lines and then told her she would have twins, which she later did.[141] When Mary Sampson was pregnant with her first child, a local woman assisted her and provided herbal remedies. However, Mary did not limit herself to this method of healthcare. She frequented a Twelve Apostles Mission Church.[142] There, she regularly took blessed water throughout her pregnancies.[143] The Twelve Apostles Mission began in 1914.[144] Micah Kodjoe George gave the government notice of the existence of a number of churches, including this one in the Western Region, in 1949.[145] The church practised divine water healing. Hannah Bowah's mother started attending in the 1940s, when many of her children were dying. She took Hannah to the church when she was young and believed that this was why she survived. Hannah attended the church when she became pregnant, that was where she went for healthcare. She was attended by her mother-in-law, who was a prophetess at the church and used Florida water and prayer to guarantee Hannah's health and the baby's safe delivery.[146] As well as water healing, other prophetesses used herbs and prayer to help women conceive and give birth.[147]

When 'Aunty' Esi's mother was giving birth in Western Region in the 1940s and 1950s, she did not attend hospital, as 'we don't have hospital here … we were always relying on local herbs.'[148] Village public health worked without colonial intervention. Indeed, as Kwame Anthony Appiah noted, for a large number of Gold Coasters, the penetration of colonialism was only ever 'shallow,' especially cognitively.[149] As Esi Praah put it, 'we were a typical village': there were no hospitals. The inference is that colonial medical systems rarely penetrated the 'typical village.'[150] Often those who needed medication or attendance during their births knew someone in their own families or in their husbands' families who could fill this role. Aba Seku, who gave birth to her first two children near Cape Coast in the early 1950s, said, 'for every woman when you are pregnant they put you in the hand[s] of an elderly person to give you medicine.'[151] Her experience suggests systemised healing based on inter-generational knowledge sharing.

Knowledge of pregnancy and childbirth was passed on through networks established outside hospitals and lecture rooms. In Gyabenkrom in Western Region, Araba Yedua started watching Maame Ashia when she was just 12 years old, around 1950. Maame Ashia attended to women in the village and was respected in the community. She was well known for her extensive knowledge of herbs, including those that would induce placental delivery and those that would give strength and prevent vomiting throughout the pregnancy. Importantly, she was remembered for particular skills, not simply a generic ability to deliver babies. Maame Ashia taught Araba herbal remedies, how to deliver children and spiritual rituals including those to be performed with the placenta following birth.[152] Although birth attendants' experiences cannot be found in the colonial archives, oral histories show that families passed down healing practices.

Community Development and Health

If medicalisation was about modernisation, it was not all about urban, large-scale projects. Women's reproductive health was not generally seen purely in medical terms or tackled principally with technologies. It was understood through a *social* lens and a moral one. As was shown in Chapter 2, participating in 'progressive' projects allowed Africans to play a part in the mission and humanitarian vision of human uplift. Indeed, Kate Skinner has argued that the perceived possession of 'good character' in Africans was central to their taking part in community development projects.[153] Reproductive health allows us to better understand development interventions by countering a history of colonial medicine which emphasises curative, technological advances. It forces us to resituate the history of medicine at the level of the community, focusing on local and social aspects. Social welfare was domesticated. It had to do with health and hygiene in the home, imagined women exclusively as mothers, and was concerned with nutrition, breastmilk and vaccination campaigns. Seeing late colonial 'development' through this lens of reproductive health emphasises the importance of looking beyond economics in our understanding of development.

The 1940s saw a shift in the colony's political structure. In 1944, the Native Authorities Ordinance was passed, making Native Authorities function more like Local Councils. They were also now supposed to include members of the 'modern elite.'[154] Due to concerns that under the indirect rule, chiefs had not provided development, local government was established as an alternative framework.[155] This brought the decentralised Native Authorities under the direct control of the central government. The Ten-Year Development Plan stressed that:

> the development of the Colony cannot proceed without the full cooperation of the Native Authorities; and if the plans for the wide expansion of health, medical and education services are to be realised, the Native Authorities will have to play an ever increasing part both in financing and administering these activities.[156]

J. K. Nsarkoh states that this new 'cool, detached administration' was needed for 'deciding policies and priorities in the age of development.'[157] But development administered by the local government did not necessarily mean it was either 'cool' or 'bureaucratic.'

The colonial government's development plans relied on 'self-help.' Colonised Africans would ideally organise locally and provide labour and materials. 'Development Committees' were established. The colonies' Chief Commissioner stated: 'financial assistance should be given first to works to which the community is prepared itself to contribute by the provision of materials or labour.' There was 'no set pattern' for these Committees; they were to adhere to local needs.[158] The policy on Community Development said that 'the acceleration of the economic and social development of the community ... by harnessing the community's own energies is the settled policy of the government.' The idea was that development originating from communities themselves, especially in rural areas, would harness real motivation to engage with development.[159] Community Development should 'raise the standard of living and ... promote development in all its forms.' Importantly, it should tackle both economic and social needs, including 'health, welfare and education.'[160]

For health services, the anticipated dynamic was increasing that local bodies would recognise and provide for local needs. Dr Turner, the Director of Medical Services (DMS) in 1947, noted that the colony's revenue would not permit the provision of sufficient hospitals and doctors, and therefore a dispensary system providing 'simple remedies' was necessary to bring 'medical aid to the whole population.'[161] Sixty-three percent of dispensers and dispensaries were provided by Native Authorities in 1947, and Turner hoped that this number would rise.[162] Midwives were encouraged to 'take up practice in the out-stations of the colony' and chiefs to contact the Midwives Board if they required a midwife and to provide her with 'decent' accommodation and wages.[163] Notably, authority over health was transferred to localised bodies usually made up almost entirely of men, shifting power and expertise away from birth attendants.

Government planners envisaged local dressing stations designed with MCH in mind. According to Dr Turner, the dressing station waiting room should double as a welfare centre. Eventually, there should be a 'small library, and possibly a stage for cinema and plays,' and accommodation for a midwife. Adjacent to the midwife's quarters should be a room where emergency cases could wait for hospital transfer.[164] A focus on maternal health was clearly pictured. Furthermore, medical officers' 'faith in the agency of education and moral uplift,' identified by Skinner and Peter Bloom, among others, is exemplified through the inclusion of educational spaces.[165] However, it should be noted that by 1957 there were only nine such health centres in existence. They did include a lecture room but not libraries or cinemas.[166]

The CPP's 1951 development plan reiterated that establishing health centres and preventative medicine must be the Local Councils' responsibility. It also noted the desirability of expanding MCH services.[167] The 1952 report, *Health Needs of the Gold Coast*, envisaged a 'modern system of local government throughout the whole country' that would oversee the construction and maintenance of health facilities including maternity homes.[168] Responsibility for health was to shift to 'local' areas, to reach a greater number of people. What is more, the creation of the new health system was framed as 'modern,' a signifier of development. Maternal and child welfare clinics, as well as health visitors, were two key areas that would be handed over to local authorities immediately, according to the report. Health centres were to provide limited antenatal and postnatal and infant care.

Looking at late colonial development through the lens of women's reproductive health alerts us to the articulation of development through moralising language. For example, when a Red Cross Sister stopped providing a clinic in a village in the Denkyira Confederacy because of a lack of local cooperation, the exasperated District Commissioner complained: 'it is high time that the Native Authority developed a sense of responsibility in such matters and it appears they will only do so by bitter experience.'[169] Colonial officials differentiated between villages based on their response to community development projects. For example, Ekumfi in Central Region was condemned for its 'inertia,' 'backward' attitude, and for being 'allergic to enumeration' qualities which exemplified a lack of cooperation with the government. On the other hand, nearby Asaafa was seen more positively, being 'anxious to start community development.'[170] This differentiation based on engagement with development projects shows that communities' progressiveness was judged by their propensity to take responsibility for health projects on the government's terms. This idea of progressiveness was carried through from concepts of development already emergent through mission and humanitarian discourse established in the interwar period and examined in earlier chapters.

Native Authorities' engagement in providing healthcare was varied. Whilst some financed and organised services, others seemed less keen or able to act. A 1949 scheme encouraged Native Authorities to send dressers for training so they could run dispensaries in rural areas upon their return. This was intended to extend health services to inaccessible areas. However, the scheme was paid for by Native Authorities, meaning that, in practice, poorer and more disconnected areas were unable to organise their own medical services.[171] There were also a number of disputes over who should benefit from maternity homes that had been constructed with particular funds.[172]

In 1953, the Chairman of Amansie District Council wrote to the Ministry for Health to report that Bekwai Maternity Clinic had 'ceased functioning' and the midwife was sent away. He emphasised that women were now travelling 'day and night' 24 miles to Kumasi for delivery, which was, he concluded, 'a sorrowful affair.'[173] In petitioning for a loan to replace the clinic, the chairman stressed that the absence of such services made the area 'backward.' Furthermore,

> 'there is a serious burden of married women's disablement and invalidism due to lack of knowledge and insufficient … midwifery attendance. Much of the damage to life and health of the women and children of this District would be got rid of if our married women … could obtain medical advice and supervision during … pregnancy and motherhood.'[174]

This form of appeal: pointing to women's ignorance and evoking of lack of progress as morally unacceptable is reminiscent of the attitudes of local leaders seen in the 1930s and suggests that this line of entreaty remained discursively relevant when applying for development funding.

Similarly, Native Authorities in Manya Krobo, near Koforidua, proposed to fund village dispensaries. They hoped to guarantee preventative measures and that the government would in turn provide 'a first-rate Hospital with Maternal Department and a Children clinic.' They proposed that 'definite steps are taken about provision for ante-natal and post-natal care of our women and children.'[175] The Native Authority argued that health was important to the district: 'several stools of this country would have very few subjects if the health of the people is not carefully looked after,' leaving the country's resources to 'lie dormant in the bowels of the Earth.' Furthermore, 'our towns, instead of *developing* and expanding into habitable *modern* places, shall deteriorate and dwindle into unpleasant spots of population decreases.'[176] The Native Authority clearly appropriated development language to pressure the colonial government to provide medical services and framed it in terms of de-population.

By 1950, it was noted that a series of development committees had been established in the cocoa-farming region between Aburi and Koforidua with 'promising' results.[177] In Mampong-Akwapim the Development Committee received a government grant in August 1951 worth £1,000 for 'development projects of benefit to cocoa farmers.' The chairman suggested that the money be used to build an antenatal clinic or 'some such enterprise which met with the approval of the cocoa farmers.'[178] This suggests that local communities of cocoa farmers saw antenatal activities as desirable. The throw-away phrasing, though, in which an antenatal clinic is placed among 'some such enterprise' suggests that clinics were imagined as signifiers of development. In Hemang, it was envisaged that the new dispensary, built and staffed under the dispensers' training scheme explained above, should become 'the nucleus for subsequent development.' It would oversee the construction of water supplies, latrines, and general village sanitation. There would grow 'a web of Child welfare and Maternity services, which could also serve as a means of dissemination of instruction on cooking and nutrition.'[179] Evidently, improvements in women's reproductive health were not only seen as a result of development but as an impetus driving it. However, there were certain difficulties in guaranteeing contributions. In 1950 in Tutu, elders were reluctant to contribute to funds because of the annual levy. Most of the money came from church communities. In Adawso, it was the young men who caused problems, refusing 'to help either with money or work.' The projects most likely to progress were school buildings, which local people would 'make sacrifices' for.[180]

Local Councils and development committees relied on a historical idea of tradition derived from Native Authorities. As Thomas Spear has argued, the authority of local political leaders in Africa was derived from 'cobbled together local customs, colonial law, Christian morality and administrative regulations.'[181] This is exemplified as Gold Coasters' discourse on community development projects included moral and social readings as well as economic and bureaucratic ones.

In the post-war period, 'development' became an important organisational tool and indicator of authority. If, as Spear argues, 'local discourse played a vital role as people continually reinterpreted and reconstructed tradition … and colonial policies often stimulated … ongoing politics of neo-traditionalism,' health and development were key to stimulation.[182] One result of this was that by transferring control of colonial health services to local groups of men, the government resituated medical authority. Furthermore, Local Councils were overwhelmingly made up of CPP members.[183] Indeed, the CPP was accused of 'monopolising' local authorities for their own political interests.[184] Previously, recourse to healing in villages and towns was not gendered, authority derived from efficacy and experience. Families were surrounded by birth attendants, herbalists and spiritualists who provided a variety of healthcare when called upon. There were intergenerational systems whereby knowledge of reproductive health was passed.

Educating Women

In 1943 the Advisory Committee on Education in the Colonies in London organised a sub-committee to investigate African girls' and women's education and develop policy. The sub-committee identified that previously, aside from the 'untiring' work of voluntary societies, there was little interest in women's education. Indeed, the proportion of girls and women with formal education in the Gold Coast was extremely low. The 1948 census showed that 2.6% of people had primary education, among which girls were a minority. Education was defined in a broad sense by the sub-committee; it perhaps referred mainly to non-academic education for women, particularly 'domestic matters and in the upbringing of children and the health of the family.'[185] Teaching women was seen to be hindered by the 'complexity' of their lives. This was understood as a barrier to 'modern' solutions. In other words, women's 'ignorance' was seen as a barrier to post-war modernity just as it had been to interwar 'progress' in the Gold Coast. The report focused on the importance of African women as biological and social reproducers. Its authors emphasised that 'girls are … instructed in their duties as members of a tribe, and particularly as future mothers of *its* children.'[186] Similarly, the report stated that husbands expected knowledge of basic healthcare from wives for 'a better chance of survival for their children.'[187] Discursively, children belonged to tribes or to men. In fact, the report concludes that 'it is unnatural to educate the woman or girl except as part of her community.'[188] Education was not encouraged for the benefit of individual women but of communities.

In fact, girls *were* educated on reproductive issues within their own communities. The report makes limited reference to this, noting that they acquired knowledge of native medicines as part of their general education. The report's authors, however, did not value this. Whilst admitting that some of these medicines were 'of therapeutic value,' they noted that 'others [were] useless or even harmful charms.'[189] Women's inability to distinguish between these categories suggested ignorance. The 1950s social development programmes stressed the value of biomedical options and the importance of knowledge on hygiene, nutrition and child-rearing originating outside women's communities. The report later states that women ought to be given some 'elementary science' lessons to warn them of the 'dangerous rites of childbirth, superstitious treatment of illness and ignorant care of children.'[190] Women's 'ignorance' continued to be blamed for their own and their children's ill health.

Schools were encouraged to teach girls 'hygiene' and childcare; domestic science was part of the curriculum by the 1940s. In 1944 groups of primary school girls were taken to PML and to the child welfare centre in Kumasi for instruction on antenatal care and childbirth.[191] By taking these girls to hospitals, the implicit location of competent motherhood shifted to a biomedical setting. Between 1950 and 1951, a series of *Notes for Housecraft Teachers and All Teachers in Girls Schools* were issued by the department of education. They covered topics including needlework, laundry, preparing food to relieve common illnesses, and providing a 'balanced diet' for children. Suggested topics for women teachers included 'feeding infants,' 'talks on midwives and their work' and 'weighing clinic; advantages of Maternity Hospitals.'[192] In other words, the subject was linked to the promotion of biomedicine. However, these kinds of schemes affected the tiny proportion of girls on the Gold Coast that regularly attended school offering domestic science.

British colonialists' enthusiasm for Mass Education dated to the post-war moment since it was linked to better cooperation with welfare agencies.[193] That is, Mass Education was a development project in itself and crucial to other social development initiatives. The Mass Education Programme was organised regionally and hierarchically. Each region was under the charge of a Community Development Officer, linked to Local Councils. Whilst fears of detribalisation and declining morality made towns a vital space for this work, so were rural areas due to their lack of development. Each region was assigned fieldworkers and a Rural Training Centre.[194] Village development was an important part of Mass Education. Village committees were responsible for deciding which social services they needed, providing communal labour and sometimes building materials. By 1954, there were 1,499 village development schemes operating. The Department of Social Welfare and Community Development report for that year noted:

> the idea of self-help is becoming firmly established in most rural areas … Village development means far more than the erection of a building … When a village development scheme is initiated, it means that a particular community has grasped the fact that progress comes from a desire for better living and the ability to work for it.[195]

Significantly, development was dependent on the desires and input of communities.

Colonial officials continued to emphasise the damaging effects of women's ignorance. In 1942, Dr Blacklock wrote *The Health of Women and Children in the Colonies*, in which she argued that the chief causes of maternal and infant mortality were 'of social origin.'[196] This made social development paramount to improving mortality rates. She claimed: 'without radical modification of these harmful social factors no great improvement … can be expected. In existing circumstances medical science can only produce palliative effect.'[197] DMS of the Gold Coast, Dr Kirk agreed. He emphasised medicine's place in the broader context of 'community service.'[198] In 1943, he wrote that 'the recognition that medical services are part of a cooperative effort of social services is timely and welcome.'[199] It was in this context that Mass Education specific to women began in Ghana: 'Work among women along home economics lines' was one of four Mass Education streams.[200] Educating women was seen as the path to a 'healthy home,' something which benefitted all. Certain courses were specifically designed around 'Preventative Medicine' and 'for illiterate women.'[201] In 1950 in Asaafa village near Saltpond, nurses joined Mass Education Officers 'to get groups of women together' to discuss childcare, nutrition and the prevention of disease.[202] Health under Mass Education was consistently gendered: seen as women's responsibility.

In 1954, the government decided to standardise women's Mass Education. A syllabus for courses was implemented, with the aid of two British Red Cross workers. In April, a three-week course was held at Axim, for 35 instructors of women's courses. They were taught 'hygiene, child care, nutrition and adult teaching techniques.' The course theme was: 'Health Education for Rural Families' implying that rural families' health was women's responsibility. Demonstrations for the course were done in Akan and Nzima, and 'charts, films and flannel-graph work … made the course vivid and real.'[203] The syllabus was used for the next few years providing a 'comprehensive training programme for village women in home economics.'[204]

Educative efforts for women and girls were by no means confined to rural areas. A number of benevolent and voluntary groups were formed during the late colonial period, by men and women responding to conditions in towns resulting from rapid urbanisation.[205] Reflecting worries over social degradation in urban life, Lady Burns, the governor's wife, established the Gold Coast Young Women's League in 1945. The aims of the League were to 'promote the spiritual, mental and physical welfare of young women.' The League opened a hostel in Accra for young women 'in need of a home life and improved living conditions but also a social, cultural and vocational centre.' The League collaborated with the Social Service department, and its warden was recruited from among the Christian missions.[206] The Federation of Gold Coast Women was inaugurated in 1953. It was a women's organisation which was autonomous from any political party.[207] It worked mainly on social welfare projects.[208] Members of the new Federation emphasised basic hygiene and nutrition. 'Family Life' was also integral to The Young Women's Christian Organisation (YWCA) 1951 work plans. Their programme emphasised the importance of housecraft institutes, antenatal clinics and health visitors.[209]

On areas in which the colonial government deemed education for women imperative was nutrition. Malnutrition was a growing and gendered concern for the government, connected especially with children and expectant mothers.[210]

Essentially, nutrition was seen as women's responsibility. It also meant that women's reproductive health became relevant beyond the medical sphere. Nutrition is related to the broad developmental needs of the colony. The development of agriculture, local resources and industry was deemed crucial for the post-war provision of 'good food.' Nutritional well-being was framed as dependent on and a symptom of development and modernity. The 1944 Purcell Report noted that 'some [agricultural development] plans may necessitate radical change in the age-long traditions of sections of the population.'[211] If the people of the Gold Coast harboured traditions that were harmful to their nutritional status, this view applied particularly to women and specifically in their roles as mothers. The rise in nutritional diseases in the 1935 Medical Report was linked to 'faulty nutrition,' in other words, Africans' lack of knowledge.[212]

By the early 1950s, concerns over nutrition had taken on a technical character, reflecting a wider pattern of scientific researchers and technical experts impacting colonial policy.[213] For example, in 1950, guidance was published for domestic science teachers emphasising the need for expectant mothers to be careful about what they ate 'otherwise both she and her child will suffer.'[214] The pamphlet goes on to explain that as a baby grows inside its mother's body, it receives all its nutrition from its mother. It notes the different types of nutrition needed: 'protein, fat, carbohydrate, minerals, vitamins and water.' It then explains what each mineral will 'build': calcium for bones and teeth, iron for blood and vitamins for general growth. It then discusses exactly which food is needed for each of these building blocks.[215] Interestingly, nutrition was also seen by some in the Gold Coast education department as a threat to fertility in the colony.[216]

Fertility

In Chapter 1, I discussed the importance of high fertility to individual communities in the 1920s. In the 1950s, people still generally wanted to have a lot of children 'so that we can grow our families and have a large community.'[217] The desire to expand the population of individual communities is described in both practical and religious terms. Nana Efua Ateifi said, 'God has even written it in the Bible that we should increase like sea sand.'[218] Martha Abena referred to the same passage: 'the Bible even said we should give birth and fill the earth like the sea sand.'[219] There were also practical benefits to individual families having many children: their labour was valued. Adua Dua, who grew up in Western Region, emphasised that despite poverty, women gave birth to many children in the 1950s.[220] Children were participants in social networks and fulfilled certain roles. Mary Boanno asked, 'for instance, if we all give birth and you refuse to give birth, whose child would you send on an errand?' She and her aunt, Martha Abena, stressed that children were needed for 'errands,' like fetching water, buying items. More importantly, though, they imply that there was shame in a childless woman asking a child to do these tasks, suggesting that women were required to add to the communal child labour pool.[221] Furthermore, in the 1950s, grants-in-aid to local authorities were based partially on the size of the population of the community.[222] It was therefore advantageous in terms of access to resources to have a larger community, especially to those in charge of these resources.

Others specified that children were necessary since they would take care of their parents in old age. Women were not guaranteed security through marriage. In Akan society, a man's wife and children did not inherit his property under customary law.[223] Even whilst living, many women testified that their children's father did not provide reliably. For example, Adua Dua's mother left her father after she was born because he was a 'drunkard.'[224] Martha Abena said that since the father of her children was not working and did not have money, she was 'the one doing everything for them.'[225] Indeed, Jean Allman and Victoria Tashjian demonstrate that divorce was quite common during the colonial period. Even as women became more beholden to their husbands because of colonial cash economies, marriage remained a fluid institution.[226] In these circumstances, relying on children appears logical.

Statistics from the 1948 census show that there was a slight change in fertility rates between generations of women previous to 1950 (Figure 3.8). Those completing their reproductive lives in 1950 had given birth to an average of 6.14 children, compared to the 6.65 children of those completing in 1930.[227] These statistics contradict the idea that African women's fertility began to rise in the

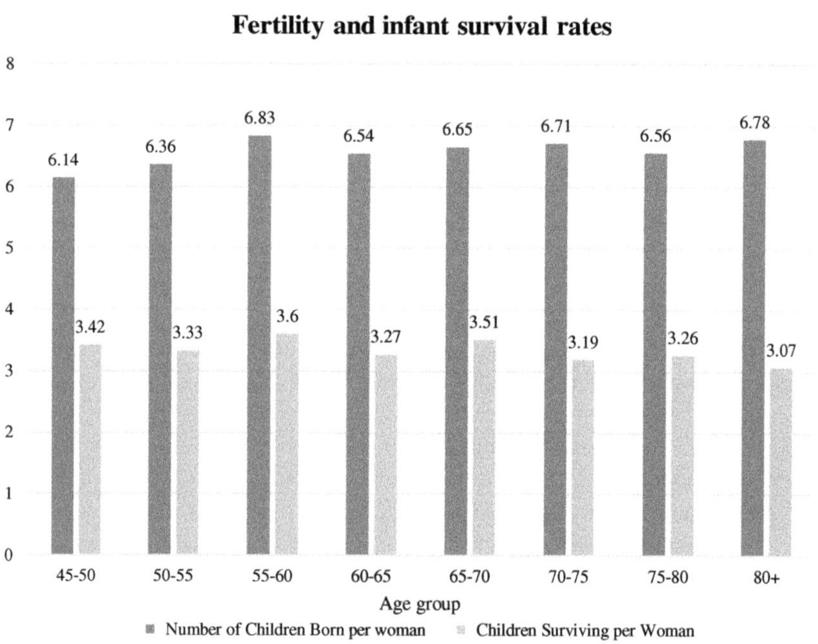

Figure 3.8 Fertility and infant survival rates by age group in 1948. PRAAD, Accra, ADM 5/2/9: The Gold Coast Census of the Population 1948. Records and Tables. Government Printing Dept., Accra, 1950, 396.

1940s, when social methods of birth spacing such as breastfeeding, abstinence within polygynous marriages and women's economic independence were threatened. Indeed, although John Iliffe explains a general rise in fertility across Africa in this way, he excludes West Africa given women's relative control over their fertility.[228] In the survey, the number of surviving children slightly increased by 1948. This suggests that as infants were more likely to survive, women chose to have fewer pregnancies. However, by 1955 birth rates were at their highest recorded levels.[229] Importantly, only about half of women's children survived on average. Esi Koffuah explained, 'in the past there was no good doctors ... so when you give [birth] some die.'[230] This further explains the need for women to bear many children.

Certain methods of contraception were available in the Gold Coast in the 1950s. Condoms were available for men to buy in some pharmacies in Accra. For the vast majority of women, birth control meant the herbal remedies discussed in previous chapters or abstinence. Most interviewees claimed that they did not know about herbal remedies, or if they did, they did not use them. Esi Praah said that she avoided sleeping with her husband at certain times during her menstrual cycle to avoid becoming pregnant. Interestingly, she specifically aimed to give birth every two years, by which time she had finished breastfeeding the previous child. She was also very conscious that early weaning would cause sickness in the child.[231] A significant number of interviewees drastically misremember or misreport birth spacing or pregnancy avoidance. Ekuah Nkrumah reported, 'It took some time but I married. After the marriage, I gave birth [every] five years.'[232] However, given that she gave birth to eleven children, this was impossible. Cecilia Fynn Essien reported that she never gave birth again until her child was 'able to put on clothes for school.' This memory reflects the changing significance of education in life cycles. Cecilia was also unable or unwilling to reflect on *how* it was that each birth was spaced by seven years. She said that '[i]t was God who did everything ... it was God who ensured when to give birth ... He makes sure that you give birth with such space in between.'[233] However, the spacing of births was normal in many Ghanaian societies through abstinence, usually in the context of polygamous marriages and couples living apart following childbirth. Like Cecilia indicates, there were certain markers for this period of pregnancy avoidance to end – rather than education though this usually happened when children's first set of teeth had come in or they were able to walk competently.[234]

Conclusion

Women's reproductive health became a significant aspect of medicalisation programmes and social development between the late 1930s and mid-1950s. This chapter has argued that late colonial development provoked the reinvention of healthcare provision on three levels. Firstly, hospitals and welfare centres, mainly based in urban spaces, constituted modernisation projects. They were settings for technological solutions to health problems, including obstetric and gynaecological medicine and were deliberate displays of modernity. As these services expanded, especially in their provision for women, more Gold Coast women came into contact with them. However, they remained limited in the 1940s and early 1950s. Despite this, women continued to be held morally responsible for accessing biomedical care. Secondly, health is delivered through social services and community development. Local level drive for healthcare became a core element of development planning. This meant that decisions over health provision were redirected into the hands of local, usually male, elites. It also placed responsibility for healthcare with communities themselves. This meant that when women did not access or seek healthcare, they continued to be blamed for moral failings. Thirdly, the social networks of health that women were part of, particularly in the context of their reproductive lives, were re-invented at this time to incorporate colonial biomedicine. This meant that women factored different elements into their choices when it came to their reproductive health. Social networks of care now included midwives, welfare workers and the challenge of transporting themselves to biomedical spaces, and new uncertainties over their care.

Notes

1 Interview with Esi Yawa. Koforidua, Central Region, 27 November 2017.
2 Sylvia Tamale, 'Ob/Gyn Experiences - Life Stories', in *African Sexualities: A Reader*, ed. Sylvia Tamale (Capetown, CA: Pambazuka Press, 2011), 377.
3 Arturo Escobar, *Encountering Development: The Making and Unmaking of the Third World* (Princeton, NJ: Princeton University Press, 1995), 1.
4 Frederick Cooper and Randall Packard, 'Introduction', in *International Development and the Social Sciences: Essays on the History and Politics of Knowledge*, ed. Frederick Cooper and Randall Packard (Berkeley, CA: University of California Press, 1998), 1.
5 Vivianne Adams and Stacey Leigh Pigg, 'Introduction: The Moral Object of Sex', in *Sex in Development: Science, Sexuality and Morality in Global Perspective*, ed. Vivianne Adams and Stacy Leigh Pigg (Durham: Duke University Press, 2005), 12.
6 Cooper and Packard, 'Introduction', 1.
7 Joanna Lewis argues that this applied across British colonies in Africa. Joanna Lewis, *Empire State-Building: War & Welfare in Kenya, 1925–52* (Athens, OH: Ohio State University Press, 2000), 23.
8 Frederick Cooper, 'Modernizing Bureaucrats, Backward Africans, and the Development Concept', in *International Development and the Social Sciences: Essays on the History and Politics of Knowledge*, ed. Frederick Cooper and Randall Packard (Berkeley, CA: University of California Press, 1998), 64–92.
9 Stephen Addae, *The History of Western Medicine in Ghana 1880–1960* (Edinburgh: The Pentland Press, 1997); K. David Patterson, *Health in Colonial Ghana: Disease, Medicine, and Socio-Economic Change, 1900–1955* (Waltham, MA: Crossroads Press, 1981).
10 Megan Vaughan, *Curing Their Ills: Colonial Power and African Illness* (Cambridge: Polity, 1991), 5.
11 Steven Feierman and John M. Janzen, 'Introduction', in *The Social Basis of Health and Healing in Africa*, ed. Steven Feierman and John M. Janzen, 30 (Berkeley, CA: University of California Press, 2009), 2.
12 Adu Boahen, 'Towards a New Categorization and Periodization of African Reactions of Responses to Colonialism', in *Africa in the Twentieth Century: The Adu Boahen*

Reader, ed. A. Adu Boahen and Toyin Falola (Trenton, NJ: Africa World Press, 2004), 345; Richard Rathbone, *Nkrumah and the Chiefs: Politics of Chieftaincy in Ghana 1951–1960* (Oxford: James Currey, 2000).

13 Dennis Austin, *Politics in Ghana, 1946–1960* (Oxford: Oxford University Press, 1964), 17–28.

14 Keri Lambert, '"It's All Work and Happiness on The Farms": Agricultural Development between the Blocs in Nkrumah's Ghana', *The Journal of African History* 60, no. 1 (March 2019): 29.

15 Morten Jerven, 'A West African Experiment: Constructing a GDP Series for Colonial Ghana, 1891–1950', *The Economic History Review* 67 (2014): 964–992; Gareth Austin, *Labour, Land and Capital in Ghana: From Slavery to Free Labour in Asante, 1807–1956* (New York: University of Rochester Press, 2009), 52.

16 Frederick Cooper, *Decolonization & African Society: The Labor Question in French and British Africa* (Cambridge: Cambridge University Press, 2008), 126–27.

17 Karl Ittmann, 'Demography as Policy Science in the British Empire, 1918–1969', *Journal of Policy History* 15, no. 4 (5 November 2003): 430.

18 Cooper, *Decolonization*, 111.

19 Ibid., 112.

20 Cooper, 'Modernizing Bureaucrats', 64–67.

21 Ibid., 81–82.

22 NA, CO 859/123/1: 'A Report to his Excellency the Governor on Social Welfare in the Gold Coast', March 1944, 1.

23 NA, CO 96/781/2: 'Extract from Confidential Collect No. 4: Letter from Acting Colonial Secretary to Members of the Gold Coast Civil Service issued by direction of the Governor', 14 September 1944, 1.

24 NA, CO 96/781/2: 'Gold Coast. Governor's despatch no. 222 of the 26 July 1944, to the Secretary of State for the Colonies', 4.

25 NA, CO 859/115/3: 'Extracts from the Gold Coast Development Plan', 1944, 10.

26 NA, CO 96/806/2: Draft *Ten Year Plan of Development and Welfare for the Gold Coast*, Gold Coast Government Printing Department, Accra, 1946, 1–2.

27 NA, CO 859/115/3: 'Extracts from the Gold Coast Development Plan', 1944, 1.

28 NA, CO 96/806/2: 'Note of a discussion with Sir Alan Burns on Thursday 19 September 1946,' 1.

29 Robert L. Tignor, *W. Arthur Lewis and the Birth of Development Economics* (Princeton, NJ: Princeton University Press, 2005), 114.

30 NA, CO 859/123/1: 'A Report to his Excellency the Governor on Social Welfare in the Gold Coast', March 1944, 1.

31 NA, CO 859/115/3: 'General Plan for Development in the Gold Coast', 1944, 1.

32 NA, CO 859/123/1: 'A Report to his Excellency the Governor on Social Welfare in the Gold Coast', March 1944, 1.

33 Lewis, *Empire State-Building*, 7, 42.

34 PRAAD, Cape Coast, ADM 23/1/1090: 'Social Security in the Colonial Territories', Printed for the Colonial Office, London, 1944, 3.

35 Gold Coast Government, *Report of the Ministry of Health 1953*, Government Printer, Accra, 1955, 16. See also: Emmanuel Akyeampong, 'Sexuality and Prostitution among the Akan of the Gold Coast c. 1650–1950', *Past & Present* 156, no. 1 (1997): 144–73.

36 Carina Ray, *Crossing the Color Line: Race, Sex, and the Contested Politics of Colonialism in Ghana* (Athens, OH: Ohio University Press, 2015), 136–37. NA, CO 859/123/1: Social Welfare in the Gold Coast: Mr Paterson's Report, 1944, 2.

37 NA, CO 859/838/12001/10: Advisory Committee on Education in the Colonies, *Report of a Sub-Committee on the Education and Welfare of Women and Girls in Africa*, Colonial Office, London, 12th February 1943, 12.

38 Escobar, *Encountering Development*, 23.

39 Missionaries had been providing some level social services in the form of education and welfare, including 'women's work', for some decades. These missions were supported in this work, financially in some cases, by the colonial government.
40 NA, CO 96/806/2: Draft *Ten Year Plan of Development and Welfare for the Gold Coast*, Gold Coast Government Printing Department, Accra, 1946, 26.
41 Frederick Cooper, *Africa since 1940: The Past of the Present* (Cambridge: Cambridge University Press, 2002), 31; Joseph M. Hodge, *Triumph of the Expert: Agrarian Doctrines of Development and the Legacies of British Colonialism* (Athens, OH: Ohio University Press, 2007), 4–5.
42 NA, CO 96/781/2: 'Gold Coast. Governor's despatch no. 222 of the 26 July 1944, to the Secretary of State for the Colonies', 4.
43 Takyiwaa Manuh, 'Building Institutions for the New Africa: The Institute of African Studies at the University of Ghana', in *Modernization as Spectacle in Africa,* ed. Peter J., Bloom, Stephan Miescher and Takyiwaa Manuh (Bloomington, IN: Indiana University Press, 2014), 268–69.
44 James Ferguson, *Expectations of Modernity: Myths and Meanings of Urban Life on the Zambian Copperbelt* (Berkeley, CA: University of California Press, 1999), 1–5.
45 NA, CO 96/806/2: Draft *Ten Year Plan of Development and Welfare for the Gold Coast*, Gold Coast Government Printing Department, Accra, 1946, 28.
46 Ibid.
47 Ibid., 29.
48 Ibid.
49 Martin Gorsky, 'Public Health in Interwar England and Wales: Did It Fail?', *Dynamis* 28 (2008): 175.
50 Gold Coast Government, *Report on the Medical Department for the Year 1950*, Accra, 1951, 17.
51 Jeff D. Grischow, 'Kwame Nkrumah, Disability, and Rehabilitation in Ghana, 1957–66', *The Journal of African History* 52, no. 2 (2011): 182.
52 Roger Gocking, *The History of Ghana* (Westport, CT: Greenwood Press, 2005), 100.
53 Ama Biney, *The Political and Social Thought of Kwame Nkrumah* (New York: Palgrave Macmillan; 2011), 57.
54 PRAAD, Accra, ADM 5/4/109: 'Report on Development Progress of the Gold Coast Apr - Dec 1953', Accra, 1954, 29–34.
55 Gold Coast Government, *Report of the Ministry of Health 1953*, Accra, 1955, 25.
56 NA, DO 35/9303: 'Press Release No. 196/59: Draft of Prime Minister's Speech on the Second Five-Year Development Plan to be Delivered before Parliament of the 4 March 1959', March 1959, 2.
57 Daniel Immerwahr, *Thinking Small: The United States and the Lure of Community Development* (Cambridge, MA: Harvard University Press, 2014), 2–14.
58 Gold Coast Government, *Report on the Medical Department for the Year 1937*, Accra, 1938, 94.
59 Ibid., 93.
60 *Report on the Medical Department for the Year 1938*, Accra, 1939, 94.
61 *Report on the Medical Department for the Year 1941*, Accra, 1942, 7.
62 Anne Hugon, *Être mère en situation coloniale: Gold Coast, 1910–1950* (Paris: Éditions de la Sorbonne, 2020), 161.
63 Gold Coast Government, *Report of the Ministry of Health 1952*, Accra, 14.
64 John S. Pobee, *The Anglican Story in Ghana: From Mission Beginnings to Province of Ghana* (Accra: Amanza Ltd., 2009), 213.
65 PRAAD, Kumasi, ARG 13/4/35: 'St Monica's Convent – Maternity Hospital', 3 August 1951.
66 PRAAD, Kumasi, ARG 13/4/35: 'Report on Mampong Midwifery Training School', 2 November 1956.

67 PRAAD, Koforidua, ADM 33/6/490: 'Inspection of Maternity Home, Aburi', 27 April 1953.
68 PRAAD, Koforidua, ADM 33/6/490: Letter to W R Hancock, Government Agent, Aburi from Red Cross HQ Organiser, Accra, 12 January 1954.
69 *Report of the Commission of Enquiry into the Health Needs of the Gold Coast*, Accra, 6.
70 Gold Coast Government, *Report of the Ministry of Health 1953*, Accra, 1955, 25.
71 Ibid., 49.
72 *Report of the Commission of Enquiry into the Health Needs of the Gold Coast*, Accra, 9.
73 Gold Coast Government, *Report of the Ministry of Health 1953*, Accra, 1955, 52.
74 PRAAD, Cape Coast, RG 1/9/2: 'Minutes of the Meeting of the Winneba Hospital Visiting Committee Held at the Hospital on the 11 June 1952 at 2.30pm', 2.
75 Ibid.
76 PRAAD, Cape Coast, ADM 23/1/1058: 'Report of the Dunkwa Visiting Committee', 23 September 1942; and 'Cape Coast Hospital Visiting Committee', 15 September 1944.
77 PRAAD, Cape Coast, RG 1/9/3: Letter from John E. Miller to Chief Commissioner, 2 February 1943.
78 Interview with Efua Ata, Abrafo, Central Region, 23 July 2019.
79 NA, CO 96/781/2: 'Gold Coast. Governor's despatch no. 222 of the 26 July, 1944, to the Secretary of State for the Colonies', 5.
80 *Report of the Commission of Enquiry into the Health Needs of the Gold Coast*, Accra, 9.
81 PRAAD, Accra, ADM 5/4/124: Gold Coast Government, *Development Progress Report, 1955*, Accra, 1956, Table 1.
82 WHO, AFR/MCH 1-17, 1957 – 1953: Poulton, E. Maclean, *A Report on a Visit to Ghana 12 July – 28 August, 1957*, WHO African Regional Office, 1957, 35–36.
83 Interview with Adjoa Ewusiwa, New Ebu, Central Region, 22 July 2019.
84 Interview with Esi Yawa, Koforidua, Central Region, 27 November 2017.
85 Interview with Aba Afrim, Nkanfoa, Central Region, 13 February 2018.
86 Interview with Efua Ata, Abrafo, Central Region, 23 July 2019.
87 Luis White has argued convincingly that, in Kenya, 'vampire stories' became idioms to express fears related to biomedical institutions. Luise White, *Speaking with Vampires: Rumor and History in Colonial Africa* (Berkeley, CA: University of California Press, 2000), 105.
88 Tamale, 'Ob/Gyn', 377.
89 Interview with Aba Afrim, Nkanfoa, Central Region, 13 February 2018.
90 Interview with Nana Efua Ateifi I, New Ebu, Central Region, 22 July 2019.
91 Gold Coast Government, *Report of the Ministry of Health, 1953*, Accra, 1955, 92.
92 Ibid., 50.
93 WHO, AFR/MCH 1-17, 1957 – 1953: Poulton, E. Maclean, *A Report on a Visit to Ghana 12 July – 28 August, 1957*, WHO African Regional Office, 1957, 5.
94 Interview with Effua Akyenoba, Aboadze, Western Region, 6 February 2018.
95 Interview with Martha Abena and Mary Boanno, Abrafo, Central Region, 23 July 2019.
96 Interview with Esi Atta, Gyabenkrom, Western Region, 27 October 2017.
97 Interview with Aunty Angela, Abakrampa, Central Region, 29 November 2017.
98 Interview with Esi Atta, Gyabenkrom, Western Region, 27 October 2017.
99 Interview with Esi Koffuah, Gyabenkrom, Western Region, 27 October 2017.
100 Gold Coast Government, *Report of the Medical Department for the Year 1945*, Accra, 1946, 13.
101 Gold Coast Government, *Report of the Ministry of Health 1953*, Accra, 1955, 13.
102 Penicillin was first used in Gold Coast in the 1940s and was used widely as part of the World Health Organization yaws campaign in the 1950s. On yaws and penicillin see: E. E. Sabben-Clare, David J. Bradley, and Kenneth Kirkwood, eds., *Health*

in Tropical Africa during the Colonial Period (Oxford: Clarendon Press, 1980), 86–94.

103 Francis K. Danquah, 'Sustaining a West African Cocoa Economy: Agricultural Science and the Swollen Shoot Contagion in Ghana, 1936–1965', *African Economic History* 31 (2003): 45–46.

104 Gold Coast Government, *Report of the Medical Department 1953*, Accra, 1954, 4: the author of this report linked the 'reduction in the loss of foetal life' to falling malaria infections.

105 See Reports of the Medical Department and Ministry of Health between 1937 and 1954. These were also principal causes mentioned by the retired midwives I interviewed.

106 The majority of women interviewed between October 2017 and July 2019 that attended ante-natal at a clinic or hospital, chose to deliver at home, or in their family homes.

107 PRAAD, Kumasi, ARG 13/4/35: Letter from Sister Miriam to Principal Medical Officer, Kumasi, 1st September, 1949.

108 NA, CO 859/838/12001/10: Advisory Committee on Education in the Colonies, *Report of a Sub-Committee on the Education and Welfare of Women and Girls in Africa*, Colonial Office, London, 12 February 1943, 7.

109 Ibid.

110 WHO, AFR/MCH 1-17, 1957 – 1953: Poulton, E. Maclean, *A Report on a Visit to Ghana 12 July – 28 August, 1957*, WHO African Regional Office, 1957, 39.

111 PRAAD, Cape Coast, ADM 23/1/3047: 'Mass Education Project in the Fante-Speaking Area of the Colony', 25 November 1950.

112 PRAAD, Accra, ADM 5/4/62: 'Welfare and Mass Education on the Gold Coast: Report 1946–51', 1951, 55.

113 PRAAD, Cape Coast, ADM 23/1/3047: 'Report on Mass Education Activities Fantiland', 1951, 2.

114 NA, CO 96/781/2: 'Gold Coast. Governor's despatch no. 222 of the 26 July 1944, to the Secretary of State for the Colonies', 4.

115 Gold Coast Government, *Report on the Medical Department for the Year 1947*, Accra, 1948, 4.

116 Interview with Cecilia Fynn Essien, Cape Coast, Central Region, 28 November 2017.

117 Ibid.

118 Reports on the Medical Department and the Ministry of Health for the years 1934–52. The Roman Catholic missions, including the one at Eikwe in Western Region mentioned by many interviewees in villages nearby, appear to have historically been exclusively for treatment of sick children. Many missions worked to provide infant and maternal healthcare which was not reporting in official figures.

119 NA, CO 859/838/12001/10: 'Advisory Committee on Education in the Colonies', 17 September 1944, 8.

120 BRC, RCC/1/31/1: Report of the Red Cross Society Overseas Branches for the year 1949, 13.

121 BRC, RCC/1/12/1/36: 'Diary of Lady Limerick, 1954', 30.

122 BRC, RCC/1/31/3: Report of the Red Cross Society Overseas Branches for the year 1951, 16.

123 BRC, RCC/1/12/1/36: 'Diary of Lady Limerick, 1954', 31.

124 Ibid., 30.

125 BRC, RCC/1/31/2: Report of the Red Cross Society Overseas Branches for the year 1950, 18.

126 BRC, RCC/1/12/1/36: 'Diary of Lady Limerick, 1954', 34.

127 Ibid., 38.

128 BRC, RCC/1/31/3: Report of the Red Cross Society Overseas Branches for the year 1951, 17.

129 BRC, RCC/1/12/1/36: 'Diary of Lady Limerick, 1954', 39.
130 Ibid., 37.
131 PRAAD, Koforidua, ERG 1/14/5: 'Minutes of the 21st Meeting of the Central Council', 13th August, 1954.
132 This is discussed more thoroughly in chapter 2.
133 Interview with Esi Kofuah, Gyabenkrom, Western Region, 27 October 2017.
134 BRC, RCC/1/12/1/36: 'Diary of Lady Limerick, 1954', 36.
135 M. J. Field, *Religion and Medicine of the Ga People* (Oxford: Oxford University Press, 1961), 162.
136 Interview with Efua Ata, Abrafo, Central Region, 23 July 2019.
137 T. E. Kyei, *Marriage and Divorce among the Asante: A Study Undertaken in the Course of the Ashanti Social Survey (1945)* (Cambridge: African Studies Centre, 1992), 40.
138 Jean Allman, 'Fathering, Mothering and Making Sense of "Ntamoba": Reflections on the Economy of Child-Rearing in Colonial Asante', *Africa: Journal of the International African Institute* 67, no. 2 (1997): 296–321.
139 BRC, RCC/1/12/1/36: 'Diary of Lady Limerick, 1954', 41.
140 Interview with Effua Akyenoba, Aboadze, Western Region, 6 February 2018.
141 Interview with Ekuah Nkrumah, Koforidua, Central Region, 27 November 2017.
142 Various women interviewed in the area referred to this Twelve Apostles Mission Church. Harriet Sekyi-Yorke who works as a midwife in the area noted that today, this church is problematic since it proffers false information about health and healing, but that often it's the only option for people in isolated villages. Interview with Harriet Sekyi-Yorke, Gyabenkrom, Western Region, 27 October 2017. PRAAD, Cape Coast, ADM 23/1/3817: 'The Twelve Apostles Church', 22 July 1954.
143 Interview with Mary Sampson, Adjumako, Western Region, 23 October 2017.
144 For more detail on the origins of this mission and its arrival in French and British West African colonies, see: David A. Shank, 'Le pentecôtisme du prophète William Wadé Harris', *Archives de Sciences Sociales Des Religions* 44, no. 105 (1999): 51–53.
145 PRAAD, Cape Coast, ADM 23/1/3817: Letter to Colonial Secretary, Accra from Micah Kodjoe George, Prophet, 21 November 1949.
146 Interview with Hannah Bowah, Mpatase, Western Region, 24 October 2017.
147 Interview with Esi Dwanwa, Koforidua, Central Region, 27 November 2017. Interview with Adua Takyiwaa, Jukwa, Central Region, 23 July 2019.
148 Interview with 'Aunty' Esi, Aboadze, Western Region, 6 February 2018.
149 Anthony Appiah, *In My Father's House: Africa in the Philosophy of Culture* (New York: Oxford University Press, 1992), 7.
150 Interview with Esi Praah, Mpatase, Western Region, 25 October 2017.
151 Interview with Aba Seku, Aboadze, Western Region, 6 February 2018.
152 Interview with Araba Yedua, Gyabenkrom, Western Region, 27 October 2017.
153 Kate Skinner, '"It Brought Some Kind of Neatness to Mankind": Mass Literacy, Community Development and Democracy in 1950s Asante', *Africa* 79, no. 04 (November 2009): 491.
154 Rathbone, *Nkrumah and the Chiefs*, 17.
155 Jeff D. Grischow, *Shaping Tradition: Civil Society, Community and Development in Colonial Northern Ghana, 1899–1957* (Leiden: Brill, 2006), 19.
156 NA, CO 96/806/2: Draft *Ten Year Plan of Development and Welfare for the Gold Coast*, Gold Coast Government Printing Department, Accra, 1946, forward.
157 J. K. Nsarkoh, *Local Government in Ghana* (Accra: Ghana Universities Press, 1964), 8.
158 PRAAD, Koforidua, ADM 29/6/393: 'Community Development and Local Development Committees', 26 September 1949, 1.
159 Ibid.
160 Ibid., 2.

161 NA, CO 96/806/2: Draft *Ten Year Plan of Development and Welfare for the Gold Coast*, Gold Coast Government Printing Department, Accra, 1946, 27.
162 Ibid.
163 PRAAD, Sekondi, WRG 15/1/522: Circular Letter from Secretary Midwives Board, 12 May 1948.
164 Cape Coast, ADM 23/1/1299: 'Rural Medical Services', 10 September 1948, 2.
165 Kate Skinner and Peter J. Bloom, 'Modernity and Danger: *The Boy Kumasenu* and the Work of the Gold Coast Film Unit', *Ghana Studies* 12/13 (2009): 124.
166 WHO, AFR/MCH 1-17, 1957 – 1953: Poulton, E. Maclean, *A Report on a Visit to Ghana 12 July – 28 August, 1957*, WHO African Regional Office, 1957, 44.
167 *The Development Plan, 1951. Being a Plan for the Economic and Social Development of the Gold Coast as Approved by the Legislative Assembly, September, 1951*, Government Printing Dept., Accra, 1951, 18.
168 *Report of the Commission of Enquiry into the Health Needs of the Gold Coast*, Accra, 1952, 13.
169 PRAAD, Cape Coast, ADM 23/1/1299: Letter from District Commissioner Dunkwa to District Commissioner Cape Coast, 13 March 1950.
170 PRAAD, Cape Coast, ADM 23/1/3047: 'Draft – Community Development Ekumfi' Enclosed in Letter to Chief Commissioner Cape Coast from District Commissioner, 2 December 1950, 2.
171 PRAAD, Cape Coast, ADM 23/1/1299: see exchange of letters of the topic of 'Rural Medical Services' beginning September 1948.
172 PRAAD, Kumasi, ARG 13/4/7: 'Amansie District Council's Intention to Take Over and Run Bekwai State Maternity Clinic', 23 March 1953 and PRAAD, Cape Coast, ADM 23/1/1387: 'Reply to Resolution from Asin Atandaso Local Council Dated 31/1/55', 19 February 1955.
173 PRAAD, Kumasi, ARG 13/4/7: Letter from Amansie District Council to Ministry of Health, Accra, 15 May 1953, 1.
174 PRAAD, Kumasi, ARG 13/4/7: Letter from Chairman Amansie District Council to Ministry of Health, Accra, 17 June 1953, 1.
175 PRAAD, Accra, CSO 21/22/182: 'Rural Health and Sanitation in Krobo,' n.d. but 1946, 2.
176 Ibid., 1. My italics.
177 PRAAD, Koforidua, ADM 29/6/393: 'Community Development and Local Development Committees,' 24 April 1950, 1.
178 PRAAD, Koforidua, ADM 29/6/393: 'Minutes of a Meeting with Akwapim State Development Committee,' 23 August 1951, 1.
179 PRAAD, Cape Coast, ADM 23/1/1299: 'Native Authority Dispensaries: Dressers and Midwives Dunkwa District,' 26 November, 1948, 1.
180 PRAAD, Koforidua, ADM 29/6/393: 'Report on Inspection of Community and Local Development Works', 25th July, 1950.
181 Thomas Spear, 'Neo-Traditionalism and the Limits of Invention in British Colonial Africa', *The Journal of African History* 44, no. 1 (2003): 3.
182 Ibid., 4.
183 Roger Gocking, *The History of Ghana*, The Greenwood Histories of the Modern Nations (Westport, CT: Greenwood Press, 2005), 99.
184 Ama Biney, *The Political and Social Thought*, 56.
185 NA, CO 859/838/12001/10: Advisory Committee on Education in the Colonies, *Report of a Sub-Committee on the Education and Welfare of Women and Girls in Africa*, Colonial Office, London, 12 February 1943, 1.
186 Ibid., 3. My italics.
187 Ibid., 17.
188 Ibid., 18.
189 Ibid., 3.

190 Ibid., 12.
191 PRAAD, Cape Coast, ADM 23/1/1090: 'Meeting of the Central Welfare Committee', 24 February 1944, 5.
192 PRAAD, Accra, RG 3/5/2060: 'Notes for Housecraft Teachers' dated between 1950 and 1951.
193 Lewis, *Empire State-Building*, 199.
194 PRAAD, Accra, ADM 5/1/401: *Annual Report of the Department of Social Welfare and Community Development for the Year 1957*, Government Printer, Accra, 1958, 12.
195 PRAAD, Accra, ADM 5/1/359: *Annual Report of the Department of Social Welfare and Community Development for the Year 1954*, Government Printer, Accra, 1955, 12.
196 NA, CO 859/77/11: Blacklock, M. G., *Colonial Office Committee on Post-War Problems. The Health of Women and Children in the Colonies*, unpublished 1942, 6–10.
197 Ibid., 8.
198 NA, CO 859/65/9: 'Certain Observations on the Memorandum Entitled Medical Policy in the Colonial Empire Miscellaneous No. 505 (Confidential)' by Dr J. B. Kirk, 7 July 1943, 3.
199 Ibid., 1.
200 PRAAD, Accra, ADM 5/1/401: *Annual Report of the Department of Social Welfare and Community Development for the Year 1957*, Government Printer, Accra, 1958, 12.
201 PRAAD, Cape Coast, ADM 23/1/3047: 'Mass Education Project in the Fante-Speaking Area of the Colony', 25 November 1950, 3.
202 PRAAD, Cape Coast, ADM 23/1/3047: 'Draft – Community Development Ekumfi' Enclosed in Letter to Chief Commissioner Cape Coast from District Commissioner, 2 December, 1950, 4.
203 PRAAD, Accra, ADM 5/1/359: *Annual Report of the Department of Social Welfare and Community Development for the Year 1954*, Government Printer, Accra, 1955, 14.
204 PRAAD, Accra, ADM 5/1/401: *Annual Report of the Department of Social Welfare and Community Development for the Year 1957*, Government Printer, Accra, 1958, 12.
205 Takyiwah Manuh, 'Women and Their Organisations during the Convention Peoples' Party Period', in *The Life and Work of Kwame Nkrumah: Papers of a Symposium Organized by the Institute of African Studies, University of Ghana, Legon*, ed. Kwame Arhin and University of Ghana (Accra: Sedco, 1991), 112.
206 PRAAD, Cape Coast, ADM 23/1/1090: 'Meeting of the Central Welfare Committee Held at Government House, Accra', 6 May 1945, 2.
207 Adwoa Opong, "Rewriting Women into Ghanaian History 1950–1966" (unpublished MPhil thesis, University of Ghana, 2012), 46.
208 Manuh, 'Women and Their Organizations during the Convention People's Party Period'.
209 PRAAD, Accra, RG 3/8/31: *Report of a Women's Conference Held at Kumasi June 22nd – 25th*, Abura Printing Works, Kumasi, 1951', 4–9.
210 For an extensive discussion of nutrition in Ghana, see: Nott, 'Between Famine and Malnutrition: Spatial Aspects of Nutritional Health during Ghana's Long Twentieth Century, c. 1896–2000' and Nott, John, '"No one may starve in the British Empire": Kwashiorkor, Protein and the Politics of Nutrition between Britain and Africa', *Social History of Medicine* 34, no. 2 (2021).
211 NA, CO 859/115/3: 'Extract from the Purcell Nutrition Report (Enclosure to Gold Coast Confidential despatch of 18 April 1944)', 1.
212 *Report on the Medical Department for the Year 1935*, Accra, 1936.
213 Joseph M. Hodge, *Triumph of the Expert: Agrarian Doctrines of Development and the Legacies of British Colonialism* (Athens, OH: Ohio University Press, 2007), 4.
214 EA: Department of Education, *Notes for Housecraft Teachers and All Teachers in Girls' Schools. Diets for Mothers*, 1950, 1.

215 Ibid.
216 NA, CO 859/115/3: Letter from Margaret Wrong, Department of Education, to Mrs Culwick, 18 October 1944.
217 Interview with Nana Efua Ateifi I, New Ebu, Central Region, 22 July 2019.
218 Ibid.
219 Interview with Martha Abena and Mary Boanno, Abrafo, Central Region, 23 July 2019.
220 Interview with Adua Dua, Abrafo, Central Region, 23 July 2019.
221 Interview with Martha Abena and Mary Boanno, Abrafo, Central Region, 23 July 2019.
222 PRAAD, Cape Coast, ADM 23/1/1358: 'Grants in Aid to Local Authorities 1953–1954', 16 March 1953.
223 Florence Abena Dolphyne, *The Emancipation of Women: An African Perspective* (Accra: Ghana Universities Press, 1991), 26–27.
224 Interview with Adua Dua, Abrafo, Central Region, 23 July 2019.
225 Interview with Martha Abena and Mary Boanno, Abrafo, Central Region, 23 July 2019.
226 Jean Allman and Victoria B. Tashjian, *I Will Not Eat Stone: A Women's History of Colonial Asante*, Social History of Africa (Portsmouth, NH: Heinemann, 2000). See chapter 2.
227 PRAAD, Accra, ADM 5/2/9: *The Gold Coast Census of the Population 1948. Records and Tables.* Government Printing Dept., Accra, 1950, 396.
228 John Iliffe, *Africans: The History of a Continent*, 2nd edition (Cambridge: Cambridge University Press, 2007), 252.
229 Statistics taken from medical reports between 1936 and 1955. The birth rate in 1955 was 42/1,000.
230 Interview with Esi Koffuah, Gyabenkrom, Western Region, 27 October 2017.
231 Interview with Esi Praah, Abra, Western Region, 25 October 2017.
232 Interview with Ekuah Nkrumah, Koforidua, Central Region, 27 November 2017.
233 Interview with Cecilia Fynn Essien, Cape Coast, Central Region, 28 November 2017.
234 MacFarlane, Deborah, Interview with Dr Fred Sai for *Smith College Population and Reproductive Health Oral History Project*, 11 March 2004, 33.

4 Reproducing the Nation in Nkrumah's Ghana, 1951–1966

In the twentieth century, Africa's population grew more than that of any other continent. It increased by about six times, rising from around 130 million at the beginning of the century to almost one billion by its end.[1] In Ghana, the 1960 census counted 6,726,820 people, which accounted for 2.6% of Africa's population on 0.8% of its surface.[2] During the 1950s and 1960s the rapid growth of Africa's population came to the attention of policymakers and activists within and beyond the continent. This included the British Colonial Office, which was coming under pressure to act from eugenicists such as Julian Huxley, and organisations like the Family Planning Association. Fears regarding 'population explosion' rippled around the world and reached Africa. This represented a significant discursive shift regarding Africa's population, which in the first half of the twentieth century, was seen as underpopulated. However, population growth did not worry the prime minister of the soon-to-be independent nation, Kwame Nkrumah. On the contrary, he embraced it. This perspective adds nuance to historiography that presents global population activism as powerful and coercive, largely unaffected by a local agency.[3] In this chapter, I explore how Nkrumah negotiated transnational and transimperial discourses of overpopulation and the results of his pronatalist policy for Ghanaian women.

In March 1957, Ghana celebrated independence from the British Empire. Kwame Nkrumah, of the Convention People's Party (CPP), who had led the African side of the diarchic government for the past six years now became prime minister of an Independent Ghana. As independence was achieved, attention to population and to health was designed to signal to former colonisers the international community and its own people that the country was developing. So it was that A. H. Reed in London's colonial office commented that development spending for the first two years of Ghana's independence was 'heaviest' in social services, with health claiming 'a fairly substantial amount.'[4] Indeed, Ghana, reported the *Ghanaian Times* in 1960, was heading towards becoming a welfare state,[5] something which was promised in the Second Five-Year Development Plan of 1959.[6] Ghanaians remember Nkrumah's era as one in which healthcare was much easier to afford and far more comprehensive than today.[7]

There were certainly no plans for population control or even provision of family planning in the new Ghanaian nation. Instead, under Nkrumah's leadership,

DOI: 10.4324/9781003274162-5

the nation took an approach to population based on gendered economic nationalism. That is, the biological and social reproduction of the nation determined women's roles within it. Women's reproductive health was subsumed into development planning, which prioritised economic growth. The Ghanaian government, led by Nkrumah, pushed for a population increase in order to drive development. Nkrumah believed that a large population would drive industrial growth and diversification and that it would constitute a show of power on a global scale. Ghanaian women were directed to play their part by birthing and rearing numerous healthy children and by accessing biomedical healthcare. A new ideology: nationalist development, was once again driving decision-making when it came to women's reproductive health in Ghana. But this wasn't simply a top-down directive. Ghanaians admired Nkrumah for this population policy, and it fit with their cultural expectations and economic needs.

'A bad bout of neo-Malthusianism'

Interest in demography in the British Empire burgeoned in the post-war period. The Economist reported in 1949 that the West was suffering a 'bad bout of neo-Malthusianism.'[8] The significance of this moment has been discussed in the previous chapter: late colonial governments in Africa attempted to maintain control over their colonies and the populations within them through 'development,' a concept that carried with it the veneer of challenging world poverty.[9] Joseph Hodge points out that 'new forms of knowledge and representation' were crucial to ongoing imperial power.[10] One of these new forms of knowledge was demography. The demographic survey written by Robert Kuczynski, whose data was explored in Chapter 1 of this book, dates to this post-war moment.[11] The study was funded by the Colonial Development and Welfare Fund and the Carnegie Corporation, which had begun to take an interest in education and demography in Africa.[12] Kuczynski was made Demographic Adviser to the Colonial Office and in this role emphasised that understanding the extent of population growth was essential to development planning. This attitude was supported by the Colonial Office.[13] As Karl Ittmann has shown, the colonial state investigated population concerns more systematically in the name of development planning.[14]

Indeed, at the Colonial Office, population growth was judged in these terms. One official noted that the reduction in infant mortality brought about by maternal and child welfare work needed to be matched by 'improvement in economic standards' in order to avoid worsening conditions for the growing population.[15] In other words, development needed to keep up with population growth. It was feared that falling mortality rates would threaten the standard of living. A paper was discussed in the colonial office, written by Professor T. H. Davey, which argued that colonial medical services would lead to unmanageable population growth globally.[16] There were varied responses. Professor Seddon suggested that colonial governments be 'forewarned' of the threat, whilst dismissing Davey's suggestion that industrialisation be used to absorb the effects.[17] Some went so far as to question whether medical services should see increased spending.[18] However, others, including Davey himself pointed to the need to reform agriculture and encourage industrialisation in order to increase output to feed growing populations.[19] In other words, the Colonial Office framed population growth as something that should be at least concurrent with development. In the spirit of demographic transition, it was then assumed that fertility would be managed as Africans chose to use resources educating their children or on consumer goods. For example, another official argued that Africans needed to be tempted by 'sophisticated wants' and consumer goods to limit their families. They must be induced to desire 'bicycles not babies, furniture instead of families.'[20]

In 1943 eugenicist Julian Huxley, who would become head of UNESCO, wrote a letter to the Colonial Office advocating birth control in West Africa:

> We are introducing health services; we are likely to encourage general prosperity. This means that the population will start shooting up ... just when all the white peoples (except the U.S.S.R.) will be starting to go down. It is ... essential that advice on Birth Control ... shall not merely be available but offered, and urged.[21]

Clearly, Huxley was invested in white supremacy and capitalism's survival. In a similar vein, supporters of population control within the Colonial Office argued for it on the grounds of avoiding immigration to the UK.[22] Professor Davey's paper mentioned above was clearly preoccupied with the expansion of non-white populations, paying attention to population growth among 'American negroes' but not the white population.[23] However, the Colonial Office was unimpressed by Huxley's arguments. The fear was that 'it would be too easy for the colonial peoples to believe that birth control was a trick of the white races to destroy the coloured peoples ... in West Africa.' Furthermore, 'generally speaking, there is room for an increase of population on the African continent.'[24] This opinion is founded on the continent's low population density. However, it also connects the need for population control to the availability of land, again making it a Malthusian, agricultural question, rather than a health one. The global population 'problem' was understood by colonial powers in relation to resources.[25] Finally, the official responding to Huxley's letter ponders: 'I don't know what method of birth control Dr Huxley would have in mind, but I am sure that primitive people would find it very hard to absorb the technique.'[26] This is a plainly derogatory attitude. More interestingly, it links the lack of familiarity with birth control to primitiveness. Controlling fertility began to be associated with modernity.

There do not appear to have been concerns about overpopulation in West Africa.[27] In response to Davey's 'Growth of Tropical Populations,' Dr Wellesley Cole pointed out at the Colonial Advisory Medical Committee meeting that West African territories had very low population density.[28] Although it was agreed that the population of African colonies was growing, officials concluded that there was not yet any problem with 'overcrowding,' again reverting to *space* as the issue. Colonial officials far more inclined to propose agricultural improvements, emigration or using the 'immense areas of land still unused by tropical Africa' to solve population pressures.[29] Furthermore, Dr Wellesley Cole added that in West Africa medical services were not yet effective enough to have caused a rapid decrease in mortality rates.[30] Members of the UK government saw the question of birth control as 'highly controversial' and sought to confine its discussion within IOs to its medical rather than sociological aspects.[31] Those in the Colonial Office largely avoided 'meddling too seriously' in the matter of birth control.[32]

In 1955, the British Secretary of State for the Colonies was asked in Parliament about the population of colonies and 'in which territories any system of teaching birth control has been established.' The Secretary did not think that any such systematic teaching existed in any British colony but wanted to be sure, anticipating the subject coming up again. The question was passed on to the Directors for Health, for Education and for Social Welfare in the Gold Coast.[33] The Director of Social Welfare confirmed that there was no systematic teaching but commented that 'Medical Officers may well give advice in this matter in the course of their normal duties.'[34] The Governor commented that 'systematic teaching ... would not be generally acceptable.'[35] We can gather from this brief exchange that education or provision of contraception was in no way supported by the government. However, there may have been individual doctors providing birth control. Indeed, Dr Bannerman, head of the Maternity Hospital in Accra 'initiated the first family planning' there in 1956.[36] In the private sphere, John Caldwell commented that condoms and spermicidal foams had 'long been on rather inconspicuous sale from pharmacies' in large towns by the early 1960s.[37] His use of the word 'inconspicuous,' however, suggests a certain condemnation of contraceptives, that they were not easily available, and that there was no systematic promotion of their use.

In the Gold Coast, colonial officials made connections between changing demographics and development. The 1948 census was taken seriously. For the first time, officials were appointed specifically to the task and a Census Office was formed under a Census Commissioner. Supervisors, enumerators and clerks were employed, and the country divided into 39 new Census Districts.[38] The census also made a separate enquiry into the fertility of women, which was published within the census report in 1950.[39] This knowledge was seen as vital in the culture of development planning.

There were concerns over demographic changes in the Gold Coast. In Accra, appalling sanitary conditions were blamed on 'too rapid growth of the town's population over the last 20 years.'[40] The concern here though was not that health was threatened by population growth per se but rather by its redistribution to urban centres. In 1950, DMS Rex Cheverton, reflected:

> The question of increase and redistribution of population must be kept in mind to provide adequate food supplies. In planning long-term projects, the reduction of mortality must go hand in hand with increased food production. The status of women in the development of community from a medical point of view is of importance and development must go forward in a balanced and coordinated manner if population trends are to be controlled.[41]

Population increase was a concern for the Medical Department in as much as it interacted with urbanisation, nutrition, the status of women and 'development.' Cheverton's outlook is neo-Malthusian: he judges population concerns according to the availability of the colony's recourse. However, we also see women's role in reproduction being considered from a health point of view.

Development planning in the Gold Coast in the late 1940s and early 1950s reflected these Malthusian understandings of demographic change. Development plans centred on the expansion and mechanisation of agriculture and co-operative farming. These plans took population growth into account. One scheme arranged for farmers from the 'over populated and over cultivated' areas of the colony, to move north, where land was more abundant.[42]

In the revised 1951 Development Plan after the CPP claimed power through diarchic government, this continued. Indeed, the plan specifically noted that as it stood, agricultural methods were 'unsuited to a population which is rapidly increasing.'[43] It was to be reformed alongside plans for economic development that included industrialisation, electrification and diversification.

However, population *growth* was generally not viewed as a problem in the Gold Coast. In 1954 in the Legislative Assembly, Mr Adomako Mensah asked the Minister for Finance: 'what are the factors that account for the smallness of the country's population?' He asked the Minister to admit that 'constant use of contraceptives and the growing practice of abortion are the evils responsible for the low rate of increase in the population.'[44] The Minister for Finance denied this completely. However, the interaction shows that there was concern over the *low* rate of population growth and that contraceptives and abortion were blamed. It also attaches negative morality to birth control. Yet there was a real and rapid population increase in Ghana.

Global Population Matters

In the 1950s, WHO and UN organisations, more broadly, began to express concern over excessive fertility in Africa for the first time. Preoccupations over population growth existed before the 1950s but did not gain significant credence internationally.[45] The League of Nations had avoided such topics due to their controversy. Now, the eyes of the global population movement turned to Africa; the population 'crisis' was linked particularly to developing countries. By the mid-twentieth century, the threat of overpopulation was ubiquitous and became a powerful prescription for action. It was thought that rapid population growth would exacerbate poverty and hinder development. Birth control was advocated as a solution. In 1962, the UN issued a Resolution that connected population directly to economic development.[46] It stated that the 'health and welfare of the family are of paramount importance, not only for obvious humanitarian reasons but also with regard to economic development and social progress.' Furthermore, the Resolution suggested action specifically in 'less-developed countries.'[47] The 'humanitarian' side of family health became secondary to development goals.

Population activism became transnational and embedded itself into developing countries training demographers and building institutions. The United States Agency for International Development (USAID) made population control a stipulation for aid. A number of philanthropic organisations began to promote the limitation of population growth in the so-called 'developing' world. They put considerable funding, expertise and political weight behind attempts to reduce fertility in the name of development.[48] Population activism was based on a global divide, in which poverty was linked with high fertility. In the early 1970s, Mahmood Mamdani argued that population control was a 'weapon of the political conservative,' because it acted as a substitute for social and economic change. Mamdani argued that overpopulation discourse contained biases that meant that controlling populations was as much to do with their 'quality' as quantity.[49] Those international and non-governmental organisations began to impact Ghana in the 1960s. The Carnegie Corporation funded a demographic survey, Population Council was responsible for funding a Demographic Unit at the University of Ghana, whilst Pathfinder Fund sent activists with contraceptives to talk to women's groups and funding to the first family planning clinic.

Nationalism and Development

Nationalist development was gendered. Scholars of nationalism emphasise the ideology's dependence on women for both the social and biological reproduction of the nation. The idea of the nation itself is deeply intertwined with certain constructions of femininity, masculinity and sexuality.[50] Whilst women's roles in the nationalist struggle in Ghana have been documented,[51] I am interested in the extent to which citizenship in Ghana has been gendered. Jeffrey Ahlman has addressed this, particularly in his study of women in the Builders' Brigade and in Ghanaian workplaces. Broadly speaking, although Nkrumah's socialist experimentation afforded women new ways to participate in nation building, they continued to be constrained by marriage and motherhood.[52] I wish to build on this to explore how gendered nationalism interacted with development discourse: in Ghana, it leads us once again to the question of reproduction. I unpick here what it meant for women to be reproducers for the nation in Nkrumah's Ghana.

Nationalism in the colony very quickly gained momentum and successes and was equally devoted to development as late imperialism. Following World War II, soldiers from the Gold Coast returned 'prepared to take any line which would better their conditions.'[53] A fierce fight for self-government was underway by 1950. British imperialists were attacked from the pages of the CPP's newspaper *The Evening News*, which depicted imperialism as 'the chief agent of Captain Lucifer.'[54] The youth of the country were called upon to do their duty to fight against it to free Ghanaians. Nationalist parties radically claimed that there were no justifiable grounds for colonialism. The fervent nationalism galvanised through Nkrumah's CPP was gendered. The leadership of the CPP and its predecessor, the United Gold Coast Convention (UGCC) were all elite males. Calls to fight for Ghana's freedom generally implied young, male, recipients of their messages.

The language used in *The Evening News* to describe the next generation of leaders in the anti-imperialist struggle was overwhelmingly masculine. However, women did take part. As Iris Berger reminds us, 'male-oriented' 'top-down' decolonisation is only part of the story.[55] Grassroots organisation, which was crucial to the anti-colonial struggle, was primary directed by women; market traders in particular mobilised their networks.[56]

Reportedly, Nkrumah encouraged women's participation in politics from the outset. From July 1950, *The Evening News* included a Women's Column in each of its issues, written by journalist and CPP activist Mabel Dove under the alias Akusia Dzatsui.[57] However, the column did not last very long. Much has been made of the installation of four female propaganda secretaries to the party in the 1950s.[58] One of these was Hannah Kudjoe, who took a leading role in the CPP both before and after independence. Jean Allman has uncovered Kudjoe's story: she acted as party organiser and secretary for UGCC, before following Nkrumah to the CPP and galvanising support through speeches, conferences and Positive Action. However, there were limited opportunities for women to take leading roles within the party, and Kudjoe and others were soon obliterated from nationalist memory.[59]

Ghana itself was frequently described as the 'motherland,' exemplifying how the nation itself was gendered. For example, in June 1950, George Asare wrote for *The Evening News*:

> My Lords I say have double patience and continue to struggle as true leaders of the DYNAMIC CONVENTION PEOPLE'S PARTY of Ghana for S. G. NOW, for the people of our fertile land – our mother land. May God bless your parents also – MOTHER GHANA.[60]

Ghana is referred to as a mother, and the national land, 'fertile.' Fertility was conjured as a gendered image. Although women did not take leading roles in the national struggle, the CPP framed it as their duty to be involved.[61] Identifying as mothers and wives allowed women to take a role in decolonisation in Ghana, and across Africa.[62]Akua Amaku appealed to women to join the struggle. 'If you are honest with yourselves,' she argued, 'you will agree … that you are not marching abreast with our men.' Amaku's final address is significant: 'Mothers of Ghana, awake, for you are the salt of the nation. On with the fight.'[63] She referred to Ghanaian women in their roles as mothers, suggesting this was women's most important role. Secondly, as the 'salt of the nation' – another biblical reference – women were expected to lead in the moral sphere.

Women's health rarely entered nationalist discourse. However, in August 1950, Gbedemah publicly posed the following question to Dr Nanka-Bruce:

> is there any truth in the allegation that Fertilol, a vitamin E restorative to sterile women which has not been declared poisonous drug has been prohibited when its use would be to the advantage to the nation, since … childbearing

> women would by its use be given the chance to bear children which tend to increase the population?

Evidently, this prominent CPP politician saw population growth as desirable and increased female fertility as a way to achieve this. Moreover, his questioning is accusatory. Gbedemah positioned the CPP as safeguarding women's fertility and population growth, as a *political* position against Dr Nanka-Bruce, who led a rival political faction. Gendered nationalist language emphasising women's role as mothers overlooked women's reproductive *health.* This problem was noted by Mabel Dove in 1950, who wrote that women 'should not be satisfied merely to be regarded as incubators for breeding purposes.'[64]

Indeed, women were expected to do their bit for the nation through their domestic roles. The *Sunday Mirror* welcomed the New Year of 1965 by encouraging women to throw off their 'purposelessness.' 'The bedrock of the current revolution is that development must be rapid,' and the 'socialist path to development has no room for [women's] vain glories.' Instead, the newspaper article encouraged women 'to be good home makers and good housewives.'[65] In other words, women's role in the socialist revolution was primarily reproductive, rather than productive. Women were supposed to be dedicated to their families, setting a 'moral example.'[66] The organisation of women was crucial under the Nkrumahist state. Ahlman argues that the CPP sought to create a 'gender revolution,' which challenged 'gender expectations and opportunities.'[67] However, in reality, women faced surveillance and ridicule upon entering the formal workforce and were constantly questioned over their ability and willingness to balance their domestic obligations with those for their jobs or their nation.[68]

Development Planning and Population

Like in many African states on the eve of independence, Ghana's nationalist politicians expected that development would be enabled by industrialisation and diversification of the economy.[69] Industrialisation led to the question of labour, and so to demography. Nkrumah demanded economic independence to fully enable political independence. This meant 'total mobilisation of … manpower resources.'[70] When the CPP formed a government in 1951, it revised the colonial government's 1946 Ten-Year Development plan, and compressed it into a new five-year period: 1951–1956.[71] It changed focus, putting more money into economic and social development. After its election in 1951, the CPP government was keen to impose a state-led economy and promote industrialisation.[72] However, the new plan noted 'that the availability of the necessary manpower may present a serious problem cannot be denied.'[73] *A Survey of Some Economic Factors* in 1952 noted that 'hitherto there has been little information available on the manpower resources of the Gold Coast, although this is one of the most important factors determining the rate of economic progress.'[74]

W. A. Lewis, a prominent Caribbean economist, was invited to the Gold Coast shortly after the election of the first CPP government to assess the country's needs for industrialisation. However, Lewis's report surprised the CPP and British colonialists. He recommended that before any programme of industrialisation was undertaken, the modernisation of agriculture should be prioritised. The lack of cheap surplus labour from agriculture meant that industrialisation would not, he said, benefit the country at this time. Lewis stated that 'there is a shortage of labour in the Gold Coast, which rapid industrialisation would aggravate.'[75] Lewis wrote that manufacturing for export depended on being able to provide labour at low cost. Land abundance and a relatively sparse labour force meant that this was not the situation in the Gold Coast.[76]

Lewis's exposé demonstrated that although Nkrumah was keen to industrialise, there was not enough surplus or skilled labour. To be clear, nowhere in his report does Lewis recommend pronatalist policies to increase the labour force. Excess labour would ideally be produced by increased efficiency in agriculture. However, this position was a far stretch from international discourses which connected overpopulation to land and food shortages and stagnating economies.[77] In this case, the opposite appeared to be the case – the Gold Coast economy was prevented from diversifying because of a *shortage* of people. It is clear then why the CPP saw little economic benefit in controlling population growth.

Demography in Ghana

Histories of development and of demography in Ghana were intimately linked. The political culture of planning for development was central in newly independent Ghana.[78] Indeed, development was the watchword of the new nation. Contradicting Arturo Escobar's interpretation of development as a victimising discourse, African politicians appropriated the idea of development for their own ends.[79] Determined that Independence should spread throughout Africa, Nkrumah moved to truly unshackle Ghana from the ties of imperialism through the 'economic kingdom.' Every Ghanaian was invited to 'Serve Ghana Now,' with hard work and engagement with development projects.[80] Attention turned to demographic matters; development planning required knowledge about the population. Louise Barré has shown for Côte d'Ivoire, methods of collecting population data were directly linked to economic development aims.[81] Similarly, the collection and dissemination of statistics was seen as key to Ghana's modernisation. As the CPP committed to the provision of health, education and industrialisation, demographic data became important.[82] Indeed Grischow and Weiss have emphasised that development planning under the CPP was based on 'concrete statistical information.'[83] Minister Mumuni Bawumia pointed out that development plans must be built on 'reliable statistics,' particularly regarding the 'population growth' of the country and its 'manpower requirements.' These comments were made in the context of a Parliamentary Debate on the registration of births, advocating the creation of more demographic data for the state.[84] These plans were formulated in an increasingly socialist, authoritarian Ghana, with 'ever-intensifying state emphasis on individual and national productivity.'[85] The goal of the 1960 census, which was overseen by UN advisers, was specifically to plan and implement the Second

Development Plan, particularly in regard to the availability of labour.[86] It was also envisaged by political leaders that this census would show off the 'progress' made in Ghana since Independence.[87]

In 1960 the Population Council made a grant to the University College of Ghana to establish a Demographic Unit including demography courses and doctoral programme.[88] One of the purposes that Population Council discussed for the Demographic Unit was the establishment of a Committee on Demographic Studies. This Committee was to 'ensure coordination between departments and individuals, and to maintain liaison with governmental and private agencies, national and international, in the field of population studies.'[89] In other words, Population Council aimed to bring Ghana into the global fold of population activism. The Council's main goal was to use scientific and technological research to promote the use of birth control globally; the establishment of the Demographic Unit was a node in the global research network it was building.

The Population Council provided a grant in 1962 to bring in demographer John Caldwell to lead the Demographic Unit. Caldwell estimated in 1963 that Ghanaian women gave birth to 7.3 children, on average, and that the population growth rate was 3.5% between 1948 and 1960. Other estimates were lower. Population growth was explained partially through immigration, and through underestimates in the 1948 census.[90] His estimate was around 1% higher than that made in the Seven-Year Development Plan.[91]

The establishment of demographics at the University was linked directly to the 1960 census. As Serra has argued, the government and IOs emphasised that the proceedings of the census be 'modern.'[92] Collection of data on the population constituted a modernisation project in the new nation. It was anticipated that the census would produce masses of data, which no Ghanaians were trained to deal with at the time.[93] This was the first census to be carried out in an independent sub-Saharan African nation. UN advisers arrived in Ghana to help with the census, led by Benjamin Gil. He provided training courses for Ghanaian statisticians at the newly created Census Office and at the Demographic Unit. African students, some of whom became census officers or consultants for IOs, were trained through this programme,[94] including Emmanuel Omaboe, who later directed Ghana's Population Policy.[95] There was also an education programme run throughout the country and F. D. Ntem acted as a Census Publicity Officer.[96] District and village level committees made up of local political and religious leaders were formed to take charge of this education and posters and pamphlets were distributed around the country.[97] Gil clearly wanted as much participation as possible from the Ghanaian public.

Those working on the Seven-Year Development Plan, directed by J. H. Mensah, utilised demographic data collated by the 1960 census. They reported high rates of population growth commenting that this could threaten economic growth. In response to this, Nkrumah set up a commission in 1964, to investigate the effects of population growth. However, no conclusions were reached before the 1966 coup.[98] The Plan mentioned high birth rates and population growth and that the labour force was 'growing very rapidly,' due to 'achievements' in lessening infant mortality and high birth rates. Rather than responding to this with suggestions on how to lower the birth rate, as later governments would, the Plan outlines how to utilise this growing workforce, arguing that 'a growing population presents an opportunity as much as a problem.'[99]

Pronatalism

The government, and most Ghanaians, maintained a pronatalist attitude, despite alarmist messages about population growth from IOs, academics, and development planners. There were three reasons for this. The first reflected Ghanaians' social and economic lives. The second is ideological, and the third linked to economic development. Firstly, it remained advantageous from the point of view of many Ghanaians to have large numbers of children. Agriculture was the main source of employment – 70% of Ghanaians lived in rural areas. Caldwell noted that, '[i]n a fully subsistence economy, where children can do much to provide their own food and other needs from a very young age, especially if the possibility of schooling does not exist, it is doubtful whether their presence imposes an extra burden.' He estimated that in rural areas, this was the situation for around one-third of families.[100] There was no 'fully' subsistence economy in Ghana,[101] and numbers attending primary school rose sharply in the 1950s and 1960s.[102] However, in the 1960s children commonly worked alongside their mothers growing food.[103]

Moreover, high birth rates remained socially desirable. Anthropologists show that Ghanaian women based their happiness and success on having large numbers of children.[104] In 1961, Margaret Field wrote that '[b]arren women, childless couples and infertile men leave no stone unturned in their earnest search for the cause and cure of their privation and often go from shrine to shrine offering extravagant gifts in exchange for a child.'[105] Both men and women were desperate to avoid infertility. Infertility can be understood not only as childlessness but also as not having the required number of children to satisfy individuals' needs and desires.[106] John Caldwell argued, based on surveys carried out in urban areas in 1967, 'most [Ghanaians were] still convinced that a rapidly growing population is *in the national good*', showing that politically, population growth was seen as positive.[107] Indeed, where the accumulation of people had historically reflected political success, now this philosophy transposed itself onto the nation. MP Mr J. D. Wireko argued that 'the people of Ghana would like our population to increase' and that it was 'shameful [to be talking] about population and not contributing towards its increase.'[108] According to Adjoa Ewusiwa, Nkrumah desired population increase because, 'he was a strong willed man … he was always thinking of us, he also loved us.'[109] Nana Efua Ateifi held a similar view. She remembered that at that time, there was family planning but 'he didn't bring it … he wanted many people … the population of Ghana was small, there were many countries with more population than us.'[110] These memories of Nkrumah's attitude tell us that he desired population increase, and that he was admired for it.

John Iliffe links demographic growth to a 'youthful, liberating momentum,' and ultimately to the success of nationalist, anti-colonial movements.[111] The limitation of population growth appeared, in this context, to be in the interests of neo-colonialists, attempting to maintain control. The Ford Foundation, which worked closely with the Ghanaian government following Independence, claimed that it had a 'strong pronatalist posture' and hoped for a 'jump' in population growth because 'population size was equated with influence in African and international affairs.'[112] Jeffrey Ahlman reminds us that in Ghana's decolonisation and nation-building process, entry onto the international stage as well as the African one was crucial for Nkrumah.[113] A large population was seen as a sign of a powerful nation, which was especially significant given Nkrumah's pan-Africanist, anti-imperialist outlook. If we accept Appiah's point that Pan-Africanism was racialised, and Nkrumah believed in Africa as a 'natural, racial, home,' negativity towards externally funded population control programmes make ideological sense.[114] Indeed, in Kenya, family planning was seen as neo-colonial, racialist, and even 'genocidal.'[115] In 1980s Namibia, health workers and patients alike expressed their distaste at the family planning programme which specifically targeted the black population.[116]

In 1960, Nkrumah gave a speech to the National Assembly, framing Africa's independence as 'a time of great danger ... but it is also a time for the greatest hope.' He called upon Africa to unite against colonial and neo-colonial forces. He said:

> The African continent consists of … almost one-quarter of the total world land area. It only, however, contains 8 ½ per cent of the world's population. This is not because, intrinsically the potential resources of the continent would not support in prosperity as large a population as other parts of the world, but because largely owing to the colonial past in Africa, African resources both in manpower and in natural products have been drained away.[117]

Evidently, Nkrumah saw population growth as a symptom of Africa's prosperity, and its limitation resultant from colonialism and underdevelopment; furthermore, Africa was capable of coping with population growth. Indeed, warnings about population growth from the Seven-Year Development plan were framed by emphasising that Ghana's economic growth could – and must – keep up with it. In other words, excess labour was not inherently problematic; it could bring prosperity.

Furthermore, Nkrumah's government was socialist, something which remained 'ill defined' at first but was fully embraced at the end of diarchic government in 1957.[118] This was especially true after 1960 and the 'lurch to the left.'[119] According to Professor Fred Sai, African leaders' 1960s socialism meant that they connected population growth to economic growth and therefore had little political interest in population control.[120] As Nkrumah got closer to Soviet leadership in the early 1960s, he started along a course of development based on socialist principles.[121] Meanwhile, in the Soviet bloc, the population was in decline. This was ideologically inconceivable in a communist state where 'women's productive and reproductive labour [was] essential to the state's growth.' As a result, Soviet leadership was decidedly pronatalist and restricted the availability of birth control.[122] In the international sphere, the USSR stood against 'neo-Malthusian tendencies.'[123] Similar ideological concerns were raised in Ghana. Mr Iddrissu, MP for Dagoma North, stated that in capitalist countries men 'indulge in bad practices' of birth control because the burden of care for children fell to individuals. In contrast, Iddrissu highlighted that in 'Russia and China,' the state provided for the care of pregnant mothers and neonates.[124] Here, the MP refers directly to policies in the USSR, highlighting the connection. The implication was that in a true socialist state, as he thought Ghana was aiming to become, there was no need for birth control.[125]

The government stressed women's place in Ghanaian nation-building in relation to their productive and reproductive roles. In this context, reproduction was specifically linked to economic development. As we saw above, Nkrumah had received warning that the country's labour force was not prepared for industrialisation. MP Victoria Nyame stated in 1963 that such was the need for labour in the new nation, that it was essential to mobilise women. She said, 'whilst calling on our women to contribute to our development programme, the State still expects them to give birth to children to swell up our population.'[126] Nyame implies a need for population increase and the *state's* expectation that this should occur. The push for population growth came from above. Nkrumah stressed the importance of 'human capital' in development projects, seeing direct labour as a way of saving money,[127] and the government pointed out that industrialisation was reliant on human resources.[128] In 1965, Mr Tedam, MP for Kassena Nankani North, argued that the government must invest in increasing the population because 'our manpower resources are not adequate.'[129] Mr Djan of Kpandu South agreed, arguing 'at present we want manpower for our industries and factories and persons who have twins and triplets are surely doing well to increase the manpower we want.'[130] These politicians linked industrialisation, the need for labour, and population increase specifically through reproduction.

The government introduced pronatalist, socialist policies such as maternity leave and day nurseries. Susana Al-Hasan, Minister of Social Welfare, described these in 1965 as

> 'laudable human arrangements which have been made by Osegyafo's forward-looking and progressive C.P.P. to grant out women various facilities related to child bearing and child care … to discharge their functions as those who have … the country's future in their bosoms.'[131]

Again women's reproductive role is emphasised as their responsibility to national development. The government also introduced a number of health policies designed to reduce child mortality. The Health Minister, J. H. Allassani, announced in 1958 that MCH was one of Local Authorities' 'most important responsibilities' noting that 'I know that the care of mothers, infants and young children is of major importance in improving the health of the people and increasing the population of the country.' He encouraged girls to take advantage of midwifery training programmes as well as an increase in maternity services overseen by his Ministry.[132] Although these campaigns had obvious humanitarian value, they were also linked to nation building. In 1963, a series of baby shows were organised as part of National Health Week. These events were directed by Margaret Martei of the National Council of Ghana Women (NCGW), an organisation affiliated with the CPP and made up of amalgamated women's organisations in 1960.[133] Baby shows are an overt example of pronatalism.

The theme for Health Week 1964 was 'Healthy Babies make a Healthy Nation': babies were not only made healthy for their own sakes, but for the sake of the nation.[134]

The consequences of pronatalism went beyond soft policies of promoting child health and providing maternity leave.[135] Sai argued that doctors could not organise to provide family planning given Nkrumah's 'ban' on contraceptives.[136] Dr Barnor also testified that family planning had to be clandestine because the government was opposed to it.[137] The law made abortion punishable by up to ten years' imprisonment.[138] Some MPs suggested that since 'Osagyefo [President Nkrumah] has asked us to produce more [children],' this punishment also be extended to those using contraceptives.[139] In other words, not only was there positive reinforcement for births, there were negative consequences to limiting them.

Maternal and Child Health in the New Nation

Reading the *Ghanaian Times*, in July 1960, one might be forgiven for thinking that all Ghanaian women gave birth in hospitals with nurses to guide them through the early days of motherhood. An article entitled: 'Tips on Child Bathing,' began: 'The excitement is over and you are back to your house with a fine bundle – a brand new baby. Alone in the house without the assistance of nurses you get scared.'[140] The article implies that women gave birth in a hospital or clinic and were alone upon returning home. Neither of these implications were realities for most Ghanaian women. Most people, especially in rural areas, lived with extended family. The 1960 census found an average of 10.6 people per house.[141] Most deliveries happened at home attended by local women. The *Ghanaian Times* image was aspirational.

When Independence came, medical services in Ghana were far from comprehensive. As the previous chapter showed, medical spending dropped in the early 1950s, and, despite growth in the availability of maternal health services, coverage was not universal by any means. The Minister for Health noted that 'infant mortality was running at an alarmingly high rate,' in 1960.[142] However, scholars John Iliffe and Ruth Prince have described this as a period of immense 'optimism' for decolonising nations, which seeped into health sectors prioritised by ideologically socialist African governments.[143] Indeed, in Ghana medical provision was free to those who could not afford to pay, with others paying a small nominal fee.[144] However, the state of medical services in Ghana between 1957 and 1966 is difficult to construct due to a scarcity of archival evidence: there were no government medical reports during this time.

Many Ghanaians remember this as a period in which healthcare was cheap and reliable. Aishutu Manuh remembered that giving birth at a hospital was free in the 1950s and 1960s, whereas now, 'if you don't have money, you can't go.'[145] Of course, the explicit comparison with today leads us to question whether these positive memories are impacted by frustrations over contemporary services. However, Aishutu was not the only interviewee to testify that healthcare under Nkrumah was good. In Georgina Hermance's town Moree, there is one clinic. She remembered that it was built 'long ago' and presumed this was during Nkrumah's time. She said that during Nkrumah's government, nurses and midwives were plentiful and they used to give instruction on pregnancy and childrearing in Moree. In comparison, 'now they are not many like in the past … now half have gone to Winneba, Kumasi, Accra.'[146] Georgina's impression was that the Nkrumah-era was a positive one for women's health. In fact, free healthcare was provided until the economic conditions of the 1970s meant that this was no longer possible and the number of health centres increased.

The 1963 Seven-Year Development Plan allocated 11% of total spending to health.[147] Compared to the 4.2% a decade earlier in 1953, this indicated prioritisation. However, despite rhetoric about schemes to expand rural health services, spending on 'regional health services' under the plan totalled around a third of funding for 'hospital services.' Dr Strudwick of WHO noted that 'the quality of care of the urban areas and coverage is much higher.' Supplies were also deficient at the local authority dispensary level, whilst they were adequate for major hospitals and health posts.[148] Despite this, the Seven-Year Development Plan boasted progress. Perhaps unsurprisingly, it stated that until the CPP was elected in the early 1950s, the Medical Service had been 'slow and spasmodic.' Since then, it stated, the 'health service has undergone a truly extensive transformation.' This included the building of rural health centres, increase of staff, and more training opportunities. There was also increased demand for services, which the government presented as a 'good sign that the population will accept health services' but conceded that it also meant it was not currently coping.[149]

In 1963 there were 6,549 hospital beds available, with a population of 6.7 million. Sixty per cent of these came under the MH, whilst government-subsidised mission hospitals still accounted for 23.5%. At Korle Bu, the largest hospital in Ghana, there were 491 beds, 37% of which belonged to the Maternity Hospital.[150] Furthermore, hospitals and health centres were not adequately staffed.[151] In 1961, WHO noted that nurses were being trained at a rate of around 32% of what was needed, annually, and the government began negotiations with the University of Ghana to provide post-basic nursing training.[152] Plans were also to expand Health Visitors' activities to include midwifery training.[153] The first training school for Community Health Nurses (CHN) opened in Tamale in May 1960. However, when Marjorie Houghton, nursing consultant, visited Ghana in 1961, she noted that there was a severe shortage in training staff. In fact, there were only three Ghanaian nurses qualified for teaching.[154] Moreover, although it was based in the Northern Region, only three of the Tamale school's cohort of 23 were from the north, indicating regional disparity.[155] In summary, although the government emphasised positive aspects, staff and equipment levels were low, and the majority of health services still situated at a distance from rural populations.

Notably, economic growth was evoked repeatedly when arguing for improvements in health services, particularly MCH. Health propaganda often utilised the notion of the nation to promote programmes. An aid appeal to USAID noted that '[a] high rate of infant mortality does not help to produce the required manpower to help in the economic growth of the country.'[156] The argument is made that 'manpower' is needed for economic growth to USAID, an agency highly invested in this topic. Its Seven-Year Development Plan also echoed this thinking. The government stated: '[q]uite apart from humanitarian reasons, capital devoted to the improvement of health services is an economic investment, for a healthy population is much more productive than an unhealthy one.'[157] National Health Week was held annually. In 1959, *Ghana Today* commented that 'public health services form a vital part of any development plan in tropical Africa. Endemic diseases ... sap energy and initiative ... lower productivity and affect the economy of the country.' As these examples show, health service provision was linked to citizens' levels of economic productivity. What is more, the *Ghana Today* article was accompanied by a picture of a plump baby sitting on a weighing scale, implying that MCH was a crucial part of this.[158] By 1965, Parliament congratulated itself, and Osagyefo, on its achievements for women's health.[159] But Patience Doris Doh, who trained as a nurse in the 1960s, somewhat cynically commented that every government worked to lower maternal mortality since high rates 'talk bad about the government.'[160] Indeed, providing health infrastructure did seem to constitute government propaganda.

There were general plans to extend the reach of MCH. CHNs were required to take a course in elementary midwifery, to enable them to do antenatal work, and were to visit pregnant and newly delivered mothers in their homes. However, the government estimated infant mortality – those that die before one-year of age – at around 10% and child mortality at 25%. Maternal mortality was estimated in 1963 at 17/1,000 live births. This was largely due to conditions such as anaemia and other 'complications,' which need not be fatal, if proper antenatal care were provided.[161] 'Disorders of pregnancy and puerperium' were listed as the eighth most common cause of death in Ghanaian hospitals.[162]

International Aid for Health

The provision of reproductive health in Ghana was delivered not only through national design, but through cooperation with global health organisations. The post-war world saw the establishment of a global bureaucracy for development, including health. The World Health Organization (WHO) was established in 1946.[163] Its constitution defined health as a 'fundamental right' as well as 'an essential factor in the attainment of security and well-being for individuals and nations.' Sunil Amrith argues that this encapsulated how post-war international health was connected to global development.[164] Whilst the idea of the 'right' to health was slow to take effect, the need for health for economic development and security was taken seriously. WHO's understanding of 'health' went beyond the absence of disease, inviting exploration of social and economic determinants.

One of WHO's earliest priorities was MCH. The International Council of Women declared their affiliation, citing their 'historical and inherent interest in children's health, maternal care, and the protection of the health of industrial workers.'[165] Although WHO is frequently presented as limited during the 1950s by allegiance to technological health solutions,[166] the field of MCH was an exception. The proposal put forward by the USA, to prioritise MCH, stated that 'among all nations there is a general recognition that children are their greatest asset in terms of human resources' and that medical care was essential to ensure children reached a healthy state of maturity.[167] In other words, MCH programmes, similarly to colonial medicine, focused on the benefits of ensuring healthy *children* explicitly, and mothers implicitly. Furthermore, healthy children are specifically valued for their economic role in global development. Jessie Bierman, head of MCH, wrote that WHO's main intervention was through training and the assignment of international personnel to work with governments.[168] WHO provided demonstrations, fellowships and research, rather than medical and health services.[169]

Scholars have argued that it was not until the era of primary health care (PHC) that WHO assisted 'national programmes' in Africa.[170] Indeed, although West Africa's Regional Director Dr Karefa-Smart, argued for increased WHO surveillance as early as 1954,[171] WHO made very few interventions in African countries in the 1950s. However, in Ghana, WHO *did* become involved in planning MCH services in the late 1950s and 1960s.

By 1957, there were ten projects either established or in preparation in Ghana, and 15 fellowships had been granted to Ghanaians.[172] At the invitation of the new Ghanaian government, within the first year of independence, five new WHO projects began. These projects dealt with malaria, bilharzia, leprosy, public health and MCH.[173] In 1957, the government invited consultant Dr Poulton to study the current state of MCH services, and to make recommendations as to how WHO and UNICEF could help improve them. Other experts visited the country. In November, an FAO representative arrived. She stayed at a Youth Centre at Anomabo, a coastal town near Cape Coast, and conducted a series of intensive courses for female Mass Education staff.[174] From its earliest days, Ghana became part of international health networks, advice and interventions, especially regarding MCH.

As of 1958, WHO and the Ghanaian government began cooperating to improve the newly independent country's health systems. A plan formulated by WHO in 1958 aimed to develop long-term rural health services by dividing the country into districts, each overseen by an MO.[175] A WHO MCH adviser was assigned and, in collaboration with the government, a project area was established in Ho, in Volta Region.[176] In addition to training staff and conducting research, a core component was community education. Project leaders would 'activate community organization and self-help.'[177] Although the project saw some progress, it was hindered by lack of staff, poor transport, and a failure to disseminate the importance of community health to local leaders.[178] In other words, it blamed its failures on a lack of local cooperation.

In 1962, negotiations began between the government, Korle Bu medical and administrative staff, and USAID to fund a Medical School and Teaching Hospital in Accra. USAID proposed to fund the project through low-interest, long-term loans, rather than a grant, to the disappointment of certain Ghanaians involved.[179] Donors, in this case, USAID, had certain control over projects and the expansion of Ghanaian healthcare. For example, the schematic for the Teaching Hospital was first proposed by USAID, only to later be signed off by the Mr Ludlam, the architect for Ghana's MH.[180] USAID also proposed that a US Dean from the Philadelphia Group of Medical Schools should run the Medical School once it was established. Dr Cruise O'Brien, Vice Chancellor of the University of Ghana, 'raised the keenest objection' to this.[181] The MH agreed, arguing that 'it would be impossible to reconcile the imperatives of Ghana as a Sovereign State with the probable implications of the School etc., being run from abroad.'[182] In the end, the Medical School officially became part of the University of Ghana. However, applications for aid emphasised that the government proposed to work 'very closely' with USAID and would 'welcome a periodical inspection.'[183]

Nevertheless, the Medical School was undoubtedly a nationalist and pan-African project. In a 1963 Development Grant application to USAID, the government stated that:

> the primary … objective of this project is the development of a Medical School which would meet the highest international standards of Medical Education … and also meet the health and medical care needs of the country and eventually help meet those of other African countries.[184]

The application included the cost of four urban health centres to be used in Medical Education, which would provide 'out-patient, ante-natal and child health services.'[185] Indeed, MCH was emphasised in the proposals; initial plans for the Teaching Hospital proposed that 14% of beds should be allocated to obstetrics and gynaecology, and another 11.5% to paediatrics.[186] Furthermore, the Medical School meant to make 'Preventative and Social Medicine the prime faculty' of the school. This would allow the health service to reach rural areas 'as yet untouched by the benefits of modern medicine.'[187] However, the school was slow to have an impact. By 1964, the first batch of medical students – 41 in total – had reached their second of seven years' training. Far more students, 630 in 1964, were in training abroad.[188] Indeed, vast numbers of medical students were trained in Soviet bloc countries during this period.[189]

Forming the Modern Ghanaian Women

The Ghanaian Woman published an article in 1960 advising women on how to keep their homes and children healthy. It was entitled: 'Your Health is Our Wealth': women's and infants' health was linked to the growth of the nation.[190] A 1962 pamphlet: 'Keeping Baby Healthy,' said: 'most babies are well and healthy when they are born, and it is the mother's duty to try to keep her baby that way.' Part of this responsibility lay in taking the baby to the welfare clinic regularly.[191] The responsibility of motherhood was mainly domestic, something that women's organisations and the department of Social Welfare gained access to on the grounds of promoting social development. Maternal solutions were once again deployed in order to achieve developmental aims.

Female Mass Education Assistants continued to be deployed. Dr Ofori-Atta described them as an asset in the *Ghanaian Times*, noting their 'great role to play' due to their contact with those most in need of 'health education.' Most important, Ofori-Atta said, was their 'training of girls … aimed at bringing up the girls as useful mothers who know their culture and the proper care of their children.'[192] In other words, women's participation in the Mass Education programme, both as teachers and learners, was directly linked to child rearing not only on the biological level but the social once since women were expected to rear children according to their 'culture.' This was about building the nation's citizenry.

Indeed, women's responsibility for the health, nutrition and reproduction of families was a cornerstone of government policy. The FAO home economics expert advising on Mass Education worked in consultation with the MH, and Ministry of Social Welfare, to revise the syllabus for women's work.[193] She led the National Women's Training Centre at Pamfokrom, alongside a Ghanaian Community Development Officer, who had trained abroad on an FAO scholarship.[194] Meanwhile, the government sent aid requests to UNICEF for support with 'Home Economics' and 'Housecraft.' In 1960, the Minister for Social Welfare made an agreement with the UNICEF representative based in Lagos, Mr Gordon, for Home Economics Women's Training Centres to be established in Ghana.[195] The project proposal, drawn up by Gordon and the Minister was entitled: 'Mothercraft and Homecraft (Women's Work in Community Development).' It worked to build up female staff at the Ministry of Social Welfare, extend home economics teaching to the villages and encourage formation of village women's clubs.[196] These development projects fixed women's place in community development as domestic and linked to motherhood. The effect of this made women-as-mothers the primary way in which they could interact with NGO projects, and their own government.

Women's Organisations

The Federation of Ghana Women (FGW) – mentioned in Chapter 3 under its previous name, the Federation of Gold Coast Women – was engaged in women's reproductive health advocacy. This was not always in ways the government may have envisaged. For example, the General Secretary wrote to the Health Minister, Imoro Igala, in February 1960 to complain about a sanitary pad tax increase, making them unaffordable to many. Given a campaign that the Federation was running on 'personal hygiene,' Amarteifio asked the Minister to 'plead on our behalf' against this raise.[197] In April 1959, the FGW invited Edith Gates, a representative from Pathfinder Fund, to give a talk at their annual conference. She spoke on the topic of 'Planned Parenthood.'[198] Given her institutional affiliation, we can assume that Gates used the opportunity to advocate the use of contraceptives to limit or space pregnancies. In late 1959, Gates reported to IPPF that the FGW was already discussing the problem of planning families for better health. She said that a committee had been formed on the subject and discussions had begun with community leaders.[199] In the pronatalist context described above, this was courageous. FGW's conferences also welcomed representatives from midwives' associations.[200] In this sense, it represented an outlet for discussion on women's reproductive rights issues that the government largely shut down with its pronatalist stance.

However, whilst women's organisations broadly aimed to 'improve the status of women,' they frequently advocated pronatalism and prescriptive gendered roles through their activities and discourse. For example, in Sekondi the FGW gave lessons in 'sewing, knitting and cookery,' elsewhere they contributed funds to a hospital, helped open a Day Nursery and visited the sick.[201] Like other nationalist associations in Africa, the FGW appealed to women as mothers.[202]

Government development plans relied on women's organisations. At the launch of the Second Development Plan, Nkrumah invited leaders of voluntary organisations to a meeting in which he explained that he was counting on their support. Delegates of the FGW enthusiastically responded with suggestions for collaboration with Social Welfare officers:

> Day Nurseries, eradication of Nudity in children, the cooperation of Chiefs in villages should be sort [sic]. The delegates of the Methodist Women's Fellowship told the meeting how they had gone to some villages to teach cleanliness; it was agreed this was very essential.[203]

These suggestions all pertained to modernity: appropriate spaces for children whilst women worked, anti-nudity,[204] and a push for cleanliness and order. Interestingly, they express the need for cooperation from chiefs, who held power locally, for women's causes.

Furthermore, after 1960, voluntary women's organisations, which had previously been non-partisan, came under government control. They formed the National Council of Ghana Women (NCGW).[205] The task of forming the NCGW was given to Tawia Adamafio, who saw it as an 'onerous and disgusting' one. Nonetheless, the Council was formed and went on to be, in his own words, an organisation with 'great promise.'[206] The NCGW Programme of Work for 1962 included 'food & nutrition,' 'household budgeting,' 'sewing and handicraft,' 'ante-natal and post-natal child care,' 'visits to local ante-natal clinics,' 'in the rural areas, resident or nearby midwife to be invited to give lectures and demonstrations,' and so on.[207] Since the object of the NCGW was to 'promote the role of women in changing the society of our country,'[208] we must assume that women's reproductive roles were central to envisaged social change. Since this organisation was now under the oversight of the CPP, opportunities for advocating for birth control or other areas of women's reproductive health were reduced to these pro-maternal activities.

Mabel Dove wrote an open letter to Ghanaian newspapers in 1961 against the White Paper Proposals on Marriage and Divorce. She argued that the proposal to create registered and unregistered wives was dangerous to men, women and the nation.[209] In the latter case, this was explicitly linked to procreation. Responsible parents were needed 'to increase our population,' and prevent children dying unnecessarily from disease and neglect. Dove's feminist discourse equated women inextricably with femininity and motherhood. She quoted Nkrumah at the opening of the NCGW, who said, 'A woman should always remain a woman.' 'It is women,' she argued,

> who go through the discomfort of pregnancy; it is women who have to care for children in their tender years. No woman in Ghana should be made to feel that a law is being proposed which gives men the whip hand over her emotions and all that makes her a woman.[210]

Whilst this essentialist discourse did nothing to break down gendered expectations of motherhood, it defended women as equal contributors to the nation through their reproductive activities. These examples of women's activism suggest two things. Firstly, that they fought explicitly for women's rights, and secondly, that they did so within limitations which linked women to their bodies and to reproduction.

Also linked to women's reproductive roles, the government established the National Food and Nutrition Board (NFNB) in 1959. The Board's aim was to accumulate knowledge about nutritional deficiencies and make recommendations to eradicate them. Its work was divided into: 'Survey and Research' and 'Education and Information.'[211] Nutritional deficiencies were explained either by food scarcity and unaffordability or 'ignorance,' which should be combatted by education. It was regarding this last issue that the NFNB targeted women. Indeed, special attention was given to the needs of pregnant and nursing mothers and to young children.[212] As investigations began in 1960, the Board found that:

> the needs of pregnant and lactating women require greater consideration. Some of our investigations show that when a woman feeds a baby she does not take the extra nourishment required and in consequence her health suffers and so does the health of future babies she may have. Furthermore, the weaning of babies is far from satisfactory … we consider that this is largely a problem of education.'[213]

The NFNB provided education through radio, film and demonstrations at clinics, schools and villages.[214] In Juabeng in Eastern Region, all mothers of 5–8 month-old babies were gathered on 21 May 1961. They were rounded up by Mr Addo, of the Nutritional Survey Team. Mr Addo had previously, along with Mrs Selby, the Regional Nutrition Officer, appealed to the town's chiefs and elders to 'urge' mothers of young children to improve their nutrition. Once mothers were gathered, the officials explained to them 'methods by which weaning diets should be improved.' Afterwards, these mothers were visited by senior school girls and Mass Education Assistants, who kept 'a close check' on the babies' weights and health.[215]

This episode in the government's early 1960s nutritional health efforts demonstrates increased surveillance of the population. Through this work, the government was increasing the 'legibility' of the state, as James Scott would put it.[216] This allowed the government to carry out large-scale modernisation projects. Indeed, a UNICEF project in Ghana specifically aimed to 'extend the work of female supervisory staff by providing them with motor transport for travel into remote areas.'[217] This affected women differently than it affected men. Women's private lives – and reproductive lives – were known about, judged, monitored and changed as the government saw fit. At the end of 1959, there were 18,805 women in classes provided by community development staff in rural areas.[218]

Family Planning

Despite the government's pronatalist attitude, local actors identified a need for birth control in Ghana. These were health professionals, including doctors, nurses and pharmacists, who formed networks of concern and, eventually, action. Exploring nascent family planning organisations in the 1960s shows us that this was not wholly imported but had roots in specific and local concerns and activism. Although Professor Sai testified to a 'ban' on contraception, there is no clear evidence for this. There were 'inconspicuous' sales of contraceptives in pharmacies in towns.[219] Furthermore, women's organisations showed an interest in family planning. In June 1959, the Federation of Ghana Women was sent 48 cartons of spermicidal foaming tablets by British Drug Houses at the request of Gates.[220] Moreover, individual doctors like Dr Bannerman were providing family planning advice, although it is unclear to what extent. Any government disapproval of contraceptives might have taken an authoritarian turn along with the general evolution of CPP rule in the mid-1960s, but if there were repercussions for doctors or pharmacies providing contraceptives, I have not found evidence of them.

On the other hand, doctors concerned with reproductive health clearly remember the state obstructing family planning. As such, there was no formal family planning association, or adoption of it under the MH in this period. But it did begin to infiltrate. The beginnings of family planning in Ghana constituted a local version of a global concern. Despite the pronatalist atmosphere, small family planning organisations began to form. They were articulated in ways that emphasised different primary concerns than those of foreign population activists. One clear example was the Medical Advice Centre (MAC) set up by the Christian Council, under the leadership of Jean Forrester-Paton, in 1961. The MAC was part of the Christian Council's Marriage and Family Life section. The clinic was explicitly for married couples.[221] Its existence was publicised through churches.[222] The IPPF highlighted its growth and the importance of education it provided given the Church community's general lack of knowledge about 'scientific contraception.'[223] It was funded by Pathfinder Fund.[224] It was only open for a few hours weekly and had trouble finding sufficient medical staff. IPPF commented on the 'international' nature of its staff – doctors hailed from Ghana, the UK and Pakistan.[225]

The MAC's primary concern was the survival and success of Christian marriages, and children's upbringing.[226] It aimed to 'investigate and treat possible causes of infertility' and to provide advice on how to space pregnancies.[227] Its aim was not to limit the number of births, or even primarily to protect the health of mothers. It was concerned with the health of Christian marriages. Infertility was regarded as a reason that marriages foundered and, alongside them, commitment to Christian, rather than 'traditional' culture. They feared that couples would turn to 'native doctors' or that men would take multiple wives in the face of fertility issues. The centre was described by Dr Bentsi-Enchill, working at Korle Bu hospital, as 'a useful bridge between those who had lost all hope and Korle Bu where ultimate investigation would probably be necessary.'[228] Indeed, the MAC took a pastoral role as well as a medical one. Doctors who worked there should, according to its directors, be best qualified in psychology, rather than family planning, since it was psychologically that infertility hit couples hardest.

In 1963, the Christian Council, which did not include the Catholic Churches in Ghana, unanimously agreed that there ought to be provision for 'family planning by scientific contraceptive methods (or abstinence if preferred) to space the birth of babies and to limit conceptions in already large families.'[229] This statement goes beyond the Christian Council's limits to recommend that family planning be available to all. It also implies that scientific methods are the most effective methods. Furthermore, the promotion of birth spacing and the limitation of births were specifically for *large* families.

In 1964, a branch of the MAC opened in Kumasi under Dr Joyce Nichols. The branch in Accra provided funds, spermicidal foam and 500 leaflets in Twi and Fanti on family planning.[230] The clinic operated for a few hours every Tuesday, although it also experienced staff shortages. Within a few months, it was reported that this clinic was 'patronised steadily.' Later, in November of the same year, Dr Moody in Ho, Volta Region, expressed a desire to set up an MAC there. She 'had shown great interest in family planning, especially through the Emko' supplied by the Christian World Service.[231] In other words, what started as a small service for certain church goers of Accra began to look like systemised provision of family planning advice and contraception. This is crucial, since it puts the role of a religious organisation at the centre of changes in women's reproductive health provision in the 1960s. Although the MAC could be criticised for only providing to married women, and only given certain conditions, it opened its doors to women and tried to understand their problems and advise them, which no other medical setting did. It went beyond family planning, women attended for a range of reproductive issues, including menopause. Furthermore, all the staff were women.

Planned Parenthood Association of Ghana (PPAG) also originated in the mid-1960s. In 1966, IPPF's Betty Hull, visited Ghana. She met with a number of health professionals who were already interested in family planning, including

Dr Barnor. In the pronatalist, and ever more security focused, atmosphere of Nkrumah's Ghana,[232] these doctors had to remain clandestine in their activities.[233] Their personal memoirs show that they were motivated to act by personal concerns over women's and children's health. Especially concerning was the high rate of self-induced abortions and prevalence of malnutrition. These doctors are remembered by those working in family planning as 'pioneers.'[234] Betty Hull invited them to the IPPF West European and Mediterranean Regional Conference in Copenhagen in 1966. Among those who attended were Drs Barnor, Bentsi-Enchill, Armar (who later became the Director of NFPP), Saakwa-Mente and de Graft Johnson (the only woman in the group).[235] The group from Ghana was one of 17 African countries represented. Dr Serwadda of Uganda noted, however, that only three of these countries were supported by their governments given the ongoing 'misconception' that family planning meant population control, and that African people were not interested in it.[236] At this conference, the Ghanaians decided to establish a family planning organisation. PPAG was inaugurated in 1967, originally run out of Dr Barnor's home, but grew to have significant impact.[237] Already by the late 1960s, it began to expand into Ghana's regions, albeit 'on a very limited scale.'[238]

Therefore, although there was no systematic family planning, contraceptives were available from pharmacies and individual doctors. However, they were generally unavailable outside urban spaces. Family planning was confined mainly to Accra and Kumasi. Interestingly, ideologies behind the origins of family planning in Ghana did not align with powerful global discourses on population control. The Church set up family planning to preserve the social reproduction of Christian families, and it was motivated by religion and the sanctity of the family. Doctors acted out of concern for women and children's health. Their motivation was preserving life; limiting fertility was a method rather than a goal. The origins of systemised family planning came before the Population Policy and NFPP. Furthermore, they stemmed from localised and religious concerns. This reading of Ghana's family planning history problematizes assumptions that it was an outside imposition.

Conclusion

Under Nkrumah, women's reproductive health was viewed through the lens of nationalist (economic) development. Nationalist rhetoric constructed the role of women as mothers for the nation. Despite the CPP's message that women were a vital part of the nation's workforce, its pronatalism and approach to social welfare show that in practice, women were imagined first and foremost as mothers. The CPP made no attempt to engage with global population activism that sought to limit fertility. Rather, it encouraged an increase in population growth. Government discourse connected the nation's power to its population size and 'human resources.' Development was presented as dependent on population growth, not threatened by it.

The CPP's rhetoric and approach to development was aspirational, and medicalisation was part of modernisation. This aspirational rhetoric continued to surround the evolution of health infrastructure. Technical assistance offered by WHO was a way for the government to promise a 'modern' health service to its citizens, especially in the realm of MCH. Nationalism seeped into the extension of health services, as we can see through rhetoric accompanying the establishment of the Medical School.

Finally, women's organisations were closely affiliated with the CPP. Their rhetoric also conceptualised national development as dependent on women's health, and particular modes of motherhood. However, women's organisations, alongside other groups, notably a faction of doctors and the Christian Council, began providing opportunities for women to access family planning for the sake of their own health and the stability of their marriages. In this sense, these groups began to advocate for women's rights, even when the state discursively narrowed women's options in the name of development. The next chapter follows the trajectory of these early family planning activists in Ghana. In 1966, following a coup which overthrew Nkrumah and the CPP, approaches to population and family planning took a U-turn, though development rhetoric was used to legitimise this reversal of policy.

Notes

1 Shane Doyle, 'Demography and Disease', in *The Oxford Handbook of Modern African History*, (Oxford: Oxford University Press; 2013), 41.
2 J. C. Caldwell, 'Population: General Characteristics', in *A Study of Contemporary Ghana. Vol. 2 Some Aspects of Social Structure*, ed. W. Birmingham, I. Neustadt, and E. Omaboe (London: London, 1967), 18.
3 Matthew Connelly, *Fatal Misconception* (Cambridge, MA: Harvard University Press, 2009).
4 NA, DO 35/9297: Note in file by A. H. Reed, 18 July 1957.
5 'Ghana Heading Towards the Welfare State Declared Quaidoo', *The Ghanaian Times*, 16 July 1960, 1.
6 NA, DO 35/9303: 'Press Release No. 196/59: Draft of Prime Minister's Speech on the Second Five-Year Development Plan to be Delivered before Parliament of the 4 March 1959', n.d. but March 1959, 1.
7 Interviews carried out between October 2017 and July 2019.
8 NA, CO 859/154/6: The Economist, *Food and People*, 14 May 1949.
9 Joseph M. Hodge, *Triumph of the Expert: Agrarian Doctrines of Development and the Legacies of British Colonialism* (Athens, OH: Ohio University Press, 2007), 3; Frederick Cooper, *Decolonization & African Society: The Labor Question in French and British Africa* (Cambridge: Cambridge University Press, 2008).
10 Hodge, *Triumph of the Expert*, 6.
11 R. R. Kuczynski, *Demographic Survey of The British Colonial Empire, Vol. 1 West Africa* (London: Oxford University Press, 1948).
12 Kuczynski, vii.
13 Karl Ittmann, *Problem of Great Importance* (Berkeley, CA: University of California Press, 2013), 107.
14 Ibid., 113.
15 NA, CO 859/154/6: Note in file, 3 March 1948.
16 NA, CO 859/154/6: 'The Growth of Tropical Populations' T. H. Davey, April, 1949.
17 NA, CO 859/154/6: 'Extracts from the Minutes of C.A.M.C. 443rd Meeting held 23.3.48', 1.
18 Ittmann, *Problem of Great Importance*, 125.

19 NA, CO 859/154/6: 'The Growth of Tropical Populations' T. H. Davey, April, 1949.
20 NA, CO 859/154/6: Note in file, 16 March 1948.
21 NA, CO 859/62/17: 'Extract from a Letter from Julian Huxley', 17 July 1943.
22 Ittmann, *Problem of Great Importance*, 132–33.
23 NA, CO 859/154/6: 'The Growth of Tropical Populations' T. H. Davey, April, 1949, 1.
24 NA, CO 859/62/17: Note in file 20 August 1943.
25 Alison Bashford, *Global Population: History, Geopolitics, and Life on Earth* (New York: Columbia University Press, 2014).
26 NA, CO 859/62/17: Note in file 20 August 1943.
27 For an intellectual history of population see: Bashford, *Global Population.* Africa was largely ignored by neo-Malthusians until much later than other continents.
28 NA, CO 859/154/6: 'Extracts from the Minutes of C.A.M.C. 443rd Meeting held 23.3.48', 1.
29 NA, CO 859/154/6: Note in file, 14 June 1948.
30 NA, CO 859/154/6: 'Extracts from the Minutes of C.A.M.C. 443rd Meeting held 23.3.48', 1.
31 NA, CO 859/154/6: 'Extract: 18. Birth Control', n.d. According to this note, the matter was to be referred to UNESCO as a priority after its establishment.
32 Nicole Bourbonnais, *Birth Control in the Decolonizing Caribbean: Reproductive Politics and Practice on Four Islands, 1930–1970* (Cambridge: Cambridge University Press, 2016), 25.
33 PRAAD, Accra, RG 3/5/1432: Savingram: 'Family Planning' from the Secretary of State for the Colonies to Government of the Gold Coast, 14 February 1955.
34 PRAAD, Accra, RG 3/5/1432: Letter from Director of Social Welfare and Community Development to the Permanent Secretary, Ministry of Education: 'Family Planning', 11 March 1955.
35 PRAAD, Accra, RG 3/5/1432: Savingram: from Governor of Gold Coast to Secretary of State for the Colonies, 21 March 1955.
36 WHO, P13/372/9: 'Letter from R H O Bannerman Chief Medical Officer for Education and Family Health, WHO to Dr Boi-Doku,' 7 December 1970.
37 J. C. Caldwell, 'Population Prospects and Policy', in *A Study of Contemporary Ghana. Vol. 2 Some Aspects of Social Structure*, ed. W. Birmingham, I. Neustadt, and E. Omaboe (London: George Allen & Unwin Ltd., 1967), 155.
38 PRAAD, ADM 5/2/9: Government of the Gold Coast, *Census of Population 1948 Report and Tables*, Government Printing Department, Accra, 1950, 7–8.
39 Ibid., 35–36.
40 *Report of the Commission of Enquiry into the Health Needs of the Gold Coast 1952*, Government Printing Dept., Accra, 9.
41 BDL, MSS.Afr.c.1872/28: 'Observations on the Medical Department Following a Tour in The Gold Coast Nov 1949–Apr 1950', 1950, 16.
42 PRAAD, Accra, ADM 5/4/69: Gold Coast Government, *Progress Report for the Period Ended 31st December 1948 on the Draft Ten-Year Plan of Development and Welfare*, Accra, 1949, 2.
43 PRAAD, Accra, ADM 5/4/84: Gold Coast Government, *The Development Plan, 1951*, Accra, 1951, 4.
44 PRAAD, Accra, ADM 14/2/83: *Legislative Council Debates*, 8 November 1954, 438.
45 Bashford, *Global Population.*
46 UN General Assembly (17th sess.: 1962) *Resolutions Adopted by the General Assembly during its 17th session, 18th September – 20 December 1962,* Resolution 1838, 18 December 1962, 25.
47 Ibid.
48 Connelly, *Fatal Misconception*; Emily Callaci, '"Injectable Development" Depo-Provera and Creation of the Global South', *Radical History Review* 131 (2018):

82–104; John Sharpless, 'Population Science, Private Foundations, and Development Aid: The Transformation of Demographic Knowledge in the United State, 1945–1965', in *International Development and the Social Sciences: Essays on the History and Politics of Knowledge*, ed. Randall Packard and Frederick Cooper (Berkeley, CA: University of California Press, 1998), 176–202.

49 Mahmood Mamdani, *The Myth of Population Control. Family, Caste and Class in and Indian Village* (New York: Monthly Review Press, 1972), 18–19.; A similar point is also made in: Randall Packard, *A History of Global Health: Interventions into the Lives of Other Peoples* (Baltimore, MD: Johns Hopkins University Press, 2016), 186.

50 There is a vast scholarship on gender and nationalism. See for example: Anne McClintock, '"No Longer in a Future Heaven": Women and Nationalism in South Africa', *Transition*, no. 51 (1991): 105; Nira Yuval-Davis, *Gender & Nation* (London: Sage Publications, 1997); Lynn M. Thomas, *Politics of the Womb: Women, Reproduction, and the State in Kenya* (Berkeley, CA: University of California Press, 2003); Sita Ranchod-Nilsson, '(Gender) Struggles for the Nation', in *Women, States and Nationalism: At Home in the Nation?*, ed. Mary Ann Tetreault and Sita Ranchod-Nilsson (London: Routledge, 2003), 168.

51 Jean Allman, 'The Disappearing of Hannah Kudjoe: Nationalism, Feminism, and the Tyrannies of History', *Journal of Women's History* 21, no. 3 (2009): 13–35; Takyiwaa Manuh, 'Women and Their Organizations during the Convention People's Party Period', in *The Ghana Reader*, ed. Kwasi Konadu and Clifford C. Campbell (Durham, NC: Duke University Press, 2016), 285–91; Edzodzinam Tsikata, 'Women's Political Organisations, 1951–1987', in *State, Development and Politics in Ghana*, ed. Emmanuel Hansen and Kwame A. Ninsin (London: CODESRIA Book Series, 1989), 73–93.

52 Jeffrey Ahlman, *Living with Nkrumahism: Nation, State, and Pan-Africanism in Ghana* (Illinois: Ohio University Press, 2017). See chapters 3 and 5.

53 Kwame Nkrumah, *The Autobiography of Kwame Nkrumah* (London: Nelson, 1957), xi.

54 'Kwame Messages Ghana Youth Spiritually,' *The Evening News*, 21 June 1950, 2.

55 Iris Berger, *Women in Twentieth Century Africa* (Cambridge: Cambridge University Press, 2016), 69.

56 Manuh, 'Women and Their Organizations'.

57 Some of these have already been published in: Stephanie Newell and Audrey Gadzekpo, eds., *Selected Writings of a Pioneer West African Feminist* (Nottingham: Trent Editions, 2004). Her first article for *The Evening News*: 'Introducing Akosia Dzatsui', *The Evening News*, 13th July, 1950, 1.

58 Tsikata, 'Women's Political Organisations, 1951–1987'.

59 Allman, 'The Disappearing of Hannah Kudjoe'.

60 'Congratulations to Our P.Gs, Vide Evenews,', *The Evening News*, 6 June 1950, 1.

61 See for example: 'Women of Ghana Organise Now! (II)', *The Evening News*, 5 July 1950, 1.

62 Iris Berger, *Women in Twentieth Century Africa*, 87.

63 'Women of Ghana Come Out', *The Evening News*, 22 June 1950, 2.

64 'Women not Incubators! Men's Mental Equals', *The Evening News*, 28 July 1950, 1.

65 'Keep Those Looks, but…', *Sunday Mirror*, 1 January 1965, 16.

66 Nate Plageman, *Highlife Saturday Night: Popular Music and Social Change in Urban Ghana* (Indianapolis, IN: Indiana University Press, 2013), 166.

67 Ahlman, *Living with Nkrumahism*, 164.

68 Ibid., 168–69.

69 Gareth Austin, Ewout Frankema, and Ewout Morten Jerven, 'Patterns of Manufacturing Growth in Sub-Saharan Africa: From Colonization to the Present' (Utrecht University, Centre for Global Economic History, 2015), 18.

70 Kwame Nkrumah, *The Autobiography*, x.

71 Jeff D. Grischow, 'Kwame Nkrumah, Disability, and Rehabilitation in Ghana, 1957–66', *The Journal of African History* 52, no. 2 (2011): 182.
72 Robert L. Tignor, *W. Arthur Lewis and the Birth of Development Economics* (Princeton, NJ: Princeton University Press, 2005), 121–23.
73 *The Development Plan, 1951. Being a Plan for the Economic and Social Development of the Gold Coast as Approved by the Legislative Assembly, September, 1951*, Government Printing Dept., Accra, 1951, 1.
74 PRAAD, Accra, ADM 7/6/14: *A Survey of Some Economic Matters. Issued by the Ministry of Finance 1952*, Printed by the Office of the Government Statistician, 2.
75 PRAAD, Accra, ADM 5/3/90: Lewis, W. A. *Industrialization and the Gold Coast Economy*, Government Printing Dept., 1953, 22.
76 Ibid., 3.
77 WHO, 1/803/1/11: 'Proposal for a Joint Action Programme of FAO/WHO to Increase World Food Production and Raise Standards of Health', 16 February 1949, 3.
78 For scholarship on the importance of a 'global history of planning', see: Valeska Huber, 'Introduction: Global Histories of Social Planning', *Journal of Contemporary History* 52, no. 1 (2017): 3–15.
79 Arturo Escobar, *Encountering Development: The Making and Unmaking of the Third World* (Princeton, NJ: Princeton University Press, 1995).
80 David Rooney, *Kwame Nkrumah: The Political Kingdom in the Third World* (London: I.B. Tauris, 1988), 136–37.
81 Louise Barré, 'Compter pour planifier: dénombrement de la population et « capitalisme d'État » en Côte d'Ivoire (1954–1967)', *Politique africaine* 145, no. 1 (27 July 2017): 109–28.
82 Gerardo Serra, '"Hail the Census Night": Trust and Political Imagination in the 1960 Population Census of Ghana', *Comparative Studies in Society and History* 60, no. 3 (July 2018): 659–60.
83 Jeff Grischow and Holger Weiss, 'Pan-Africanism, Socialism and the Future: Development Planning in Ghana, 1951–66', in *The Struggle for the Long-Term in Transnational Science and Politics: Forging the Future*, ed. Jenny Andersson and Eglė Rindzevičiūtė (New York: Routledge, Taylor & Francis Group, 2015), 230.
84 PRAAD, Accra, ADM 14/2/126: *Parliamentary Debates Official Report Contents Thursday, 26th August 1965*, col. 232.
85 Ahlman, *Living with Nkrumahism*, 150.
86 UN, S-0175-0480-03: 'The 1960 Population Census of Ghana – Its Objectives and Methods (by Dr. Benjamin Gil), 12 December 1959, 1.
87 *The Ghanaian Times*, Dickson: Census Will Determine Ghana's Progress, October 2, 1959.
88 RAC, Population Council Papers, Box 15, Folder 246: 'Demographic Grant', 1962, 1.
89 RAC, Population Council Collection, Box 15 Folder 246: 'Proposal for a Programme of Studies in Demography at the University College of Ghana', 1959, 2.
90 E. V. T. Engmann, *Population of Ghana, 1850–1960* (Accra: Published for the University of Cape Coast by Ghana Universities Press, 1986), 106.
91 J. C. Caldwell, 'Population Change', in *A Study of Contemporary Ghana. Vol. 2 Some Aspects of Social Structure*, ed. W. Birmingham, I. Neustadt, and E. Omaboe (London: Allen & Unwin, 1967), 81.
92 Gerardo Serra, '"Hail the Census Night"', 666.
93 RAC, Population Council, Box 45, Folder 640: 'A Proposal for a Programme of Teaching and Research in Demography', 16 October 1959, 1.
94 RAC, Population Council Collection, Box 46 Folder 646: 'Student Data', 1963.
95 RAC, Population Council Collection, Box 46 Folder 646: Letter from J C Caldwell, 17 July 1962.
96 UN, S-0175-0480-03: 'Monthly Progress Report No. 7 Covering the Period September – November 1959', 12 December 1959, 1.

97 Ibid., 4.
98 Perdita Huston, *Motherhood by Choice: Pioneers in Women's Health and Family Planning* (New York: Feminist Press at CUNY, 1992), 141.
99 PRAAD, Accra, 7/5/89: 'The Seven-Year Development Plan 1963/64 to 1970/71', Accra, 1964, 7–8.
100 Caldwell, 'Population: General Characteristics', 39.
101 E. Omaboe, 'An Introductory Survey', in *A Study of Contemporary Ghana*, ed. W. Birmingham, I. Neustadt, and E. Omaboe, vol. 1 The Economy of Ghana (London: George Allen & Unwin Ltd, 1967), 20.
102 There were 653,400 children in total attending school in 1959, this number rose to 1,028,800 by 1963. See: G. E. Hurd in *A Study of Contemporary Ghana*, 227.
103 Interview with Mary Boanno and Martha Abena. Abrafo, Central Region, 23 July 2019.
104 Wolf Bleek, 'Family and Family Planning in Southern Ghana', in *Sex Roles, Population and Development in West Africa: Policy-Related Studies on Work and Demographic Issues / Edited by Christine Oppong*, ed. Christine Oppong (Portsmouth, NH: Heinemann, 1987), 143; Florence Abena Dolphyne, *The Emancipation of Women: An African Perspective* (Accra: Ghana Universities Press, 1991), 30–34.
105 M. J. Field, *Search for Security: An Ethno-Psychiatric Study of Rural Ghana* (London: Faber and Faber, 1960), 121.
106 Johanne Sundby, 'Infertility and Health Care in Countries with Less Resources', in *Infertility around the Globe: New Thinking on Childlessness, Gender, and Reproductive Technologies*, ed. Marcia Claire Inhorn and Frank van Balen (Berkeley, CA: University of California Press, 2002), 248. See also: Akosua Adomako Ampofo, 'Whose "Unmet Need"? Dis/Agreement about Childbearing among Ghanaian Couples', in *Rethinking Sexualities in Africa*, ed. Signe Arnfred (Uppsala: Almqvist & Wiksell Tryckeri AB, 2004), 115–34.
107 Caldwell, 'Population Prospects and Policy', 152.
108 Republic of Ghana, National Assembly, *Parliamentary Debates*, 10 March 1965, col. 1302.
109 Interview with Adjoa Ewusiwa. New Ebu, Central Region, 22 July 2019.
110 Interview with Nana Efua Ateifi I. New Ebu, Central Region, 22 July 2019.
111 John Iliffe, *Africans: The History of a Continent*, 2nd edition (Cambridge: Cambridge University Press, 2007), 251.
112 RAC, Ford Foundation Collection, Box 390: 'At least two roads to Rome: the evolution of population policy and programs in Ghana and Thailand (Reports 009436)', Working Draft, June 1972, 6.
113 Ahlman, *Living with Nkrumahism*, 3.
114 Anthony Appiah, *In My Father's House: Africa in the Philosophy of Culture* (New York: Oxford University Press, 1992), 20.
115 Lynn M. Thomas, *Politics of the Womb: Women, Reproduction, and the State in Kenya* (Berkeley, CA: University of California Press, 2003), 179.
116 Jennie Lindsay, 'The Politics of Population Control in Namibia', *Review of African Political Economy* 36 (1986): 59.
117 PRAAD, Accra, ADM 16/1/25: 'Osagyefo Speaks to the National Assembly on Africa's Challenge', 1960, 2.
118 Ama Biney, *The Political and Social Thought of Kwame Nkrumah* (New York: Palgrave Macmilla, 2011), 47, 56.
119 David Rooney, *Kwame Nkrumah: The Political Kingdom in the Third World* (London: I.B. Tauris, 1988), 169–77; Youry Petchenkine, *Ghana: In Search of Stability, 1957–1992* (Westport, CT: Praeger, 1993), 16.
120 MacFarlane, Deborah, Interview with Dr Fred Sai for *Smith College Population and Reproductive Health Oral History Project*, 11 March 2004, 21–22.
121 Grischow and Weiss, 'Pan-Africanism, Socialism and the Future', 228–29.

122 Yuliya Hilevych and Chizu Sato, 'Popular Medical Discourses on Birth Control in the Soviet Union during the Cold War: Shifting Responsibilities and Relational Values', in *Children by Choice?: Changing Values, Reproduction, and Family Planning in the 20th Century*, ed. Ann-Katrin Gembries, Theresia Theuke, and Isabel Heinemann (Boston, MA: Walter de Gruyter, 2018), 4–5.
123 WHO, P13/86/2/9: 'Report on the 9th Session of the UN Population Commission', 4 February 1957.
124 Republic of Ghana, National Assembly, *Parliamentary Debates*, 10 March 1965, col. 1301.
125 Ibid., col. 1298–99.
126 Republic of Ghana, National Assembly, *Parliamentary Debates*, 16 December 1965, col. 139.
127 Republic of Ghana, National Assembly, *Parliamentary Debates,* 18 March 1964, col. 263.
128 Republic of Ghana, National Assembly, *Parliamentary Debates*, 16th December, 1965, col. 136.
129 Republic of Ghana, National Assembly, *Parliamentary Debates*, 10 March 1965, col. 1308.
130 Ibid., col. 1311.
131 Republic of Ghana, National Assembly, *Parliamentary Debates*, 16 December 1965, col. 136.
132 NA, DO 95/9272: 'Speech to be Delivered by the Honourable J. H. Allassini, M. P. Minister for Health at Meetings to be Held with the Chiefs of Kpandu and Anfoega', 9 August 1958, 2.
133 PRAAD, Kumasi, ARG 2/8/43: 'Proposed National Baby Show – 9 November 1963 – National Health Week,' 4 April 1953.
134 Republic of Ghana, National Assembly, *Parliamentary Debates*, 17 March 1964, col. 207.
135 Maternity leave was not always welcomed by men in the workplace. For a more extensive discussion on women entering the workforce and responses to their taking sick leave or maternity leave see: Ahlman, *Living with Nkrumahism*, 164–67.
136 Frederick T. Sai, *With Heart and Voice: Fred Sai Remembers* (Cambridge: Barton, 2010), 81.
137 M. A. Barnor, *A Socio-Medical Adventure in Ghana: Autobiography of Dr. M.A. Barnor* (Accra: Vieso Universal, 2001), 255–57.
138 This came under Act no. 29 of 1960, Criminal Offenses Act, sections 58–60.
139 Republic of Ghana, National Assembly, *Parliamentary Debates*, 10 March 1965, col. 1298–99.
140 'Tips on Child Bathing', *The Ghanaian Times*, 13 July 1960, 16.
141 Caldwell, 'Population: General Characteristics', 63.
142 PRAAD, Accra, ADM 13/2/68: 'Proposed Health Nursing Service' by the Minister for Health and Social Welfare, 15 January 1960, 1.
143 Iliffe, *Africans* (see chapter 11); Ruth J. Prince, 'Situating Health and the Public in Africa: Historical and Anthropological Perspectives', in *Making and Unmaking Public Health in Africa: Ethnographic and Historical Perspectives,* ed. Rebecca Marsland and Ruth Prince (Ohio: Ohio University Press, 2013), 3.
144 WHO, M2/372/3 GHA: Letter from Dr Strudwick, WHO AFRO Representative in Ghana, to S. Falkland Public Health Administration. Enclosure: 'Special Report P.H.A./B.H.S. Ghana-1', 20th November, 1964, 6.
145 Interview with Aishutu Manuh, Adjumako, Western Region, 23 October 2017.
146 Interview with Georgina Hermance, Moree, Central Region, 28 November 2017.
147 KBMS, Box 19 Item 82: 'Application to the Agency for International Development by the Government of the Republic of Ghana', 2 January 1963, 6.

148 WHO, M2/372/3 GHA: Letter from Dr Strudwick, WHO AFRO Representative in Ghana, to S. Falkland Public Health Administration. Enclosure: 'Special Report P.H.A./B.H.S. Ghana-1', 20 November 1964, 20, 22.
149 PRAAD, Accra, 7/5/89: 'The Seven-Year Development Plan 1963/64 to 1970/71', Accra, 1964, 175.
150 KBMS, Box 19 Item 82: 'Application to the Agency for International Development by the Government of the Republic of Ghana', 2 January 1963, 3.
151 Ibid., 5.
152 KBMS, Box 19 Item 84: Letter from K. Saakwa-Mente, Chief Medical Officer, to The Registrar of the University of Ghana, Legon. Enclosure: 'Plan of Operation for a Post-Basic Nursing Education Project in Ghana', October, 1961, 1.
153 PRAAD, Accra, ADM 13/2/68: 'Proposed Health Nursing Service' by the Minister for Health and Social Welfare, 15 January 1960, 2.
154 KBMS, Box 19 Item 84: 'Report on a Visit to Ghana, 23 March to 24 May 1961', 4.
155 WHO, AFR/NURS/27: 'Report on a Visit to Ghana 12–20 October, 1960 by Louise M. Bell, Regional Office for Africa', 4.
156 KBMS, Box 19 Item 82: 'Application to the Agency for International Development by the Government of the Republic of Ghana', 2 January 1963, 5.
157 PRAAD, Accra, 7/5/89: 'The Seven-Year Development Plan 1963/64 to 1970/71', Accra, 1964, 176.
158 'Building a Future' *Ghana Today* 3, no. 3 (1959): 16.
159 Republic of Ghana, National Assembly, *Parliamentary Debates*, 16 December 1965, col. 136.
160 Interview with Patience Doris Doh, Koforidua, Eastern Region, 24 January 2019.
161 PRAAD, Accra, 7/5/89: 'The Seven-Year Development Plan 1963/64 to 1970/71', Accra, 1964, 180.
162 WHO, M2/372/3 GHA: Letter from Dr Strudwick, WHO AFRO Representative in Ghana, to S. Falkland Public Health Administration. Enclosure: 'Special Report P.H.A./B.H.S. Ghana-1', 20 November 1964, Table VIII.
163 For more information on this organisation see: Nitsan Chorev, *World Health Organization Between North and South* (Ithaca, NY: Cornell University Press, 2012); Javed Siddiqi, *World Health and World Politics: The World Health Organization and the UN System* (London: Hurst, 1995).
164 Amrith, *Decolonizing International Health*, 74.
165 WHO, 1/400/2/48: 'Fifth Session. Committee of Relations with the International Council of Women', 8th January 1948, 2.
166 John Manton and Martin Gorsky, 'Health Planning in 1960s Africa: International Health Organisations and the Post-Colonial State', *Medical History* 62, no. 4 (October 2018): 427.
167 WHO, 1/2/2/26/2: 'World Health Organization Interim Commission. Fifth Session', 28 January 1948, 1.
168 WHO, Jessie M. Bierman, *Maternal and Child Health in the Developing Countries*, Chronicle of the World Health Organization, vol. 12, no. 11 (November, 1958): 361.
169 WHO, 1/605/1/6: Letter from Dr R. Gautier to Director General, WHO, Geneva 12 August 1948, 1.
170 Manton and Gorsky, 'Health Planning in 1960s Africa', 435.
171 WHO, AFR/QR/1 (1954): 'Report for the First Quarter 1954. 1 January – 31 March 1954', 9.
172 WHO, AFR/RC8/3: 'rapport annuel du directeur general 1 julliet 1957 – 30 juin 1958', 15 August 1958, Map 'Region d'Afrique.'
173 WHO, AFR/RC8/3: 'Rapport Annuel du Directeur General 1 julliet 1957 – 30 juin 1958', 15 August 1958, 153–56.

174 PRAAD, Accra, ADM 5/1/359: *Annual Report of the Department of Social Welfare and Community Development for the Year 1954*, Government Printer, Accra, 1955, 12.
175 WHO, GHANA-3: Letter to Regional Director AFRO, Dr P. P. Clément: 'Plan of Operations for a Rural Health Project with Special Reference to MCH Services in Ghana', 5 February 1959.
176 WHO, AFR/MCH/45: 'Assignment Report Maternal and Child Health Services by Dr P. Bhinder', 31 March 1969, 1.
177 Ibid., 2.
178 WHO, GHANA-3: WHO Quarterly Field Report by Denis Pirrie, 25 March 1964, 1.
179 KBMS, Box 19 Item 82: Letter from E. Affia Addo, Ministry of Health, to Mr William Lawles, Director of USAID, 5 October 1962.
180 KBMS, Box 19 Item 82: 'Proposed Medical School and Teaching Hospital, Minutes of a Meeting, August', 1962, 3.
181 PRAAD, Accra, ADM 13/2/102: 'Cabinet Memorandum by the Minister for Health Subject: The Ghana Medical Center', 1963, 1.
182 Ibid., 2.
183 KBMS, Box 19 Item 82: 'Application to the Agency for International Development by the Government of the Republic of Ghana', 2 January 1963, 7.
184 Ibid., 2.
185 Ibid., 4.
186 KBMS, Box 19 Item 82: 'Proposed University Medical School', 1.
187 KBMS, Box 19 Item 82: 'Application to the Agency for International Development by the Government of the Republic of Ghana', 2 January 1963, 8.
188 WHO, M2/372/3 GHA: Letter from Dr Strudwick, WHO AFRO Representative in Ghana, to S. Falkland Public Health Administration. Enclosure: 'Special Report P.H.A./B.H.S. Ghana-1', 20 November 1964, 18.
189 For more insight into this see: Adell Patton, *Physicians, Colonial Racism, and Diaspora in West Africa* (Gainesville, FL: University Press of Florida, 1996).
190 'Your Health is Our Wealth', *The Ghanaian Woman* 1, no. 3 (1960): 6.
191 *Keeping Baby Healthy*, Health Education Unit, Ministry of Health, Accra, 1962, 3–5.
192 'Dr Ofori Atta Stresses Role of Our Women', *The Ghanaian Times*, 25 July 1960, 1.
193 PRAAD, Accra, ADM 5/1/441: *Annual Report of the Department of Social Welfare and Community Development for the Year 1959*, Government Printer, Accra, 1960, 22.
194 PRAAD, Accra, ADM 13/2/75: Cabinet Minutes 717 (60) Memorandum by the Minister for Social Welfare: 'Plan of Operations for Assistance from UNICEF in the Development of Home Economics Amongst the Women of Ghana', Enclosure: 'Mothercraft and Homecraft (Women's Work in Community Development)', 1960, 2.
195 Ibid., 1.
196 Ibid.
197 EA: Letter to Mr Imoro Igala: 'Increase of Duty on Sanitary Pads', 29 February 1960.
198 EA: 'National Federation of Ghana Women. Quarter Delegates Conference - 9 and 10 April 1959', 1.
199 Wellcome, A 10/8: 'International Planned Parenthood Federation: Report on Central, East and West Africa', 8 April 1960, 3.
200 EA: 'Minutes of the Quarterly Delegates Conference at the Accra Community Centre on the 9th and 10 July1959', 3.
201 Ibid., 6.
202 Iris Berger, *Women in Twentieth-Century Africa*, New Approaches to African History 10 (Cambridge: University Press, 2016), 67.
203 EA: 'Minutes of the Quarterly Delegates Conference at the Accra Community Centre on the 9 and 10 July 1959', 4.
204 For more on anti-nudity campaigns in Nkrumah's Ghana see: Jessica Cammaert, *Undesirable Practices: Women, Children, and the Politics of the Body in Northern Ghana, 1930–1972* (Lincoln, NE: University of Nebraska Press, 2016), chapter 5.

205 Manuh, 'Women and Their Organizations, 125.
206 Tawia Adamafio, *By Nkrumah's Side: The Labour and the Wounds* (Accra; London: Westcoast PubHouse in association with Collings, 1982), 117–20.
207 PRAAD, Kumasi, ARG 2/8/43: 'National Council of Ghana Women. Programme of Work for 1962', 25 May 1962.
208 Ibid., 2.
209 For more detail on this and others surrounding women's legal status see: Kate Skinner, 'Gendering Citizenship and Decolonizing Justice in 1960s Ghana: Revisiting the Struggle for Family Law Reform', *American Journal of Legal History* 60, no. 3 (1 September 2020): 357–87.
210 PRAAD, Kumasi, ARG 2/8/43: 'An Open Letter to My Countrymen and Women of Ghana on the White Paper Proposals on Marriage and Divorce' by Mabel Dove, 1961, 2.
211 EA: 'Organisation and Arrangement of Technical Work of the Board', 12 April 1961, 1.
212 Private Papers of Evelyn Amarteifio: 'A Brief Note on the Aims and Objectives of the National Food and Nutrition `Board of the Government of Ghana', c. 1959, 1.
213 EA: 'National Food and Nutrition Board: Report for the Period 1/10/1960 - 4/1960', 3.
214 EA: 'Organisation and Arrangement of Technical Work of the Board,' 12 April 1961, 1.
215 EA: 'Executive Secretary's Report for the Month of May, 1961', 1–2.
216 Scott, *Seeing Like a State*, 183.
217 PRAAD, Accra, ADM 13/2/75: Cabinet Minutes 717 (60) Memorandum by the Minister for Social Welfare: 'Plan of Operations for Assistance from UNICEF in the Development of Home Economics Amongst the Women of Ghana', Enclosure: 'Mothercraft and Homecraft (Women's Work in Community Development)', 1960, 2.
218 PRAAD, Accra, ADM 5/1/441: *Annual Report of the Department of Social Welfare and Community Development for the Year 1959*, Government Printer, Accra, 1960, 21.
219 J. C. Caldwell, 'Population Prospects and Policy,' 155.
220 EA: Letter from L. W. Russell, The British Drug Houses, to Evelyn Amarteifio, Federation of Ghanaian Women, 3 June 1959.
221 NCL, 1/2.1: 'The Churches' Marriage and Family Life Programme', written by Jean Forrester-Patton, n.d., 23.
222 NCL, 1 /2.1: 'Christian Council of Ghana. Committee on Marriage and Family Life. Minutes of a Meeting Held on Tuesday 30 October 1962', 1.
223 Ghana', *International Planned Parenthood News*, No. 123, March, 1964, 3.
224 NCL, 1 /2.1: 'Christian Council of Ghana. Committee on Marriage and Family Life. Minutes of a Meeting Held on Tuesday 4 June 1963', 2.
225 'Ghana', *International Planned Parenthood News*, No. 123, March, 1964, 3.
226 Holly Rose Ashford, 'The Christian Council, Moral Citizenship and Sex Education in Ghana, 1951 – 1966', *History of Education* 51, no. 1 (2022): 1–23.
227 NCL, 1/2.1: 'The Churches' Marriage and Family Life Programme', written by Jean Forrester-Patton, n.d., 23.
228 NCL, 1 /2.1: 'Christian Council of Ghana. Committee on Marriage and Family Life. Minutes of a Meeting Held on Monday 18 November 1963', 1.
229 NCL, 1 /1.2: 'Christian Council of Ghana. Committee on Marriage and Family Life. Minutes of a Meeting Held on Friday 27 June 1963', 1.
230 NCL, 1 /2.1: 'Christian Council of Ghana. Committee on Marriage and Family Life. Minutes of a Meeting Held on Monday 18 November 1963', 1.
231 NCL, 1 /2.1: 'Christian Council of Ghana. Committee on Marriage and Family Life. Minutes of a Meeting Held on Monday 3 November 1964', 2.
232 Ahlman, *Living with Nkrumahism*, 148–57.
233 Barnor, *A Socio-Medical Adventure in Ghana*, 258.
234 Interview with Sabina Mensah, Anaji, Western Region, 5 February 2018.
235 Huston, *Motherhood by Choice*, chapter 11.

236 'Ugandan Doctor Calls for More Co-operation in Africa', *International Planned Parenthood Association News*, No. 154, December, 1966, 1.
237 Dawson-Amoah, Catherine, 'The PPAG Story', unpublished presentation given in Accra.
238 PRAAD, Koforidua, ERG 5/1/41: 'Letter Planned Parenthood Activities from Dr R Y B Karikari', 13 May 1969.

5 Establishing the National Family Planning Programme, 1966–1974

Rapid population growth, like the uncontrolled growth of cells in the body, can be dangerous. It can jeopardise national aspirations for economic and social development and adversely affect the welfare of families and the health of individuals.

Population Planning for National Progress and Prosperity, March 1969

When Nkrumah was overthrown in a coup in 1966, a less noted outcome was significant changes to reproductive health services. For those working in the field the shift was dramatic. For women in urban centres, there was hugely increased availability of contraception which meant that they could reliably limit their pregnancies. For vast numbers of women though, contraception remained an unknown or simply undesirable. The National Family Planning Programme (NFPP) was not for everyone, but family planning was linked to 'modern' citizenship and discursively presented as a necessity for national economic and social development.

The circumstances leading to the launch of NFPP between 1966 and 1970 are fascinating since they rest on a political shift that appears to be out of sync with contemporary emerging theories of global economic inequity. The implementation of a Population Policy and NFPP in Ghana was not simply a matter of international imposition, nor local initiative, but a combination of the two united under development discourses. We also see that whilst global concerns over population growth were impactful in Ghana, local organisation and behavioural codes governed how family planning played out. NFPP was not conceived by the new Ghanaian military government – the National Liberation Council (NLC) – alone. Input from donors was integral throughout. The Ford Foundation, Population Council and IPPF were involved. Indeed, most of the information about NFPP in this chapter comes from Ford Foundation records, since there is so little in Ghana itself. Unfortunately, this means that data ends in 1974, when the Foundation pulled programme funding.

The Progress Party (PP) was elected in 1969 and governed the country until January 1972, when it was overthrown in another military coup. The leader of this party was Dr Kofi Abrefa Busia. He was arguably less keen on implementing NFPP, which remained a 'controversial' move in 1969.[1] However, the structures

DOI: 10.4324/9781003274162-6

put in place during military rule meant that it was all but inevitable by the time he took power. NFPP was a tool for implementing the Population Policy paper, which was released in March 1969: the first national policy on population in Africa. This policy was developmental. Examining the first years of NFPP implementation, it is evident that the programme followed gendered and socio-economic assumptions. Women's part in aspirational development was judged, partly, through their approach to family planning.

Given the importance of demographics in African history, NFPP should be a significant event for historians. For John Iliffe, rapid population growth in the second half of the twentieth century was one of the most important factors in African history.[2] However, NFPP qualifies his observation that family planning was 'not generally accepted by governments until the 1980s.'[3] This chapter asks how far family planning in Ghana was meant to improve women's health or increase women's reproductive rights and how far it was an attempt to mould the country's demographics for economic development. Whilst both sides came into play, the latter was clearly the priority.

Planned Parenthood before NFPP

Continuing where we left the previous chapter, we know that Dr Barnor had formed part of a network of doctors and midwives who were concerned over malnutrition, high abortion rates and women's poor reproductive health. They had begun to see family planning as essential. So far though, the CPP government had forced them to act clandestinely, offering limited, private services. After the coup, IPPF's Betty Hull asked Dr Barnor whether there might be an opportunity to form an IPPF-affiliated association in Ghana. He responded positively. PPAG was launched in 1967 at the 'fully packed' YWCA hall in Accra. It had four initial aims: 'improvement of socio-economic life of the population,' improvement of 'physical and mental health … especially through … spacing of births,' to provide education on family life, and to cooperate with the Ministry of Health.[4]

Already by the late 1960s, PPAG began to expand slowly into the regions in Ghana.[5] It acted as a forerunner for NFPP, launched in 1970. Arguably, PPAG established structures and demand for family planning that allowed NFPP to quickly function coherently. PPAG became a contact point for medical staff interested in family planning. Dr Armar was stationed in Kumasi and ensured that PPAG there was 'running neck to neck' with that in Accra.[6] Fieldwork was led by Rosina Konuah, a pharmacist who organised the first 'on the ground' promotional activities in Accra.[7] Forrester-Paton of the Christian Council volunteered, as did Letitia Omaboe, wife of NLC Commissioner for Economic and Financial Planning, and midwives and non-medical professionals in Accra and Kumasi.[8] In Koforidua, a branch was established in June 1969 by Dr Comfort Akrofi, who was head of the Government Midwives' School there.[9] From these regional branches, interest extended to smaller towns and villages. In 1969 midwife Gladys George wrote on behalf of the town she served, proposing to run a clinic there if PPAG could support her. She thought 'the inmates of the town would enjoy such Planned Parenthood' following Christian Home Week, when she had held discussions on limiting births, sex and contraception. She reported that 'people were delighted and asked interesting questions.'[10] The organisation grew as more doctors took interest and volunteers joined. In Western Region, Dr Mensah returned from Hungary, where he had been working, with a training certificate from IPPF. He showed this to nurses in Sekondi, which generated enthusiasm among them to attend family planning training. Soon a lively and vibrant PPAG network was established in the region.[11]

The MH began working with PPAG to expand family planning. In January 1969 members of PPAG met with Dr de Heer, Senior MO, for MCH and nutrition. They discussed plans for the integration of family planning into MCH. They decided that each regional MCH officer should take charge of family planning activities. Furthermore, planned parenthood 'should always proceed apace with the availability of doctors, public health nursing staff and midwives.'[12] Significantly, the availability of MCH support staff was seen as essential. The meeting's participants envisaged that women would access family planning for *medical* reasons. These included 'kwashiorkor child' or having five or more children already. A separate category of people would be referred through the social welfare department if they had a 'socio-economic problem making it difficult for normal family life.'[13] *Normal* family life was not expected to involve contraception. Family planning was envisaged by PPAG and the MH, before the launch of NFPP, as a health measure. Midwives would arrange for 'persons or families' to be seen by trained doctors who would prescribe appropriate contraceptives. Following the meeting, Dr de Heer sent a circular to Regional MOs offering to equip them with contraceptive pills, IUDs and a set of equipment for the insertion of IUDs in clinics.[14] These particular technologies meant women rather than men were expected to attend clinics. Evidently, foams, jellies and condoms were not favoured.

These activities, and PPAG, came under NFPP after May 1970. However, PPAG remained a distinct and prominent organisation. Its independence was guaranteed through support from IPPF.[15] Although PPAG started as a group of doctors responding to local women's health needs, it is important to note that their worries were harnessed by a global organisation, IPPF. IPPF was keen to promote the formation of associations across Africa. The Ghanaian association was the eighth on the continent and, according to IPPF's magazine, reflected 'increasing momentum in family planning in Africa.'[16] This meant that matters beyond the original health concerns were brought into play. For example, when the doctors attended the IPPF conference in Copenhagen in 1966, 'topics were the effect of population on development, employment and the creation of jobs in less economically developed countries.'[17] Moreover, IPPF made new forms of contraceptives widely available. Before PPAG, only spermicide jellies and foams and the diaphragm were available in Ghana.[18]

The United Nations and the 'Status of Women'

An Economic and Social Council (ECOSOC) resolution, adopted by the UN General Assembly in 1963, led to the establishment in Ghana, and elsewhere, of national Committees on the Status of Women. These committees were supposed to improve conditions for women in their respective countries and allow them to take part in economic and social development. In 1965 funds were provided and a Committee was established in Ghana. One of the Committee's tasks was 'the formulation and elaboration of national policies directed towards the evaluation of the opportunities, needs and problems of women.'[19] Ghanaian women took the possibilities afforded by this Committee seriously. They submitted a document protesting the lack of opportunities for women under the NLC. They complained that women were not consulted on policy making and were disregarded in national politics, and even women's columns in newspapers were edited by men.[20] However, initially, the Committee was ignored; it 'was thought that women wanted more for themselves than they deserved.'[21]

It was revived in 1968 when ECOSOC resolved that national surveys should be undertaken on the 'status of women and family planning.' These investigations would consider the effect of population growth on economic and social development, how fertility affected the status of women, and how family size affected MCH. ECOSOC framed family planning as a human right. This resolution reached Ghana in 1969 through the Commission on the Status of Women delegate, Florence Addison. It was circulated around the Ministries of Social Welfare, Education, the YWCA and the Committee on the Status of Women, led by Janet Tay.[22]

This Committee produced the memorandum: 'Suggestions for a National Family Planning Program for Ghana.' It emphasised the need to reduce population growth, whilst acknowledging other tangential benefits of family planning. The principal objective, 'to reduce the birth rate as rapidly as possible,' would be achieved by 'convincing' as many couples as possible to 'space or limit pregnancies.' This was deemed necessary by the Committee for 'optimal … national development.' In other words, it reiterated discourses linking population to development. In fact, the committee recommended the public declaration of a Population Policy as a priority, and that government endorsement and financing be made readily available to enact it.[23]

The Committee estimated 24,000 women gave birth annually in the country's largest hospitals, and it was this group that should be targeted, effectively limiting family planning to the socio-economic substratum that delivered their babies in hospital. In hospitals women were arguably removed from their social context and decision-making networks. The Committee also recommended training courses for family planning staff, information programmes and widespread commercial sale of contraception. Interestingly, they rejected ideas that commercial sales would encourage promiscuity, arguing that 'if young people are going to experiment with sex—as some of them undoubtedly are—perhaps it is better if they are able to avoid venereal disease or an illegitimate pregnancy and birth.' This was a pragmatic and liberal point of view. The Committee's final point was that 'low fertility is not yet well established as an ideal or norm in Ghana and vigorous, imaginative efforts are needed to popularize it.'[24] It is significant that this body, supposedly dedicated to the status of *women*, propagated militant discourse on population control.

As well as promoting the status of women, the UN pushed the idea of population control in Africa. Mr Gille of the UN demographic mission to the Economic Commission for Africa (ECA) stressed that, although population density was seemingly low, it was in fact the rate of growth that mattered. This stood at 2.6% growth annually, justifying the UN's concern in the region.[25] In the late 1960s, the ECA began collecting and consolidating demographic data throughout Africa to promote population control programmes.[26] In 1971, a regional standing body on population was established. Numerous conferences were planned as well as an ongoing programme (1971–1976) to provide assistance to governments on the demographic aspects of economic and social development.[27] This activity shows us that population control had become a core issue for the UN in Africa through ECA and WHO's regional office. The widespread collection of data, especially on fertility, recalls the idea of African states becoming more legible, in this case, to IOs.

Mothercraft in the Late 1960s

Until 1969 'women's work' came under the remit of the Department of Social Welfare and Community Development. After this, it was transferred to the new Department of Rural Development, and would include 'home economics, mothercraft and social advancement, women's welfare centres and family planning,' the latter clearly being a recent addition and became part of a series of reforms women were expected to make in motherhood.[28] Women's groups were to report monthly. In 1968, group membership ran into the thousands across the country and continued to grow. For example, in Greater Accra, there were 1,058 women members in August 1968, and 1,430 by November.[29] Women's work continued to refer almost entirely to women's domestic work. This included health, which was seen as women's responsibility. *The New Ghana* implied this by publishing advice on 'Keeping Baby Healthy' and 'Feeding Baby' on its 'Women's Page,' it was not alone in this approach.[30]

It was typical for social welfare to focus on babies and nutrition. However, some took *women's* health needs into account. A programme in Central Region included a 'simple explanation of pregnancy' and emphasised the 'need for regular visits to a midwife or doctor, reporting discomforts or for advice.' A midwife was also invited to 'give a talk on antenatal care and the use of clinics.'[31] As this example shows, social services promoted basic antenatal care for women. It is interesting that the course included a 'simple explanation of pregnancy.' Most women, despite having witnessed pregnancies constantly throughout their early lives, had little *medical* knowledge of their reproductive systems.[32]

Meanwhile, NCGW was dismantled during the coup, as it had been affiliated with the CPP. It was relaunched in 1969 under a new name: the Ghana Assembly of Women (GAW).[33] GAW formed following a 1968 UN meeting in Addis Ababa on the Role of Women in National Development. This meeting called for countries to form women's organisations that 'cover all sections of the country… cater for literate and illiterate women and take account of the needs of women in rural and urban areas.' The preamble to their formation cites the UN promise for 'equal rights of women and men.' The Assembly's objectives were to promote women's work through education, vocational training, literacy, community development and children's welfare. They also specifically sought to tackle 'customs and traditions which militate against the advancement of women and their families.'[34] GAW was affiliated with a number of women's organisations in Ghana. These were mainly religious but also included the Ghana Registered Midwives Association and the Ghana Registered Nurses' Association.[35]

By the late 1960s, most women in rural areas of Western and Central Regions described attendance at an antenatal clinic as a regular part of their pregnancies. In towns, this was almost obligatory. Gertrude Engmann, living in Takoradi in 1972 during her first pregnancy, testified that every woman knew to go to an antenatal clinic when she suspected pregnancy.[36] However, it was still not standard practice for women to deliver in hospital.[37] In 1967, there were 523,201 recorded attendances at antenatal clinics, and 47,059 at postnatal clinics, indicating a preference for care before babies were born. Using population and birth-rate estimates, we can calculate that there were around 400,000 births in 1967.[38] Assuming that women attended antenatal clinics regularly during pregnancy, 523,201 attendances represent around 100,000 women, or a quarter of all births in 1967. Ford Foundation also estimated that one quarter of pregnant women in 1970 went through the MCH system.[39]

Women attending antenatal clinics underwent a series of tests and were given lifestyle advice by a midwife. At Korle Bu in 1973 for example, Dr Otchere remembers that women had blood tests for anaemia, chest X-rays to look for tuberculosis, swabs to look for STIs. Midwives advised women on nutrition and exercises. They told them not to go to the 'old women and the old midwives' when the time came for delivery, 'because if you go there and something happens you will lose your life.'[40] Nevertheless, the pattern of delivering babies in women's homes continued. Women were usually attended by older women, and occasionally men, during childbirth. They could certainly rely on others to direct them to herbal medicines during pregnancy. The next chapter will delve further into the experiences of, what came to be known as 'traditional birth attendants' or TBAs.

Fertility rates in Ghana remained high throughout the 1960s. Doubtless connected to their economic benefit, children had high cultural and were status markers for both men and women. Sister Doh, who qualified from nursing training in 1969 remembered that in the 1960s, Ghanaians 'want plenty children to have a broad family, so many women wasn't [*sic*] interested' in birth control.[41] In 1965 Caldwell estimated the fertility rate at 7.3 children per woman. He found that although fertility transition was taking place in urban spaces in Ghana, the same could not be said of rural areas.[42] Furthermore, before NFPP, contraceptives and information on family planning were scarce. The Ghanaian government claimed that the fertility rate had not changed since the census of 1921.[43] However, there remained a problem with data reliability. There were still only 42 registration areas and in Tamale registration area, for example, only around 20% of births and deaths were registered. This means that there was little reliable data.[44] Continuities in women's reproductive lives outweighed changes.

Writing the Population Policy

Almost as soon as the NLC took power, work on a Population Policy began. It was headed by Emmanuel Omaboe, Commissioner for Economic Finance and Planning. He had a personal interest in the matter, according to colleagues.[45] Dr Mensah, who worked with PPAG in Western Region, remembers that attitudes changed quickly when the NLC took over and saw that 'the population was exploding.' They immediately set about intensifying family planning.[46] On Omaboe's team were Ford Foundation economists including Lyle Saunders and Gordon Perkin.[47] He also asked Dr Fred Sai, one of the 'pioneer' family planning doctors, to advise.[48] The NLC was far more inclined than the CPP had been to turn to Western assistance in development planning and financing.[49] This allowed Ford Foundation to become instrumental in the formation and implementation of the Population Policy in Ghana; it already provided funding to PPAG.[50] Indeed, by 1970 half of its total funds were directed towards population control.[51]

Ford worked with the conviction that *controlling* population growth was necessary for social and economic growth across the 'third world.' In its annual report 1970-1971, it reflected that '[a]lthough concern with excessive population growth has increased enormously throughout the world in recent years, few developing countries have been successful in limiting their fertility.' The report blames this lack of success in Africa on the shortage of contraceptives and 'deficiencies in the management of population programs.'[52] This created a discursive divide between African countries, unable to control fertility levels due to poor management, and organisations such as their own, which recognised the overpopulation problem and took effective steps to tackle it.

Given that Ford provided economic advisers to the Ghanaian government throughout the 1960s, it is possible that they pushed the NLC towards a Population Policy. Ford advisers in Accra were certainly integral to writing the Policy. Saunders describes 'putting pressure' on Ghanaian governments at crucial junctures to make sure that momentum continued for the policy and NFPP.[53] Ford advisers encouraged the Policy's authors to use more empirical evidence, providing statistics and facts to include in the paper's second section, outlining the dangers of population growth. They pushed for the policy paper to be more 'dramatic' and 'forceful' in its argument.[54] This policy would not have existed, in this form, at this time, without global overpopulation discourse. The ubiquity of fears over population growth globally was cause for action and philanthropic population activists played specific roles in establishing Ghana's family planning.

However, clearly there was also impetus from the military government to introduce family planning systematically. The fact that its policy was framed as a *Population* Policy immediately signals that it went further than a health issue. The NLC saw the policy as part of its 'ambitious programme of planning and development.' It argued vividly that development was threatened by the rate of population growth:

> [r]apid population growth, like the uncontrolled growth of cells in the body, can be dangerous. It can jeopardise national aspirations for economic and social development and adversely affect the welfare of families and the health of individuals.[55]

Although linking population growth to national development, the NLC took a more insular approach to the issue than Nkrumah had. As we have seen, Nkrumah saw population on a global level and blamed any lack of economic growth in Ghana on its periphery status in a *global* economy and its inequities. NLC moved away from this global view by attributing the nation's poverty to high birth rates and looking for solutions there. This does not chime with the simultaneous emergence of a dependency theory for Africa.[56]

The Population Policy established a clear cause for population growth in Ghana. The Policy did address immigration. It coincided with fears over high levels of immigration and the Aliens Compliance Order, which sought to expel immigrants.[57] A larger part, however, dealt with fertility. The authors of the paper promised: 'unlike some other types of development projects, a fertility limitation programme can be relatively inexpensive and the benefits begin to appear rather quickly.'[58] It was therefore seen as, and sold as, a quick fix for economic problems. After all, the coup had been justified by the worsening economic situation of the mid-1960s.[59]

Like Nkrumah's pronatalism, the Population Policy was based on nationalism and an understanding that human resources were crucial for development. Development planning in Ghana had taken place since early colonial rule, but by the postcolonial period it had clearly become ingrained in political culture.[60] Omaboe wrote in the preface of the paper that 'we are moving into an age where quality rather than quantity determines the power of nations'; a clear rebuttal of Nkrumahist ideology that Ghana's international influence could be measured by her population and that numbers were needed for industrialisation.[61] It is also a dismissal of ingrained political culture whereby chiefs measured their power through the populations they controlled. Indeed, the policy is very clear about the desirability of modernity and the rejection of tradition. It stated: 'high fertility is almost an anachronism in the modern world, it was appropriate in a pre-industrial age when survival was difficult and uncertain. It has no place in a century in which people aspire to something more than subsistence.'[62] Population control was equated with modernity and development and high fertility with primitive concerns.

The Population Policy is written in three sections. The first emphasises rapid population growth, mainly due to high fertility and decreased mortality. The second section turns its attention to the consequences of this, which are described as overwhelmingly negative. It contains the empirical data Ford pushed for, proving that jobs, healthcare, education and economic growth could not keep up with population growth. It briefly mentions the negative effects of repeated childbearing on individual women. The final section outlines the plan to reduce fertility in Ghana. It discursively leaves Ghanaians with little choice but to opt for family planning if they want prosperity for their families and nation. Throughout is an impression of certainty that high fertility threatens economic development.

Significantly, the Population Policy and NFPP were handled by economic and finance ministries. It was under these ministries that the National Population Council was established as a committee to oversee the policy.[63] They were specifically framed as part of planning for development. Population growth was characterised unequivocally as a 'problem,' contrary to Nkrumahist ideology, which presented it as an opportunity.

The National Family Planning Programme

The NFPP, launched in May 1970, aimed to reduce fertility. Its launch was accompanied by developmentalist rhetoric and promises that it would lead to better health for women, prosperity for families and success for the nation. The government published a leaflet: 'Family Planning. Why?' It stated that 'the very rapid increase in the number of people in Ghana is a threat to their health, welfare and happiness.' And therefore that:

> the government believes that for the good of the nation as well as for the better health and welfare of families, *women* should know how they can have fewer pregnancies and have only the number of children they want and can really care for.[64]

Limiting Ghanaian women's fertility was clearly framed as in the national interest, as well as that of individual families. Indeed, the two were connected. Ghana was threatened, according to ministers, by population growth that was outstripping economic growth, meaning that the country would not be able to provide public services for future generations. What is more, at NFPP's launch, the new Minister for Finance and Economic Planning, J. H. Mensah, said that overpopulation was 'one of the greatest threats to mankind' and that Ghana must respond to a problem that 'no nation can ignore.'[65] This reflects the *global* understanding of the threat. This push for fewer pregnancies changed the pace at which family planning was executed; the approach of securing enough MCH staff to support it broke down.

NFPP consistently depended on diverse sources of funding. Ford granted it \$76,000 in 1970 and a further \$134,000 in 1971, which was paid in monthly instalments.[66] In 1971, this represented around 15% of total foreign aid to NFPP. Other donors included USAID, the Canadian International Development Agency, the British Overseas Development Agency, IPPF, Population Council and UNFPA. The Foundation acted as an 'unofficial coordinator' for these agencies' donations.[67] These agencies provided costs for programme trials, conferences, equipment and commodities, whilst the government provided regular 'local' costs.[68] Contraceptives also came from foreign organisations. IPPF supplied all contraceptives to PPAG, Population Council provided them to their Postpartum Program and Ford gave foams and jellies to Korle Bu.[69] Meanwhile, UNFPA and USAID also gave a grant for 'commodity requirements.'[70] Ghana was therefore dependent on aid for functioning family planning services. As NFPP grew, it contacted IOs for support. In 1972 its director made an appeal to WHO for funding for 'the development of ... maternal and child health services including family planning activities in particular.'[71]

Given the strong advisory role that Ford Foundation took on in the NFPP's early years, it became a truly transnational Programme. Its record card came from Pakistan, the method for distributing the pill was copied from Costa Rica, training materials that were developed in Thailand were adopted and, finally, the Programme's symbol – the red triangle – came from India. This was partly due to travel grants awarded to Ghanaians to observe family planning practice in Asia, the US and Latin America.[72] It was due to Ford's network that Ghanaians were facilitated in becoming part of a global movement for family planning. Indeed, this was a period in which the influence of non-governmental organisations grew in the field of population and family planning, relative to governmental power.[73]

NFPP was launched under the new civilian government led by Busia. It began operating through clinics situated at existing health facilities. Meanwhile PPAG was run through stand-alone clinics. Although PPAG was an independent organisation, its first aim was to 'assist in national efforts aimed at improving the quality of the population': in line with NFPP.[74] NFPP had three strands: the MH, PPAG and the 'other' category, which was made up of Christian organisations and private practitioners. The 'other' category was the smallest by far. Finally, NFPP subsidised businesses, especially pharmacies, to sell contraceptives.

The Programme began with 46 clinics in May 1970. It aimed to 'establish family planning services in all existing government hospitals, health centres and health posts as rapidly as possible.'[75] Indeed, it achieved early expansion. By December 1970 there were 63 clinics in operation and 80 by March 1971, meaning it almost doubled in its first year.[76] There were 139 institutions registered with NFPP by November 1972.[77] Attendances grew: at Korle Bu, numbers went from 15 to 20 attendances per clinic to around 90 by March 1971, according to NFPP reports.[78] However, the spread of family planning services was uneven. When the Programme was launched, 20% of all clinics were located in Accra (Figure 5.1).[79] In April 1971, one year after the launch of NFPP, family planning remained overwhelmingly situated in southern urban areas. This reflects general biases in Ghana's postcolonial health systems.[80] In that month, just 2.6% of 'acceptors' were in Northern Region, and 0.1% in Upper.[81] Before December 1970, there were no clinics at all in Upper Region, and just two reporting to the Programme from Northern Region.[82]

By April 1971, 39,858 people had already accepted some form of contraception from clinics. This represented a tiny group from a population of around 8.5 million. However, numbers attending clinics grew significantly in the first four years (Figure 5.2). What is more, MH-run clinics were rising in proportion to

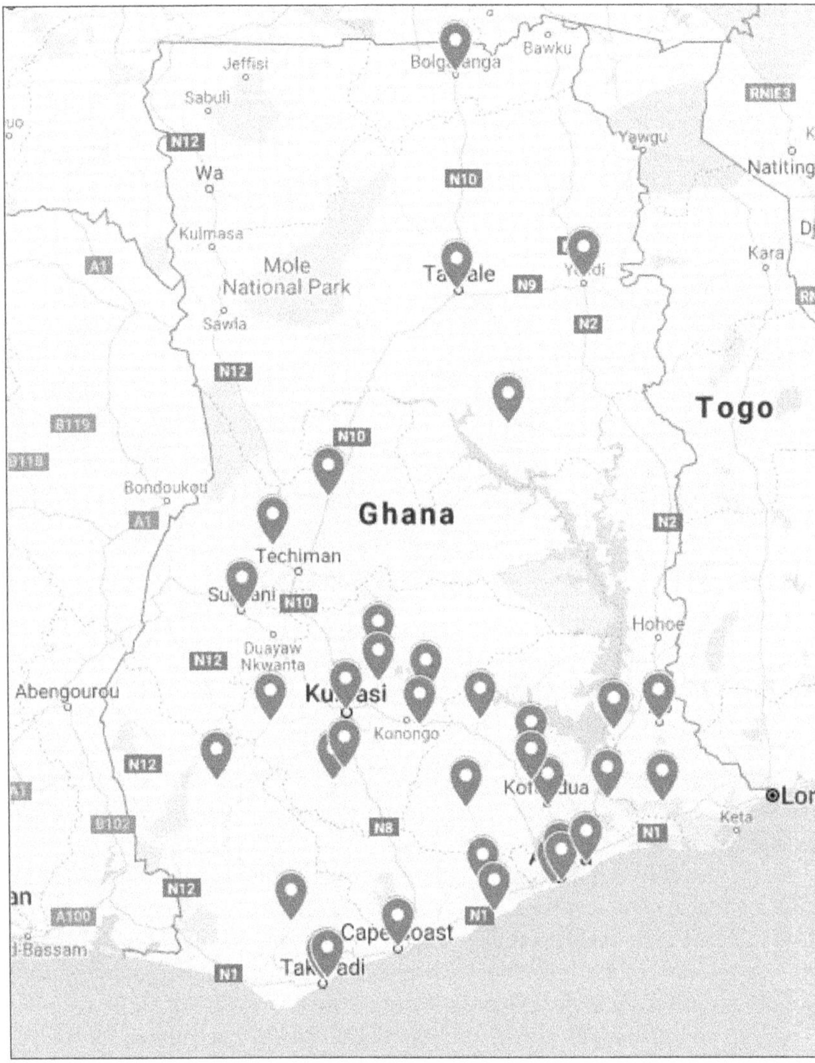

Figure 5.1 Locations of family planning clinics, May 1970. Source: PRAAD, Koforidua, ERG 5/1/41: 'Family Planning Services in Ghana May 1970,' Enclosure in Circular from Dr A. A. Armar to Regional Officers of Health, 20 May 1970.

PPAG clinics (Figure 5.3), which had been established slightly earlier. There was also a push 'from below' for family planning, as health workers contacted NFPP to request equipment and to register as providers with the Programme: Dr Bruce-Kennuah wrote in 1970 requesting contraceptives at Tafo hospital;[83] the Koforidua MO received requests from Akim Oda, requesting materials to set up

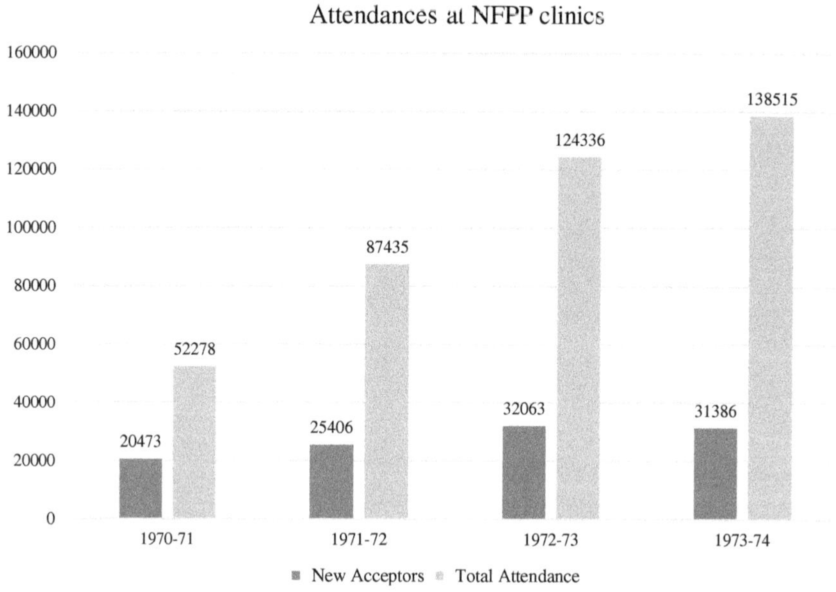

Figure 5.2 Attendances at clinics, 1970–1974. Source: RAC, Ford Foundation Collection, Grant #07090496, Reel 4048: 'Ghana National Family Planning Programme Fourth Annual Report (July 1973–June 1974),' n.d. but 1974, 26, Table 1.

family planning clinics in their hospitals.[84] Fieldworkers expanded their reach into villages and gave talks on family planning there, emphasising economic advantages.

The data also shows that although attendances at clinics were rising, numbers committing to use contraceptives, was much slower to rise. Ford's prediction of a 'tenfold increase in couples practicing contraception' was disappointed.[85] Despite NFPP's promotion of the pill and IUD as effective methods of contraception, other methods proved popular (Figure 5.4). In the first two years of NFPP records, only 20% of contraceptives given out were IUDs. The pill accounted for 41.5% and 'other,' including jellies, foams, diaphragms and condoms made up 38.5%.[86] This was due to three factors. Firstly, there was a lack of health infrastructure to support long-term contraceptives. It was not practical for women to travel long distances to hospitals to have an IUD inserted, checked or removed. This was also true of the pill, which required medical follow-up.

Secondly, family planning fieldworkers' attitudes towards 'illiterate' women governed what contraceptives they offered. This also reflected stark urban/rural divisions. Laura Briggs showed that in Puerto Rico, philanthropists stopped providing women with the diaphragm because they thought them too ignorant to use it. Instead, they provided jellies and foams that were considerably less effective.[87] There is evidence of a similar pattern in Ghana. In Winneba, a project was

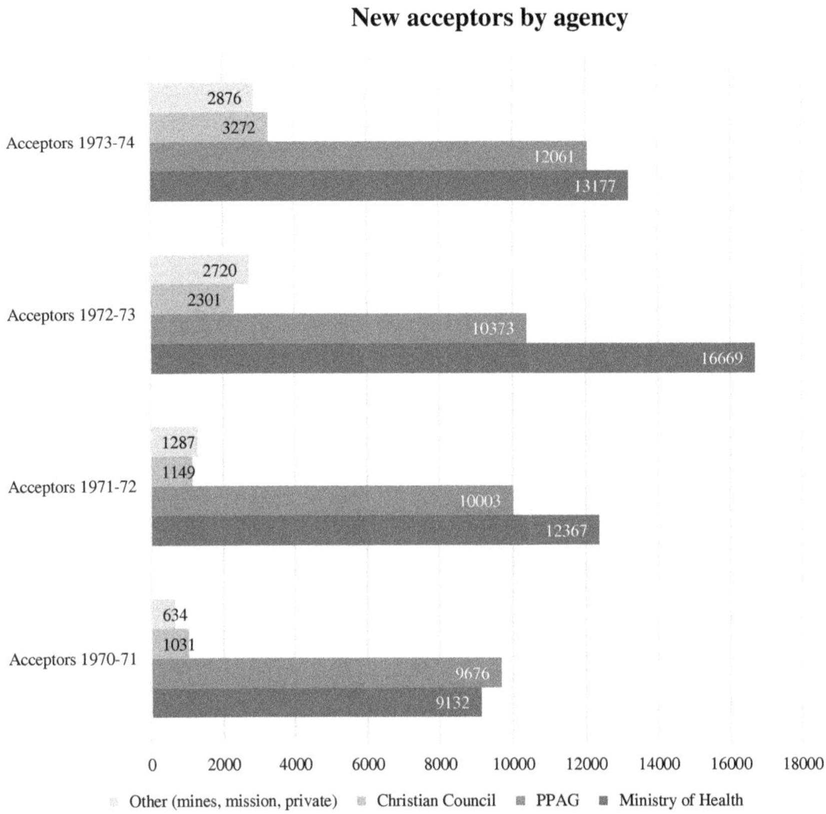

Figure 5.3 New acceptors of contraception by agency, 1970–1974. Source: RAC, Ford Foundation Collection, Grant #07090496, Reel 4048: 'Ghana National Family Planning Programme Fourth Annual Report (July 1973 – June 1974),' n.d. but 1974, 27, Table 2.

designed to test how effective Rural Development Assistants (RDAs) were in promoting family planning, compared to family planning workers in towns. The project was managed by Winneba District Rural Development Officer, as opposed to a Ministry of Health official. It was funded by Ford. The project is interesting because of the attitudes displayed towards rural people – women in particular – and because of the methods it employed. Fieldworkers were given payments for each 'client recruited.'[88] At first, these payments so exceeded what was expected that they caused severe budgetary concerns.[89] Fieldworkers were given 40 pesewas for 'clients' taking up the pill or IUD but, after the first six months, only 10p for those opting for a foam or condoms. The results of this showed that when monetary incentives reduced for condoms and foams but continued for the IUD and pill, many of the fieldworkers nonetheless stuck to promoting the former, since this had been their main form of revenue. This was explained by pointing

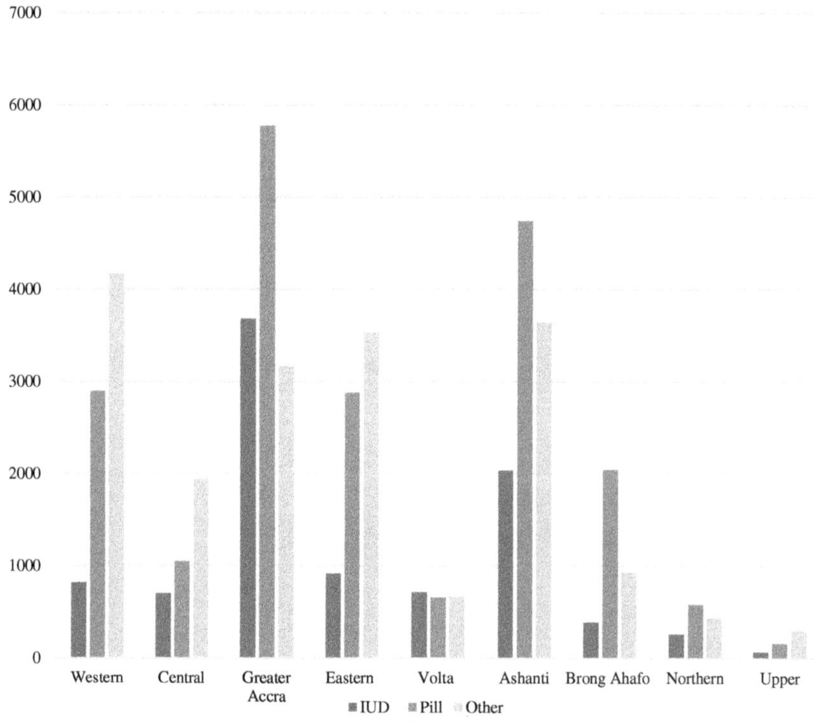

Figure 5.4 Acceptors by region and method, June 1970–July 1972. Source: RAC, Ford Foundation Collection, Grant #07090496, Reel 4048: 'Ghana National Family Planning Programme. Monthly Report on Family Planning Acceptors July, 1972,' Evaluation and Research Unit, Accra, n.d. but 1972, 3.

out that the people they worked with were not 'city folk' and also that they did not have sufficient proximity to clinics for IUDs or the pill to be practicable.[90] After a few months the rules were changed again so that clients had to be seen by a family planning nurse. This, coupled with late payments, was enough to reduce fieldworkers' incentives drastically and new acceptors dried up.[91]

Finally, the IUD sparked numerous rumours. Some thought it would 'clamp the heart,'[92] others that it could wander from the uterus around the body, causing harm.[93] In Kumasi, Population Council reported that after the death of a woman using the IUD in 1972, use of this method plummeted.[94] Indeed, data shows a significantly lower proportion of IUD users in Kumasi's hospital compared to Korle Bu and Effia Nkwanta in 1973.[95] Other fears included that menstruation would be worsened, the IUD would 'disappear into the body,' and most importantly, that it caused permanent infertility. There were reports of women 'broadcasting' ill effects and rumours to younger women, including the wife of a pastor – a woman of considerable influence – who claimed that the IUD disappeared into her body.[96] The IUD was the least popular contraceptive in almost all regions from 1970 to 1972.

Fears and rumours about the IUD emphasise that despite NFPP's rapid growth, it was not universally welcomed. As retired nurse Munirata Yahaya reflected, it was something new, 'it takes time for people to understand.' She explained that an effective way to spread the benefits of family planning was to ask a mother who had practised it for a few years to share her experiences.[97] This would take time. The majority of rural women interviewed in Central and Western Regions reported that there was no family planning in the 1970s, that it came much later. Given the small number of people attending clinics, and its urban bias, this is perhaps unsurprising. Those who did hear of NFPP or family planning in the 1970s were generally either uninterested or afraid.[98] Those who feared using contraceptives usually gave an example of an incident in which someone had suffered or died as a result of using them. For example, Esi Praah said: 'I [was] scared if they inject something into my body and it might result in my death … I have seen four people that … injection has resulted in their death.'[99]

Population Council partnered with NFPP through its Postpartum Program, which aimed to promote family planning though countries' MCH systems. Population Council believed that women who had just given birth, or whose pregnancies had terminated, would likely want contraceptives. Attendance at hospital for deliveries was still low in proportion to births. However, Korle Bu saw 20,000 deliveries in 1968, for example, which meant, as they saw it, 20,000 potential acceptors.[100] The Postpartum Program was established in three regional hospitals: Korle Bu, Effia Nkwanta in Sekondi and Komfo Anokye in Kumasi. Records suggest that Population Council's experience with Ghana was mainly frustrating. Reporting was consistently incomplete. Worse, records that were produced showed 67% Ghanaian women in the programme were 'indirect' rather than 'direct' acceptors in 1970. That is, they started using contraception more than three months after their pregnancies.[101] This was not the point. Population Council blamed local doctors for their lack of effort persuading women to accept birth control.[102] Dr Bentsi-Enchill, in charge of the programme at Korle Bu, explained that the delay in acceptance was because 'women want more time to discuss family planning with their husbands.'[103] This attitude reflected gendered norms of decision-making around reproduction, which Population Council hoped to circumvent.

NFPP also comprised non-medical aspects. These included limiting maternity leave, as well as education and information measures throughout the country. Sister Doh said that NFPP was 'well known' because of information shared through radio and churches.[104] Although this is not reflected in most interviews with rural women, archival evidence shows that there was a proliferation of information produced by NFPP. Those who do recall the beginning of NFPP state that the programme was promoted through the radio.[105] Not all information materials were well distributed. Ford consultants complained that comic strips and films they developed were not followed up by NFPP organisers.[106] Other forms of information, education and propaganda though, were more visible, for example extensive regional launch programmes and 'Family Planning Week', which involved many festivities and speeches.[107]

Who Was NFPP For?

Government rhetoric suggested that family planning should be widespread to achieve a significant reduction in the birth rate, although no specific targets were given. But it was clear from the outset that NFPP was not for everyone but for specific target groups. Four NFPP targets were families, men, women and urban dwellers.

Families

NFPP was sold as a path to prosperity for families. Ghanaian governments argued that families should act as responsible citizens, planning their lives to benefit from government development programmes.[108] The very label that was given to services providing contraception – *family planning* – encapsulates the ideology behind it. Furthermore, as the quote at the beginning of this chapter illustrates, it discursively connected the prosperity of individual families to that of the nation. Recalling NFPP's message in the early 1970s, Sister Doh said: 'the essence of family planning [was] for yourself, the family, the community and the nation.'[109] In other words, individuals' prosperity could be linked in a chain all the way up to the nation and could be achieved through family planning. This idea was used by fieldworkers to promote it.

However, the government was at pains to emphasise that NFPP was voluntary and would not act as 'an instrument for regulating the private lives and reproductive habits of Ghanaian people.' The launch was marked with newspaper articles carrying large headlines 'Family Planning is Voluntary.'[110] Ministers saw that threatening individuals' right to bear children would be unacceptable. There was continued respect for the importance of reproduction. Indeed, family planning was envisaged primarily for those who already had children. One woman writing into the *Sunday Mirror* for contraception advice in 1974 emphasised that she had already had four children. This established, she was advised to go to her local family planning clinic and enquire about the IUD.[111] Newspapers promoted women's roles as mothers through 'Mainly for Women' pages, which predominantly constituted advice on domestic and childrearing tasks. Indeed, in public discourse, women's roles as mothers were emphasised particularly in the context of family planning.

At its launch, NFPP organisers feared that men would see contraceptives as evidence of women's promiscuity.[112] Sabina Mensah remembers: 'male motivation was necessary because…he kicks against [family planning], because they thought that women would be promiscuous.'[113] Family planning fieldworkers had to work hard to deny this. In fact, PPAG put restrictions on single women's access to contraceptives. Contraception was 'on no account' to be promoted at teacher training colleges or university campuses. It was not envisaged as a means for single, professional women to become sexually liberated. Unmarried women – particularly women under twenty-one – were only provided with contraceptives at clinics if they already had children or terminated pregnancies. Female higher education students and teenagers had to be accompanied to clinics by parents and were only permitted to use the diaphragm or foams.[114] Hierarchies of authority in which parents controlled daughters' sexuality were maintained. This also shows a lack of awareness – or willingness to engage with – a high incidence of extra or pre-marital sex.[115]

Family planning programmes therefore discouraged young, single women from becoming sexually active or accessing contraceptives. This applied particularly to girls and women in education. In Kumasi in 1973 the Regional Youth Committee organised a talk on family planning for young women including 'nurses, teachers, office and factory workers.' It stipulated,

> like all our programmes on this subject, I may mention that the participants are neither going to be exposed to the methods and techniques of family planning nor be made agents for peddling drugs and other birth control devices.[116]

The concern was that women in positions of authority might pass on knowledge or commodities and for the morality of young, educated women, which was safeguarded by keeping certain knowledge from them.[117] This was despite the fact that a major cause of school drop-out among girls was due to unplanned pregnancy.[118]

However, we cannot know how strictly restrictions were enforced. It might be that the practice was more pragmatic than the theory. Dr Mensah, the gynaecologist working with PPAG, stated that he never prescribed contraceptives to women without their husbands' consent. However, he acknowledged that since women came alone to clinics, he had no way of knowing whether consent had been given.[119] Some women certainly went behind their husbands' backs to acquire contraception.[120]

The importance of family planning to families is explained, almost idiomatically, through its connection with education. The Population Policy paper said that education was one aspect of social development that was threatened by population growth. The paper explained that, due to 'modern technology,' workers needed more skills so that education needed to be modernised for the sake of development. This was impossible if 'larger and larger numbers of children' entered the system.[121] The connection with education went deeper still. In this period, educating children became more possible than ever before[122] but still represented a way to improve the entire family's prospects. Nkrumah had sold education as the key to development and prosperity for families. G. E. Hurd wrote in 1967 that 'in the social sphere, the educational system operates as a mechanism of social selection, and as a means of determining which individuals become socially mobile.'[123] In interviews, this comes across in relation to family planning. Sabina Mensah thought that she missed out on the opportunity of higher education because her mother had seventeen children; in response, she 'banned' her brothers and sisters from having more than four children and became a family planning fieldworker.[124] Adua Dua remembered:

> People gave birth to the number they can cater for. During that time, children were intelligent. People struggled to send their children to school so when they were taught, they are taught well … Elementary [school] then and people were abroad. Now they complete university and they are seated here.[125]

Adua connects people having a responsible number of children with their eventual success. Importantly, education was central to responsible parenthood in her idealised past.

Men

Men's roles in sexual and reproductive health have been consistently underestimated.[126] Interestingly, NFPP identified men as a primary target group and women as a secondary group, contrary to critiques that men's roles were not foregrounded.[127] This seems counterintuitive as most contraceptive methods were specifically for women. The press directed family planning messages to women. Women were seen as mothers and responsible for all aspects of that role. Still, men were the presumed decision-makers in Ghanaian society. As Dr Mensah's testimony above shows, men's authority was valued by medical staff. When NFPP was reviewed in the 1980s, observers stressed that women would not accept contraception when their husbands disapproved. One study found that men were 'instrumental in determining whether a wife or girlfriend would use a modern family planning method. In cases where husbands disliked family planning methods, wives dared not use a contraceptive device.'[128] Indeed, scholars continued to observe this dynamic into the twenty-first century.[129] NFPP planners assumed men would be resistant to family planning, since they had less to benefit from it. Children were status markers for men as much as women; in fact, Dr Mensah said, 'with our culture, the men would like to have a lot of children, so they prevent their wives' from using contraceptives.'[130] Additionally, Juliana Brown, Director for PPAG in Central Region, said that in the 1970s, men thought God had 'given them a mandate to reproduce.'[131]

Fieldworkers noted that women deferred to men in many cases. Midwife Magdalene Ackuah recounted the case of a woman who had presented many times after delivery, haemorrhaging. After their ninth child was born, Ackuah told the couple to avoid further pregnancies for the sake of the woman's health. However, her husband rejected the idea of using contraception and she dared not go ahead without him for fear that he would take another wife. The result was another pregnancy and another extremely dangerous birth ending with hospitalisation and hysterectomy. The possibility of polygamous marriage was a threat to many women. Religion was also an issue. For those in monogamous marriages due to strict Christian beliefs, the pressure to provide children fell on one wife. It is surprising how little attention NFPP plans gave to religious differences. There was a decided emphasis on the Christian population. For example, information and education activities for 1973–74 targeted Church groups, Church singing bands and the YWCA. Around half of the activities planned for Family Planning Week in Koforidua were held in Christian churches and none in Islamic spaces.[132] Similarly, Kumasi's 1975 Family Planning Week was organised through 'various churches.'[133] NFPP was promoted through Christian Home Week, and the report referenced 'talks in the pulpits.'[134] Meanwhile, there was no mention of targeting Islamic groups, which made up 10–15% of the population, nor the 45% that belonged to neither of these.[135]

Sister Ackuah testified that, frequently, when family planning was explained to men in the early years 'you have caused an abomination … they don't want to hear the word vasectomy, it means we are coming to castrate them!'[136] Sabina Mensah agreed, stating that men often associated family planning with castration or impotence.[137] Then there was the fear of contraception leading to promiscuity.[138] Women's frequent refrain regarding family planning, Sister Ackuah reported, was 'let me talk to my master [i.e., husband] first.'[139] Men's identities were built around their gender and sexuality. Indeed, fatherhood is crucial to the achievement of senior masculinity and social adulthood in Ghana.[140] Panic at impotence and castration show that men feared threats against their sexuality as much as any other aspect of family planning. Furthermore, fears of women's promiscuity demonstrate that controlling women's sexuality was a crucial aspect of men's gendered identities. Meanwhile, it was through women's bodies that proof of men's fertility was produced. As Ampofo, Okyerefo and Pervarah put it, 'one sure sign of manhood is the ability of the male organ.'[141]

PPAG also targeted men. One of their early campaigning techniques was to visit 'industrial or commercial concerns,' delivering education to workers during breaks or after work. These visits were 'aimed mainly at the male population to make them aware of benefits to be derived from planned parenthood.'[142] PPAG showed films to audiences in Eastern Ghana, including 'My Brother's Children,' produced in Nigeria. The film showed two brothers' choices regarding the number of children they have and the consequences of that choice. The message is that individual family prosperity is dependent on limiting births. Notably though, the film ends by showing the two sisters-in-law entering a family planning clinic. The implication is that although men make decisions about family planning, it is women who carry the practical burden.[143] Programmes directed at men were driven by those working on the ground. Fieldworker Sabina Mensah reported that she soon saw the importance of getting men on board in the Western Region. She targeted palm oil factories, organising football matches where she gave out free condoms. From there she gradually moved to water works and garages across the region. Her programme grew into the Male Motivation Project and spread all over Africa.[144]

In practical terms, NFPP's focus on men meant that contraception campaigns outside clinics focused on condoms and foams, accompanied by the slogan: 'safe, simple, sensible.'[145] In 1974, for example, around 500,000 condoms were sold through commercial distribution.[146] We have no way of knowing whether men or women were buying condoms, although NFPP assumed it was men. Its 1973 report commented that men chose brands of condoms based on their 'sensitivity.'[147] Danfa, a joint US and Ghanaian rural health and family planning NGO, expressed surprise that 57% of its acceptors were men. This figure probably does not reflect uptake in the general population, since Danfa ran intense, village-level campaigns. Importantly though, its 1974 report implies that men were not using contraception with their wives.[148] Similarly, in 1972, NFPP disregarded condom sales as part of their estimates for the years' 'acceptors,' since there was no way of connecting their use to women.[149] Organisations struggled to frame condom use as part of *family* planning and emphasised contraceptives used by women such as foam, the pill and the IUD.

The Population Policy explicitly directed itself to men. It stated:

> the official policy will be aimed at educating the individual so that *he* can make *his* choice bearing in mind *his* family's interests and its economic and social circumstances. If *he* decides to plan the size of *his* family, the government will be ready to offer the necessary supporting services.[150]

Although the use of the male pronoun could be interpreted as neutral, at the least it implies that family planning was not for single women.

Women

Women's fertility was highlighted as the main cause of population growth, implicitly laying 'blame' with women. Indeed, NFPP expected women to attend clinics and take charge of contraception; it promoted long-acting contraceptives that necessitated clinic attendance. There is some evidence that women were more inclined to use contraceptives because they were the ones facing pregnancy-related health issues. In early 1970s Ghana, Dr Mensah remembers that women who gave birth frequently became anaemic, weak and had low immune resistance.[151] Midwife Harriet Sekyi-Yorke reported that before women had access to family planning, they frequently attempted to abort pregnancies themselves.[152] However, if women did not know about contraception, they would not attempt to access it. Interviews suggest that women's understanding of family planning in the 1970s was incomplete. This was true even if they attended antenatal clinics during their pregnancies, suggesting that either clinics were not directing women to family planning, or that they were ignoring information. A survey in 1979 suggested that 30.9% of Ghanaian women had no knowledge of 'effective' contraceptive methods.[153] Furthermore, knowledge of contraception was much more common among women in their 20s and educated women. Perhaps unsurprisingly, this was truest where those categories overlapped.[154] However, Jennifer Johnson-Hanks argues that higher education levels might indicate more sexual freedom for women, and higher extramarital birth rates.[155] Bledsoe shows Gambian women's knowledge about contraception was used to *increase* their number of surviving children.[156] These observations complicate assumptions that contraceptive knowledge, or simply education, would necessarily mean lower birth rates.

Motherhood was important in most Ghanaian cultures. Clare Robertson interviewed market women in Accra in the late 1970s; one stated: 'marriage becomes fulfilled when a child arrives. Nothing surpasses the joy of a woman having her own child.'[157] Prime Minister Busia stated, when launching the National Population Council in 1971, that 'the greatest contribution a woman as a wife and mother can make to the health and stability of our country is to give the best nurture and the best education to her children.'[158] It was therefore *through* their roles as mothers that women were expected to contribute to population control. Providing 'the best' for children now involved not having too many of them. However, this idea was slow to filter through. There were reports of women being laughed out of family planning clinics by other outpatients labelling them as 'women who do not want to increase their households.'[159]

As mothers, women were responsible for healthy, happy families. We can see this through a glance at newspapers' 'women's pages' and the government's 'women's work' programme. In the popular press, women appeared almost exclusively in their roles as mothers, wives or connected with appropriate women's organisations. A 1969 *Ghanaian Times* article stated that 'the mental health of society depends on the quality of mothering each individual receives.'[160] Under NFPP, this healthy, happy family took on a new characteristic, which women were also responsible for: it ought to be appropriately sized. As Akosua Adomako Ampofo has demonstrated, models for family planning categorise contraceptive 'unmet need' according to '*women's* fertility goals and their contraceptive practice' alone. Therefore, women having children despite an apparent 'unmet need' for contraception were depicted as 'irrational, or simply ignorant.'[161] These perspectives failed to acknowledge the influence of the male partner, despite their importance in decision-making, as outlined above.

The Population Policy discussed high fertility as harmful to development aspirations. It stated that 'Ghanaian women … produce between six and seven children … this ranks the Ghanaian female as among the most fertile in the world.'[162] This assessment of fertility in Ghana places the agency for the production of children with women. Furthermore, the label 'the Ghanaian female' dehumanises women, especially given the definite article: *the*. It detaches women from their social and economic context, making it appear as if Ghanaian women randomly decide to have numerous children. Simultaneously, this phrase blames Ghanaian women, but takes away their agency.

Women were publicly encouraged to limit their family size. One women's newspaper column stated that 'family planning is necessary for survival' and that women should not give in to social pressure and embark on 'thoughtless parenthood.'[163] In other words, women should act as barriers to pressures from traditional authority figures. Indeed, women were supposed to embody modernity through the way they chose to have their children. Newspapers pitted young women against older female relatives. A newspaper article entitled 'The Five Stages of Women' argued that a woman no longer had to be 'in fear of old wives tales,' nor 'in pawn to her glands and hormones,' thanks to synthetic hormones.[164] Another told the story of a young woman about to give birth for the first time, juxtaposing her grandmother's 'terrifying' stories with the advice of midwives at clinics.[165] These articles contrast modern, young women's attitudes with the older generation. Both rely on science to legitimise modern methods.

Similarly, one doctor wrote that women engaging in unhealthy nutritional practices during pregnancy did so because 'books cannot pass on information since most people are illiterate. Grannie is the Book of words.'[166] In other words, women – especially illiterate women – succumbed to traditional, harmful beliefs passed on by older women. Some women were influenced by others who derided them for wanting to limit the number of children they had. As may be expected, certain elders saw family planning as a route to immorality. Others, for example Hope Richardson, noted the health benefits of family planning and, interestingly, improvements to their looks. Comfort Appiah noted how well-treated by nurses the women in her area felt – despite losing their referral cards![167]

Urban

The skewing of family planning clinics towards urban centres was driven by the fact that planners believed there was demand in towns and cities. John Caldwell explained Ghana's rapid population growth culturally. He argued that the 'urban elite' being caught up in a 'headlong rush to *modernity*' would naturally lead the way in family planning. Furthermore, this group 'must necessarily be concerned with population questions … [because] their literacy and education make it possible for them to understand the problems of economic development.'[168] By arguing that the urban elite saw the necessity of population control because of their cultural modernity and awareness of the intricacies of economic development, Caldwell presented fertility transition as already taking place in Ghana.

Demographic transition theory argued that modernity should lead to reduced fertility. By the end of the 1940s, the chief authors of this theory had already started to view it as 'practical policy' so that population growth needed to be slowed for the benefits of economic development to be felt.[169]

NFPP planners expected that the 'urban elite' would set an example for rural people. It stated that 'urban knowledge will flow to rural areas.'[170] Targeting those more inclined to hear the message in the hope that it spread makes sense. NFPP planners' attitudes went beyond this though: the 'progress' embodied by urban people was assumed to be influential due to their educated, elite status. As we saw above, urban women were also expected to be 'modern women.' Anthropologist Wolf Bleek described one family planning leaflet that showed a 'well furnished home' arguing that the presentation of such affluence led most Ghanaians to 'take it that family planning is for the élite and none of their business.'[171] Frequently, newspapers pitted Ghanaians against their ancestors. One newspaper article in the *Ghanaian Times* in 1969 argued that Ghana had 'suffered a great deal from the ravages of things our ancestors did not do well,' including bad family planning.

However, the article stated that now, women lived in a 'civilized world' whereby they had access to the technologies and information to make better choices.[172]

As we have seen family planning facilities were overwhelmingly based in urban areas, reflecting historical patterns in health services. Figure 5.5 shows the ten most visited NFPP clinics in July 1972. In fact, there were 1,100 attendances at the Harper Road clinic in Kumasi, compared with Korle Bu's 653. However, NFPP statisticians weighted Korle Bu higher because more women there opted for the IUD. The top clinics were within a very limited geographical area. Three were located in Accra, three in Kumasi and one in each of Tamale, Tema, Koforidua and Takoradi, some of the largest towns in Ghana. Of these one is in Northern Region and one in Western Region. As well as the urban bias, there was a regional one. NFPP envisaged different 'education and information' activities for each

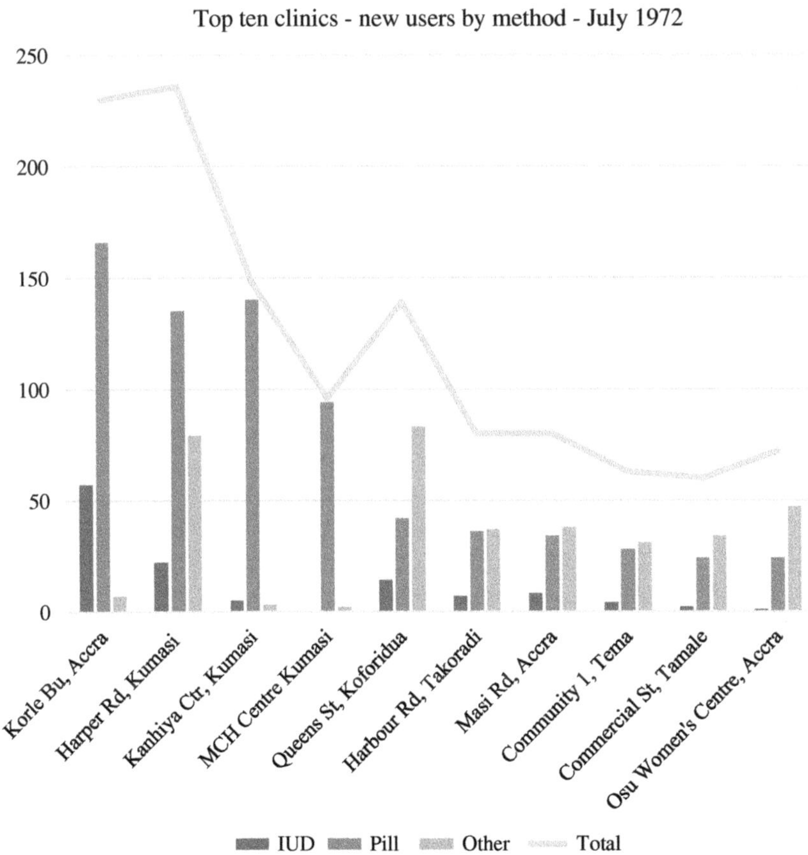

Figure 5.5 Top ten most visited clinics by method, July 1972. Source: RAC, Ford Foundation Collection, Grant #07090496, Reel 4048: 'Ghana National Family Planning Programme. Monthly Report of Family Planning Acceptors July, 1972,' Evaluation and Research Unit, NFPP, Accra, n.d. but 1972, 5.

region. Western Region was described as difficult to access because of its 'thickly forested area.'[173] This might explain why none of the women I interviewed in this region had heard about NFPP in the 1970s.

The few women who had heard of family planning in the 1970s said they did not engage with it and thought it was something for later generations or other people. In some cases, they argued that economic conditions today discourage larger families.[174] Indeed, Shane Doyle has pointed out that fertility decline in Africa as a whole was eventually linked to 'exceptionally negative' circumstances of economic downturn and poverty.[175] This older generation's perception of an economic need to limit family size now, rather than in their reproductive years, could also be explained demographically. Support that women received from extended families may no longer be accessible due to urbanisation. Others maintained that it was for God to decide how many children they had.[176] Queen mother of a village in the Central Region, Nana Efua Ateifi, said, 'maybe they thought [of family planning] in the big cities,' linking it specifically to urban life.[177] Although this reflects the availability of services, it was also related to economic structures in rural areas whereby large families remained more desirable. For some women, the very notion of 'family planning' did not fit with the structure their lives would follow. Marriage was a flexible institution, which meant that women were more likely to have a series of sexual partners which would all ideally result in children. This made it difficult for women to plan families in a way that the Programme envisaged.[178]

However, rural women's higher fertility was often linked to 'tradition' and the uptake of contraceptives was perceived as a signifier of 'modernity.' The Population Policy stated that in rural areas 'aspirations are low' and 'traditional expectations defined the value of women largely in terms of their ability to bear children.' On the other hand, it assumed women 'among the more affluent,' living in cities, had other aspirations.[179] PPAG's Dr Mensah said that urban women were more 'enlightened and educated.' In his experience, 'illiterate' women from villages had to be persuaded to take up family planning since they believed they should have more children.[180] Furthermore, they depended on herbalists to provide enemas which they did not know the content of and could be harmful.[181] He saw herbalists' knowledge as unreliable and dispensable.

Despite the problematic way that this was expressed, the idea that rural women had more pregnancies was not necessarily untrue. NFPP organisers were aware that rural areas were neglected. Rural people were grouped together with the 'non-literate,' and it was noted that 'modern' communication methods would be useless for reaching them, aside from the radio.[182] Minister J. H. Mensah also singled out rural women during a speech launching NFPP in 1970. He stated that family planning would save them from 'a precarious reproductive career.'[183] Despite this, in its early years, NFPP did little to reach rural or illiterate parts of the population. One exception to this was the Fieldworker Pilot Project in Winneba, mentioned above. However, practical problems remained: for example, women who travelled considerable distances to clinics for the pill or IUD were turned away as they should begin these immediately after menstruating. Many simply gave up rather than make the journey again given the long journey and expensive lorry fare.[184]

Conclusion

At the beginning of the 1970s, Ghana saw its first systematic national family planning services. These services were limited, to be sure, but they were growing, and they represented a side of women's reproductive health that had not been available to the vast majority of women before. Importantly though, NFPP was not seen first and foremost as a health service. It was framed as part of a development programme. Discursively, family planning was subsumed under population control, which was linked inextricably to economic development. This was partly due to global population activism that reached Ghana through IOs and US philanthropy and partly to a new Ghanaian government in the late 1960s, which was equally keen on the idea of development and differentiating itself from Nkrumah. Family planning was sold to Ghanaians as an opportunity for family prosperity that would also benefit the nation. This was in a context in which education was more widespread than ever and the opportunities for families to look to children's 'quality' rather than 'quantity' were a reality for a greater number of people. Women in Ghana were expected to engage with development through embracing the characteristics of modern motherhood. However, although these ideas were rife in public discourse – especially in urban areas – they did not reflect the reality for many women. The next chapter will shift its focus to more rural areas. In the 1970s, MCH and family planning reached further as population control gave way to PHC in international policy and in Ghana.

Notes

1 RAC, Ford Foundation Collection, Grant #07090496, Reel 4048: 'Address by the Rt. Hon. The Prime Minister Dr K. A. Busia, on the Occasion of the Inauguration of the National Family Planning Council,' 19 March 1971, 1.
2 John Iliffe, *Africans: The History of a Continent* (Cambridge: Cambridge University Press, 2007).
3 Ibid., 310.
4 M. A. Barnor, *A Socio-Medical Adventure in Ghana: Autobiography of Dr. M.A. Barnor* (Accra: Vieso Universal, 2001), 261.
5 PRAAD, Koforidua, ERG 5/1/41: Letter 'Planned Parenthood Activities' from Dr R. Y. B. Karikari, Medical Officer, to Regional Medical Officer of Health, 13 May 1969.
6 Barnor, *A Socio-Medical Adventure*, 258.
7 Ibid., 264.
8 Ibid., 261.
9 Ibid., 267.
10 PRAAD, Koforidua, ERG 5/1/41: Letter from Gladys George, Midwifery Superintendent, to Medical Officer of Health, Koforidua, March 1969.
11 Interview with Dr Patrick Mensah, Takoradi, Western Region, 26 October 2017.
12 PRAAD, Koforidua, ERG 5/1/41: 'Minutes of the Working Party of the MCH Sub-Committee on Planned Parent Hood,' January 1969, 1.
13 Ibid., Appendix A.

14 PRAAD, Koforidua, ERG 5/1/41: Circular from Dr de Heer, Senior Medical Officer of MCH and Nutrition, to all Regional Medical Officers of Health, 28 February 1969.
15 MacFarlane, Deborah, Interview with Professor Fred Sai, *Smith College Population and Reproductive Health Oral History Project*, 11 March 2004, 17.
16 Wellcome: 'Two New African Associations Join IPPF,' *International Planned Parenthood News*, No. 167, January 1968, 1.
17 Barnor, *A Socio-Medical Adventure*, 259.
18 MacFarlane, Deborah, Interview with Professor Fred Sai, 13.
19 PRAAD, Accra, RG 3/8/292: Memorandum by the Minister of Social Welfare and Community Development: 'Establishment of a National Commission on the Status of Women' enclosed in letter from J. E. K. Aggrey-Orleans, UN and IOs Dept., to Chief Social Welfare and C. D. Officer, 30 November 1965.
20 PRAAD, Accra, RG 3/8/292: 'Recommendations for the Advancement of the Status of Ghanaian Women, the Development of Their Potentialities and Their Role in the National Reconstruction,' September 1966, 2.
21 PRAAD, Accra, RG 3/8/292: 'Third Meeting of the Ad-Hoc Committee on UN Seminar on Civic and Political Education for Women held at the State House – Wed 19th June, 1968 at 3pm. Chaired by Justice Annie Jiagge,' 1968, 4.
22 PRAAD, Accra, RG 3/8/292: Circular from J A Boateng, Principal Secretary United Nations Division, 9 January 1969. For the ECOSOC resolutions and recommendations, see attached documents.
23 PRAAD, Accra, RG 3/8/292: 'Suggestions for a National Family Planning Program for Ghana,' 1969, 1.
24 Ibid., 7–13.
25 WHO, P13/372/3/AF: Memorandum: Mr Gille UN Demographic Mission ECA, 22 May 1968, 2.
26 See file WHO P13/522/6: 'ECA Regional Working Group on Fertility Studies and Evaluation of Population Programmes – Addis Ababa, January, 1970.' Preparations for this meeting involved the collection of data from across Africa. The agenda for the meeting focused especially on fertility rates and trends.
27 WHO, N72/372/2: 'List of ECA's Projects on Population, 1971–1976, Indicating Interest of United Nations Organizations, Tentatively Ascertained,' 22 April 1971.
28 PRAAD, Sekondi, WRG 34/1/22: Circular: 'The Department of Rural Development,' 21 November 1969, 1.
29 PRAAD, Accra, RG 3/8/345: Women's Work Reports 1967–1970.
30 'Keeping a Baby Healthy,' *The New Ghana* 12, no. 10 (1968): 11.
31 PRAAD, Accra, RG 3/8/351: 'Programme of Work – Urban Women's Work Central Region 1st Quarter January–March 1970,' 1.
32 Interview with Patience Doris Doh, Koforidua, Eastern Region, 24 January 2018; Interview with Rosina Apraku, 25 January 2018
33 EA, 'Ghana Assembly of Women Foreword by Mrs Grace Nelson,' 9 August 1969.
34 EA, 'Objectives of the Ghana Assembly of Women,' 23 June 1969, 1.
35 EA, 'Ghana Assembly of Women,' 9 August 1969, 17–26.
36 Interview with Gertrude Engmann, Sekondi, Western Region, 30 January 2018.
37 Interview with Dr Daniel Otchere, Takoradi, Western Region, 31 January 2018.
38 PRAAD, Accra, ADM 5/1/573: *Annual Report of the Medical Services of Ghana, 1967*, E. Akwei, Director of Medical Services, 2.
39 RAC, Population Council Collection, Box 234 Folder 2176: 'Family Planning Within and Beyond Maternal and Child Health' by G. Perkin, 28 October 1970, 3.
40 Interview with Dr Daniel Otchere, Takoradi, Western Region, 31 January 2018.
41 Interview with Patience Doris Doh, Koforidua, Eastern Region, 24 January 2018.
42 J. C. Caldwell, 'Family Formation and Limitation in Ghana: A Study of the Residents of Economically Superior Urban Areas,' in *Family Planning and Population Programs: A Review of World Developments*, ed. Bernard Berelson (Chicago, IL: University of Chicago Press, 1966), 595–613.

43 PRAAD, Accra, ADM 5/2/13: *Population Planning for National Progress and Prosperity*, Accra, March 1969, 7.
44 PRAAD, Accra, ADM 5/1/573: *Annual Report of the Medical Services of Ghana, 1967*, E. Akwei, Director of Medical Services, 2.
45 RAC, Ford Foundation Collection, Grant #07090496, Reel 4048: 'Inter-Office Memorandum to David Bell from Lyle Saunders,' 4 November 1969. Gordon Perkin, Ford Foundation adviser in Ghana, described NFPP as 'Omaboe's baby,' 1.
46 Interview with Dr Mensah, Takoradi, Western Region, 26 October 2017.
47 RAC, Ford Foundation Collection, Grant #07090496, Reel 4048: FAP Grant Action for Family Planning in Ghana, 4 June 1970. Enclosed grant action request, 3.
48 MacFarlane, Deborah, Interview with Dr Fred Sai, *Smith College Population and Reproductive Health Oral History Project*, 11 March 2004, 14.
49 J. D. Esseks, 'Economic Policies,' in *Politicians and Soldiers in Ghana, 1966–1972*, ed. Dennis Austin and Robin Luckham (London: Frank Cass and Co. Ltd., 1975), 43; Bianca Murillo, *Market Encounters: Consumer Cultures in Twentieth-Century Ghana*, New African Histories (Athens: Ohio University Press, 2017), 116–27.
50 PRAAD, Accra, ADM 5/1/587: *Fourth Annual Report 1970–1971 Planned Parenthood Association of Ghana*, Accra, 1971, 7.
51 PRAAD, Accra, RG 8/2/617: *The Ford Foundation Annual Report, October 1, 1970 to September 30 1971*, New York, 31 December 1971, 82.
52 Ibid., 81–82.
53 RAC, Ford Foundation Collection, Grant #07090496, Reel 4048: 'Inter-Office Memorandum to David Bell from Lyle Saunders,' 4 November 1969, 1–2.
54 RAC, Ford Foundation Collection, Catalogued Reports: 'Suggestions on "a Population Policy for Ghana" (Reports 004247),' 15 August 1968, 1.
55 PRAAD, Accra, ADM 5/2/13: *Population Planning for National Progress and Prosperity*, Accra, March 1969, Preface.
56 Walter Rodney, *How Europe Underdeveloped Africa* (Abuja: Panaf Publishing Inc., 2012); Samir Amin, 'Underdevelopment and Dependency in Black Africa: Origins and Contemporary Forms,' *Journal of Modern African Studies* 10, no. 4 (1972): 503–24.
57 For more on immigration and citizenship, including this Order, see Ousman Kobo, '"We Are Citizens Too": The Politics of Citizenship in Independent Ghana,' *The Journal of Modern African Studies* 48, no. 1 (2010): 67–94.
58 PRAAD, Accra, ADM 5/2/13: *Population Planning for National Progress and Prosperity*, Accra, March 1969, 17.
59 Dennis Austin and Robin Luckham, eds., *Politicians and Soldiers in Ghana, 1966–1972* (London: Frank Cass and Co. Ltd., 1975). For the political and economic situation surrounding the coup, see particularly the introduction to this book.
60 Valeska Huber, 'Introduction: Global Histories of Social Planning,' *Journal of Contemporary History* 52, no. 1 (2017): 3–15.
61 PRAAD, Accra, ADM 5/2/13: *Population Planning for National Progress and Prosperity*, Accra, March 1969, Preface.
62 Ibid., Preface.
63 MacFarlane, Deborah, Interview with Dr Fred Sai for *Smith College Population and Reproductive Health Oral History Project*, 11 March 2004, 60.
64 PRAAD, Kumasi, ARG 2/14/10: 'Family Planning Why?,' Ghana Publishing Corporation, March 1969. My italics.
65 PRAAD, Koforidua, ERG 5/1/41: 'Address by J H Mensah … on … Formal Launching of National Family Planning Programme,' 22 May 1970, 1.
66 See RAC, Ford Foundation Collection, Grant #07090496, Reel 4048: Programme Action Ford Foundation 'Assistance to Family Planning Activities in Ghana,' 16 July 1974.
67 RAC, Ford Foundation Collection, Grant #07090496, Reel 4048: Request-no. ID-1059 Foundation-administered project: 'Background and Justification,' 23 July 1971, 5.

68 RAC, Ford Foundation Collection, Grant #07090496, Reel 4048: Report to Mr McGeorge Bundy from Mr David Bell, Grant Report 'Assistance to Family Planning Activities in Ghana,' 4 June 1970, 5.

69 RAC, Population Council Collection, Box 581 Folder 5630: 'Site Visit to Korle Bu Hospital, Accra,' June 1970, 5.

70 RAC, Ford Foundation Collection, Grant #07090496, Reel 4048: 'National Family Planning Programme: Progress Report, March 1971,' 1971, 5.

71 WHO, P13/372/9 GHA: Letter sent by Dr A. A. Armar: 'Request for UNFPA Support for the Ghana National Family Planning Programme,' 10 December 1972.

72 RAC, Ford Foundation Collection, Grant #07090496, Reel 4048: FAP Grant Action for Family Planning in Ghana, 4 June 1970. Enclosed grant action request, 4–5.

73 MacFarlane, Deborah, Interview with Dr Fred Sai for *Smith College Population and Reproductive Health Oral History Project*, 11 March 2004, 40.

74 RAC, Ford Foundation Collection, Grant #07090496, Reel 4048: 'Planned Parenthood Association of Ghana Five Year Plan,' n.d. but 1972, 1.

75 RAC, Ford Foundation Collection, Grant #07090496, Reel 4048: 'Ghana National Family Planning Programme Progress Report – March 1971,' 3.

76 Ibid.

77 PRAAD, Kumasi, ARG 2/14/10: 'Ghana National Family Planning Programme Monthly Report on Family Planning Acceptors, November 1972,' Evaluation and Research Unit, Accra, 1973, 1.

78 RAC, Ford Foundation Collection, Grant #07090496, Reel 4048: 'Ghana National Family Planning Programme Progress Report – March 1971,' 3.

79 PRAAD, Koforidua, ERG 5/1/41: 'Family Planning Services in Ghana May 1970,' Enclosure in Circular from Dr A. A. Armar to Regional Officers of Health, 20 May 1970.

80 Kodjo Senah, 'Problems of the Health Care Delivery System,' in *State, Development and Politics in Ghana*, ed. Emmanuel Hansen and Kwame A. Ninsin (London: CODESRIA Book Series, 1989), 242–67.

81 PRAAD, Koforidua, ERG 5/1/41: Ghana National Family Planning Programme Monthly Report on Family Planning Acceptors, April 1971, Evaluation and Research Unit GNFPP, Accra, 1971, 3.

82 PRAAD, Koforidua, ERG 5/1/41: Ghana National Family Planning Programme Monthly Report on Family Planning Acceptors, December 1970, Enclosed in Letter to Regional Medical Officer of Health, Koforidua, 30 January 1971, Table 1.

83 PRAAD, Koforidua, ERG 5/1/41: Letter from Dr Bruce-Kennuah to Planned Parenthood Association of Ghana, 24 August 1970.

84 PRAAD, Koforidua, ERG 5/1/41: Letter from Medical Officer in Charge of Health, Dr S. K. Chatterjee, to Senior Medical Officer in Charge, Akim Oda, 9 September 1970.

85 RAC, Ford Foundation Collection, Grant #07090496, Reel 4048: Request-no. ID-1059 Foundation-administered project: 'Background and Justification' 23 July 1971, 3.

86 Ibid., 28, Table 4.

87 Laura Briggs, *Reproducing Empire: Race, Sex, Science and U.S. Imperialism in Puerto Rico* (Berkeley: University of California Press, 2003), 102–3.

88 RAC, Ford Foundation Collection, Grant #07090496, Reel 4048: Memorandum to Renate Jacob from Bruce Carlson 'Report on Fieldworker Pilot Project: Winneba (709-0496),' 18 December 1973, 1.

89 Ibid., 2.

90 Ibid., 3.

91 Ibid., 4.

92 Interview with Munirata Lardi Yahaya, Cape Coast, Central Region, 14 February 2018.

93 Interview with Juliana Brown, Aburi, Cape Coast, Central Region, 9 February 2018.
94 RAC, Population Council Collection, Box 579 Folder 5562: 'Recent Performance Trends for the Postpartum Program,' 20 June 1972, 6.
95 RAC, Population Council Collection, Box 645 Folder 5: 'International Postpartum Program Annual Report, 1973,' 29 March 1974, 44.
96 RAC, Ford Foundation Collection, Grant #07090496, Reel 4048: Memorandum to Renate Jacob from Bruce Carlson 'Report on Fieldworker Pilot Project: Winneba (709-0496),' 18 December 1973. Enclosure: Interview of Field Staff, 1.
97 Interview with Munirata Lardi Yahaya, Cape Coast, Central Region, 14 February 2018.
98 Of all of those I interviewed, only one said that she had heard of NFPP and used contraceptives regularly (although not until 1988 after she had had five children): Interview with Akua Nkwiwah, Abra, Western Region, 25 October 2017.
99 Interview with Esi Praah, Abra, Western Region, 25 October 2017.
100 RAC, Population Council Collection, Box 644 Folder 7: 'Postpartum Programs Supported by the Population Council,' 30 April 1969, see Table.
101 RAC, Population Council Collection, Box 581 Folder 5630: 'Site Visit to Korle Bu Hospital, Accra,' June 1970, 4.
102 RAC, Population Council Collection, Box 77 Folder 725: Letter from Dr Benjamin Major to Wright, 18 February 1971.
103 RAC, Population Council Collection, Box 581 Folder 5630: 'Site Visit to Korle Bu Hospital, Accra,' June 1970, 4.
104 Interview with Patience Doris Doh, Koforidua, Eastern Region, 24 January 2018.
105 Interview with Adjoa Ewusiwa, New Ebu, Central Region, 22 July 2019.
106 RAC, Ford Foundation Collection, Grant #07090496, Reel 4048: Inter-office Memorandum from John Lowthian to Mr. Haldore Hanson 'Report on Assignment, Ghana. National Family Planning Programme,' 30 March 1971, 3.
107 See files: PRAAD, Kumasi, ARG 2/14/10; PRAAD, Koforidua, ERG 5/1/41.
108 'Family Planning Helps Parents,' *Ghanaian Times*, 28 January 1969, 4.
109 Interview with Patience Doris Doh, Koforidua, Eastern Region, 24 January 2018.
110 'Family Planning Is Voluntary,' *Daily Graphic*, 25 May 1970, 11.
111 'Mother and Child Care,' *Sunday Mirror*, 10 May 1974, 6.
112 RAC, Ford Foundation Collection, Grant #07090496, Reel 4048: 'Ghana: Family Planning Communications, A Programme Status Report' by W. O. Sweeny, May 1971.
113 Interview with Sabina Mensah, Anaji, Western Region, 2 February 2018.
114 RAC, Ford Foundation Collection, Grant #07090496, Reel 4048: 'Planned Parenthood Association of Ghana. Work Programme 1972–1976,' February 1972, 20–21.
115 Wolf Bleek, 'Family and Family Planning in Southern Ghana,' in *Sex Roles, Population and Development in West Africa: Policy-Related Studies on Work and Demographic*, ed. Christine Oppong (Portsmouth, NH: Heinemann, 1987), 147.
116 PRAAD, Kumasi, ARG 2/14/10: Letter from J. Micah Amuah, Ashanti Regional Youth Committee to Ashanti Regional Development Corporation, 14 August 1973.
117 For an extended discussion on sex education in Ghana in the 1960s, see Holly Rose Ashford, 'The Christian Council, Moral Citizenship and Sex Education in Ghana, 1951–1966,' *History of Education* 51, no. 1 (2022): 1–23.
118 Felix Odei Akuffo, 'Teenage Pregnancies and School Drop-Outs: The Relevance of Family Life Education and Vocational Training to Girls' Employment Opportunities,' in *Sex Roles, Population and Development in West Africa: Policy Related Studies on Work and Demographic Issues*, ed. Christine Oppong (Portsmouth, NH: Heinemann, 1987), 154–64.
119 Interview with Dr Mensah, Takoradi, Western Region, 26 October 2017.
120 Interview with Patience Doris Doh, Koforidua, Eastern Region, 24 January 2018.
121 PRAAD, Accra, ADM 5/2/13: *Population Planning for National Progress and Prosperity*, Accra, March 1969, 11.

122 Jeffrey Ahlman, *Living with Nkrumahism: Nation, State, and Pan-Africanism in Ghana* (Illinois: Ohio University Press, 2017), 55.
123 G. E. Hurd, 'Education,' in *A Study of Contemporary Ghana. Vol.2 Some Aspects of Social Structure*, ed. W. Birmingham, I. Neustadt, and E. Omaboe (London: George Allen & Unwin Ltd., 1967), 229.
124 Interview with Sabina Mensah, Anaji, Western Region, 2 February 2018.
125 Interview with Adua Dua, Abrafo, Central Region, 23 July 2019.
126 Akosua Adomako Ampofo, '"When Men Speak Women Listen": Gender Socialisation and Young Adolescents' Attitudes to Sexual and Reproductive Issues,' *African Journal of Reproductive Health* 5, no. 3 (December 2001): 197.
127 Christine Oppong, 'Responsible Fatherhood and Birth Planning,' in *Sex Roles, Population and Development in West Africa: Policy-Related Studies on Work and Demographic Issues*, ed. Christine Oppong and World Employment Programme (Portsmouth, NH: Heinemann, 1987), 165.
128 *National Conference on Population and National Reconstruction. April 7–10, 1986*, Vol II: Contributed Papers, Population Impact Project, University of Ghana, Legon, 1987, 245–46.
129 Akosua Adomako Ampofo, Michael Perry Kweku Okyerefo and Micheal Pervarah, 'Phallic Competence: Fatherhood and the Making of Men in Ghana,' *Culture, Society & Masculinity* 1, no. 1 (2009): 61.
130 Interview with Dr Mensah, Takoradi, Western Region, 26 October 2017.
131 Interview with Juliana Brown, Abura, Central Region, 9 February 2018.
132 PRAAD, Koforidua, ERG 5/1/41: 'Planned Parenthood Association of Ghana. Family Planning Week – 27th September–3rd October. Programme,' n.d. 1970.
133 PRAAD, Kumasi, ARG 2/14/10: 'Meeting of Planning Committee for National Family Planning Week Held in the Regional Office on 8th May, 1975,' 1.
134 RAC, Ford Foundation Collection, Grant #07090496, Reel 4048: 'Ghana National Family Planning Programme.' Fourth Annual Report (July 1973 –June 1974), n.d. but 1974, 13–15.
135 C. G. Baeta, 'Aspects of Religion,' in *A Study of Contemporary Ghana. Vol.2 Some Aspects of Social Structure*, ed. W. Birmingham, I. Neustadt and E. Omaboe (London: George Allen & Unwin Ltd, 1967), 249.
136 Interview with Magdanele Juliet Ackuah, Cape Coast, Central Region, 9 February 2018.
137 Interview with Sabina Mensah, Anaji, Western Region, 2 February 2018.
138 RAC, Ford Foundation Collection, Grant #07090496, Reel 4048: 'Ghana: Family Planning Communications, A Programme Status Report' by W. O. Sweeny, May 1971.
139 Interview with Magdanele Juliet Ackuah, Cape Coast, Central Region, 9 February 2018.
140 Ampofo et al., 'Phallic Competence,' 65; Stephan F. Miescher, *Making Men in Ghana* (Indianapolis: Indiana University Press, 2005).
141 Ibid.
142 PRAAD, Accra, ADM 5/1/587: 'Fourth Annual Report 1970–1971 Planned Parenthood Association of Ghana, 1971,' Accra, 1971, 12.
143 Ibid., 6.
144 Interview with Sabina Mensah, Anaji, Western Region, 2 February 2018.
145 RAC, Ford Foundation Collection, Grant #07090496, Reel 4048: 'Ghana: Family Planning Communications, A Programme Status Report' by W. O. Sweeny, May 1971.
146 RAC, Ford Foundation Collection, Grant #07090496, Reel 4048: 'Ghana National Family Planning Programme.' Fourth Annual Report (July 1973–June 1974), n.d. but 1974, 10. Similar figures were reported for the year 1971–1972.

147 RAC, Ford Foundation Collection, Grant #07090496, Reel 4048: 'Ghana National Family Planning Programme.' Third Report (July 1972 – June 1973),' n.d. but 1973, 6.
148 WHO: *Danfa Comprehensive Rural Health & Family Planning Project: Ghana. UCLA Annual Progress Report. January–December 1974*, by Alfred Neumann, UCLA, 4.
149 RAC, Ford Foundation Collection, Grant #07090496, Reel 4048: 'Ghana National Family Planning Programme Progress Report, June 1972,' NFPP Secretariat, Accra, 3.
150 PRAAD, Accra, ADM 5/2/13: *Population Planning for National Progress and Prosperity*, Accra, March 1969, Preface. My italics.
151 Interview with Dr Mensah, Takoradi, Western Region, 26 October 2017.
152 Interview with Harriet Sekyi-Yorke, Gyabenkrom, Western Region, 27 October 2017.
153 The survey differentiated between 'effective' methods, such as pill, IUD, foams, jellies, diaphragms, and 'traditional' methods, such as abstinence, withdrawal.
154 PRAAD, Accra, RG 8/2/661: *Ghana Fertility Survey 1979–1980 First Report*, vol. II Statistical Tables, Central Bureau of Statistics, Accra, 1983, 219–21.
155 J. Johnson-Hanks, 'Éducation, ethnicité et pratiques reproductives au Cameroun,' *Population* 58, no. 2 (2003): 171–200.
156 Caroline H. Bledsoe and Fatoumatta Banja, *Contingent Lives: Fertility, Time, and Aging in West Africa* (Chicago, IL: University of Chicago Press, 2002).
157 Claire C. Robertson, *Sharing the Same Bowl: A Socioeconomic History of Women and Class in Accra, Ghana* (Indianapolis: Indiana University Press, 1984), 230.
158 RAC, Ford Foundation Collection, Grant #07090496, Reel 4048: 'Address by the Rt. Hon. The Prime Minister Dr K. A. Busia, on the Occasion of the Inauguration of the National Family Planning Council,' 19 March 1971, 1.
159 RAC, Ford Foundation Collection, Grant #07090496, Reel 4048: Memorandum to Renate Jacob from Bruce Carlson 'Report on Fieldworker Pilot Project: Winneba (709-0496),' 18 December 1973. Enclosure: Interview of Field Staff, 1.
160 'Child's Attachment to Mother,' *Ghanaian Times*, 21 January 1969.
161 Akosua Adomako Ampofo, 'Whose "Unmet Need"? Dis/Agreement about Childbearing among Ghanaian Couples,' in *Re-Thinking Sexualities in Africa*, ed. Signe Arnfred (Uppsala: Nordic Africa Institute, 2004), 118.
162 PRAAD, Accra, ADM 5/2/13: *Population Planning for National Progress and Prosperity*, Accra, March 1969, 7.
163 'Mainly for Women,' *Ghanaian Times*, 28 October 1969, 4.
164 'Five Stages of a Woman,' *Ghanaian* Times, 9 December 1969, 4.
165 'Mother and Child Care,' *Sunday Mirror*, 10 May 1974, 5.
166 Susan B. G. Ofori-Atta, 'Nutritional Deficiencies and Maternal and Child Health in Africa,' *Journal of the National Medical Association* 52, no. 1 (January 1960): 42.
167 RAC, Ford Foundation Collection, Grant #07090496, Reel 4048: Memorandum to Renate Jacob from Bruce Carlson 'Report on Fieldworker Pilot Project: Winneba (709-0496),' 18 December 1973. Enclosure: Interview of Field Staff, 2.
168 John C. Caldwell, *Population Growth and Family Change in Africa: The New Urban Elite in Ghana* (Canberra: Australian National University Press, 1968), 16–17. My italics.
169 Simon Szreter, 'The Idea of Demographic Transition and the Study of Fertility Change: A Critical Intellectual History,' *Population and Development Review* 19, no. 4 (December 1993): 672.
170 RAC, Ford Foundation Collection, Grant #07090496, Reel 4048: 'Ghana: Family Planning Communications, A Programme Status Report' by W. O. Sweeny, May 1971.
171 Bleek, 'Family and Family Planning in Southern Ghana,' 148.
172 'Family Planning Helps Parents,' *Ghanaian Times*, 28 January 1969, 4.

173 PRAAD, Kumasi, ARG 2/14/10: Letter from NFPP Executive Director to the regions, 17 July 1975.

174 Interview with Mary Sampson, Adjumako, Western Region, 23 October 2017.

175 Shane Doyle, 'Demography and Disease,' in *The Oxford Handbook of Modern African History*, 1 October 2013, 47.

176 Interview with Ekua Mensah, Ekua Amah, Efua Kaya, Esi Adjumah and Comfort Kwenu, Barabadze, Central Region, 30 November 2017.

177 Interview with Nana Efua Ateifi I, New Ebu, Western Region, 22 July 2019.

178 Monica Das Gupta, 'Kinship Systems and Demographic Regimes,' in *Anthropological Demography: Toward a New Synthesis*, ed. David I. Kertzer and Thomas E. Fricke, Population and Development (Conference on Anthropological Demography, Chicago, IL: University of Chicago Press, 1997), 44; Bleek, 'Family and Family Planning in Southern Ghana,' 138.

179 PRAAD, Accra, ADM 5/2/13: *Population Planning for National Progress and Prosperity*, Accra, March 1969, 15.

180 Interview with Dr Mensah, Takoradi, Western Region, 26 October 2017.

181 Ibid.

182 RAC, Ford Foundation Collection, Grant #07090496, Reel 4048: 'Ghana: Family Planning Communications, A Programme Status Report' by W. O. Sweeny, May 1971.

183 PRAAD, Koforidua, ERG 5/1/41: 'Address by J H Mensah … on … Formal Launching of National Family Planning Programme,' 22 May 1970, 3.

184 RAC, Ford Foundation Collection, Grant #07090496, Reel 4048: Memorandum to Renate Jacob from Bruce Carlson 'Report on Fieldworker Pilot Project: Winneba (709-0496),' 18 December 1973. Enclosure: Interview of Field Staff, 1–2.

6 From Population Control to Primary Healthcare?

Rural Health Interventions in Ghana, 1969–1982

We have seen that, at times, women struggled to access reproductive healthcare. This might be because of their distance from health facilities, the costs associated, the constraints on them because of their gender or because of assumptions made about their 'rural' or uneducated status. I delve into this further in this chapter, exploring what it meant to be labelled as 'traditional' or 'rural' in terms of health. This became especially pertinent given shifts in attention to rural development, primary healthcare (PHC) and international debates over the integration of family planning into broader Maternal and Child Health (MCH) services. Primary healthcare centred MCH. But it also simultaneously relied on rural women to carry out crucial healthcare roles and treated women as victims lacking agency. We see here continuities from discourses of 'self-help' and 'women's work' that had placed the burden of healthcare on social and biological reproduction with women for decades. We also see new formulations of 'tradition' as birth attendants were harnessed for MCH.

Focus on rural health projects exposes a different perspective on reproductive health to the stand-alone population control programme we saw in the previous chapter. I pay attention to community development projects, as distinct from the larger modernisation project of NFPP. I investigate, as Daniel Immerwahr has argued historians should, community development and 'localism' as a distinct strain in the history of development. This approach allows us to understand the history of development beyond a march of modernisation.[1] I rely heavily on WHO-archived documents to investigate this, given a scarcity of health-related materials for the 1970s in Ghana's national archives.

PHC was a community development project, grounded in communities assessing their own needs and providing their own solutions. It aimed to expand health networks, especially to rural areas, and provide health equity, recognising the need to challenge social and economic determinants of health.[2] The 1970s turn to the New International Economic Order (NIEO) and PHC occurred in the context of decolonising nations gaining power within international organisations. NIEO was a set of proposals made by developing countries within the UN system, which aimed to reduce economic inequality through fairer global trade deals and greater development assistance. It also saw developing countries commit to 'self-reliance.'[3] A global overhaul of development strategies recognised that '[t]he

DOI: 10.4324/9781003274162-7

development decade had … produced growth without development.'[4] Poverty and inequality persisted.

Ghana's health policy moved towards PHC implementation but struggled with several limitations. Firstly, the worsening economic situation of the 1970s, which did not see improvements until around 1984.[5] Ghana's GDP fell dramatically and consistently between 1971 and 1983.[6] Secondly, PHC projects and services were gendered. MCH, including family planning, was a core aspect of community-based services. In accordance with long-standing attitudes reflecting women's responsibility as reproducers, this put women at the centre of community healthcare. I show, primarily through investigating the role of TBAs, that women's adherence to tradition continued to be framed as problematic, even as it was supposedly incorporated into PHC. Finally, the focus of – especially NGOs' – MCH programmes remained fertility limitation. I demonstrate this particularly through exploring Danfa Rural Health and Family Planning Project (Danfa). Like Ferguson, I do not evaluate rural health projects by their success or failure, but I ask what development practice 'does.'[7] This also allows investigation into projects' standards and goals. Despite arguments that family planning should be part of PHC, and basic health infrastructure available for all, a disproportionate focus on fertility limitation meant that aspects such as poverty, access to healthcare and women's rights were overlooked.[8]

By focusing on gender and family planning, I build on historical studies of PHC and its limitations. Martin Gorsky and Christopher Sirrs track the idea of 'health for all' to the 1920s. They point out that '"universal" has never straightforwardly signified the whole population.'[9] Indeed, reflections on Ghana's contemporary Community-based Health Planning and Services highlight continued inequities in provision. Particularly, costs continue to hinder participation.[10] In other words, wealth affects access to healthcare. Gender is another core determinant in how healthcare is accessed and experienced. Women are leaned on excessively for their labour in healthcare.[11] This is not new. Earlier chapters have shown how 'women's work' was intimately connected with domesticity, nutrition and healthcare under the colonial government and in post-independence Ghana. The 1970s though was a decade when women's roles in development were explicitly being debated.[12] In this context, projects sought to acknowledge women's contributions – real or potential – to development. However, this often had the result of increasing expectations for women's labour. By asserting that healthcare should derive from communities, gendered expectations were perpetuated. As mothers and as 'traditional birth attendants' (TBAs), women were responsible for maternal and child health.

Pre-Alma-Ata Shifts towards Primary Healthcare

Economic trends are essential in order to understand patterns in the provision of social services.[13] When officially adopting PHC in 1978, Ghana's government observed that the costs were 'well within' the government's means, indicating that the low cost of PHC made it attractive.[14] In the 1970s, Ghana experienced an economic downturn, which successive governments failed to deal with. Instead, according to Jennifer Hart, governments looked for scapegoats.[15] Tendencies to shift responsibility for the nation's prosperity onto individual families also suggest scapegoating, as does the promise of family planning as a 'quick fix.' In rural policies, the 'self-help' mantra could be seen as a mechanism to displace responsibility from the state to individual communities. Furthermore, the language of self-help contains moral messages and makes citizenship conditional on participating in development, much like the dynamic that was seen among elite citizens involved in MCH in the 1930s.

Although PHC became integral to international health policy, its implementation in Ghana could equally be viewed as a response to failures of earlier modernisation projects. Indeed, in 1978 the government admitted that 'in spite of huge infusions of resources ... there has been little improvement in the general health status of the nation in the last 15 years.'[16] At a time when Ghana was experiencing political instability following years of CPP rule which had largely embraced modernisation, industrialisation and technology as development, it made sense to look for alternative methods.[17]

Indeed, renewed efforts to improve and extend the reach of health infrastructure – especially MCH – began contemporaneously with the launch of the Population Policy. In fact, almost as soon as the NLC came to power, it promised a decentralisation of health and prioritisation of locally derived authority.[18] In the late 1960s, there were 242 MCH clinics in Ghana. More than a quarter of these were in Greater Accra and Eastern Region, and another fifth in Ashanti.[19] Ghana had a hospital bed capacity of 9,628 by 1967, as well as six urban health centres and 38 rural health centres.[20] This reflected historic biases in health systems favouring urban areas. Numbers of midwives qualifying rose steadily every year, reaching 1,941 by 1967.[21]

In 1967, the NLC proposed to build health posts to extend health services. It planned to expand a WHO project which established nine health posts in Volta Region nationally.[22] Some health posts were built using communal labour organised by the Department of Social Welfare and Community Development.[23] This policy of extending into rural areas continued under the Progress Party (PP) government. In June 1971, the maternity home and dressing station at Fanti Nyankumasi was transformed into a government health post. The Omanhene, Nana Tsibu Darku, referred to this as a 'self-help' project, in which every village would contribute to the running and extension of the health post.[24] Of the 26 villages it served, a committee of 11 men and 11 women was formed in June 1971 to see to its 'proper running ... and to organise voluntary self-help activities.'[25] The gender equity of this committee suggests it was deliberate and that health committees routinely included both sexes. However, given women's workload both in and outside the home, they may have been unable to participate in decision-making in *practice*.

The PP aimed to quickly develop Basic Health Services (BHS) throughout the country. The idea of BHS dated back to a WHO declaration of 1953 and was promised after independence in 1957. However, its implementation was extremely limited until the late 1960s.[26] The PP government intended to establish a system of urban and rural health posts, and health centres, which would reach the entire population, especially peripheral areas.[27] In 1967, WHO and UNICEF supported a BHS project in Brong-Ahafo beginning. The project aimed to plan and implement a healthcare delivery system in this area, which could then extend elsewhere.[28] Crucially, it was to '[improve] … the health and status of the rural population.' To that end, projects were to be 'decided on, organized and performed by the communities themselves as an integral part of rural community development.'[29] The government undertook widespread planning of BHS in the early 1970s.[30] In July 1971 the Central Region's Officer of Health sent plans to the central government detailing that he expected 17 further health posts to be functioning in the region by the year's end. This is especially ambitious considering that at the time there were only two.[31] The Kintampo Rural Health Training School was opened in 1969, mainly for training medical auxiliaries, nutrition experts and disease control technicians to work in rural areas.[32]

This surge of 'self-help' style health initiatives could be seen as exploiting voluntary rural labour. However, communities campaigned for BHS locally. For example, a letter addressed to the Central Region Chief Executive opened with:

> We members of the Nyakrom Development Association … are aware of the Government's concern for the health needs of the people, and in particular of rural communities. Resulting from this concern it has been the government's laudable policy to provide a Health Post for each Constituency.[33]

This was one of many similar petitions to the MH to provide health posts in Central Region, that adopt the same tone, and refer to the government's claim to be working on providing rural health services. Another letter pointedly petitioned the ministry on the grounds that 'we are aware that, unlike the previous Governments … it is not the present Government's intention to site such Health Centres at inaccessible places to cause hardship.'[34] These petitions generally came from village committees.[35] The small amount of funding from the government for these development projects was evidently welcome.

Rural health posts were run by local communities, following PHC principles.[36] The Fanti Nyankumasi health post, mentioned above, included quarters for a midwife, a clinic and an antenatal ward for inpatients. MCH was repeatedly emphasised as central to BHS and PHC. Plans in the late 1970s to establish PHC referred to central focal points: pregnancy management, child welfare, disease control, family planning, nutrition and health education.[37] Not only did these priorities reflect continuities from past rural health plans, but they also emphasised the gendered nature of PHC as they were linked to domesticity, reproduction and childrearing.

The fact that the Fanti Nyankumasi post covered 26 towns and villages highlights the limitations of healthcare coverage. In 1978 the government estimated that due to the 'passive' and 'static' nature of health services, 70% of Ghanaians could not use them.[38] A request from Assin Jakai, a village six miles from Fanti

Nyankumasi, was denied its request for its own post on the grounds that they had health services 'nearby.'[39] The Development Committee of Assin Jakai saw things differently, claiming that 'transportation is very difficult and scarce.'[40] A woman at Assin Jakai making antenatal visits to the Fanti Nyankumasi health post would have been unable to walk there in labour. Indeed, this decision against Assin Jakai was not unanimous in the ministry; Yaw Sam demanded: 'what happens when someone needs medical attention urgently and he cannot walk 6 miles [?]'[41] His appeal was rejected. Elsewhere, at Twifu Praso, a health centre, including Maternity Block, was opened in June 1971, but lacked a generator and water tank. Despite this, staff saw 6,000 patients in its first two months. Cases that needed more sophisticated medical attention, though, had to be sent to Cape Coast hospital, 48 miles, or a three-hour journey, away, due to bad roads.[42]

Meanwhile, a second military coup brought Colonel Acheampong and the National Redemption Council (NRC) to power in January 1972. After 1975, General Acheampong – as he now entitled himself – formed and headed the Supreme Military Council (SMC). The NRC was preoccupied with the desire to become self-sufficient and in many ways reflected Nkrumahist principles. They rejected foreign interference and neocolonial control. They had an ambiguous attitude to family planning, claiming that population growth was not a 'major problem' for Africa, but continued to support the NFPP, at least rhetorically.[43] In the context of discussing the country's economic revival, Acheampong declared:

> to the whole world ... that we have the will power and the human and material resources to be self-reliant ... we will have to adopt a revolutionary attitude to our whole manner of living. In short, we have to be truly independent and self-reliant in all respects.[44]

This rhetoric chimed with self-help, in which community-based healthcare made sense. WHO reported in 1974 that the 'principle of community involvement [in health] appears to be strongly endorsed in Ghana where there is a national commitment to self-help and self-reliance applied to a broad range of national and local needs.'[45] Shifting responsibility to communities arguably reduced the government's accountability.

The NRC founded a Department for Rural Development, with a special emphasis on 'self-help projects.' Health posts now came under this Department's remit. Under the new Rural Development department, the Home Science Extension programme was established. It was 'geared at teaching rural folk, especially women, how to build up strong and happy homes.'[46] Despite the self-proclaimed revolutionary nature of the NRC, its imagination when it came to women's roles was limited, overwhelmingly connected to the domestic sphere. The idea that women should 'build up' strength in their homes was linked to the NRC's demands for dedicated labour from Ghanaians.

The NRC continued a building programme of health posts. At one post's inauguration in 1972, in a speech mirroring the earlier discourse of government responsibility to rural areas, the local chief stated: 'This has ... shown that the

NRC has deep interest in the rural population for fair distribution of projects.'[47] Given the government's limited resources, and evidence of disputes over health posts' placement above, the word 'fair' might be used here to defend the decision to locate it in his dominion. Previously, hospitals had been a focus of health development programmes as symbols of modernity and providers for the elite.[48] The NRC diverted funds from building *new* hospitals to improving the existing ones. In the 1975 Five-Year Development Plan, it announced that its core health goal was 'the equitable redistribution of health facilities' to make them more accessible to all.[49]

In the early 1970s, the government recruited women for Community Health Nursing (CHN) training, a course which took just two years. Advertisements for courses were sent to chiefs and elders in remote villages as well as newspapers.[50] One woman who underwent CHN training was Munirata Yahaya. She explained that CHNs' work was mainly preventative: teaching about hygiene, nutrition and minor ailments and making home visits. She decided to become a nurse to alleviate the suffering she witnessed in her village.[51] Florence Boateng also became a CHN because she 'want[ed] to take care of mothers, babies' and described her role: 'we look after pregnant women, we look after children, we weigh them, we give them immunisations, we look after old age.' She described examining pregnant women and giving them advice for a healthy pregnancy, especially on nutrition.[52] Again, these testimonies highlight the prominence of MCH in community health work.

People in rural areas depended on roles like CHNs since hospitals were often inaccessible. Martha Abena lived in Abrafo in Central Region; the nearest hospital in the 1970s was Cape Coast, 30km away. She said that in an emergency, for example a haemorrhage, women could not get there. Instead, Martha administered 'first aid.' This consisted of 'plantain … we cut it and beat it nicely and let the woman sit on it.' She herself had a 'terrible experience' when, 12 hours into labour with twins she was still unable to find transport to Cape Coast hospital. In the end, a passing tractor took her but by the time she arrived, it was too late to save one of the twins, which had to be delivered by caesarean section.[53] Likewise, Munirata saw women in labour on the backs of bicycles trying to reach hospital, because it was the only available transport. CHNs were trained in performing emergency deliveries so that they could help women they found in second-stage labour as they travelled from village to village.[54]

The push for rural services included family planning. During a 1975 training course 'to improve the quality of rural life,' S. K. Kwafo, NFPP leader, referred to the 1969 Population Policy. He stated that this policy linked the limitation of population growth to development. However, he argued, development meant nothing if it left behind rural people: the majority of Ghanaians. Rather, family planning should 'constitute a significant component of the social infrastructure to be provided in the rural sector.' Kwafo reiterated that Ghana could not cope with the current scale of population growth. He called for the 'expansion of existing health and social welfare services throughout the country' to allow for the effective implementation of family planning.[55] In other words, family planning should neither be stand-alone, nor urban in character. This rhetoric was based on a vision of family planning as a part of improving community development.

Following the 1978 Alma-Ata International Conference on Primary Health Care, the SMC announced that it would implement a PHC policy in Ghana, providing each district at least one hospital and each local council one health post.[56] The emphasis was to shift from curative to preventative medicine.[57] Dr Atobrah remembered that when he worked at Effia Nkwanta Hospital in Western Region in 1979, radio programmes were played through mobile vans in the villages to promote MCH and encourage women to attend clinics. As well as mobile information vans, 'the government ensured we had small clinics at vantage points giving … [MCH and health education] to the people.'[58] The promise of extending preventative, and rural, health infrastructure reappeared in an almost circular fashion from the colonial period onwards. Interestingly, in 1981, there was some resistance against establishing community health posts rather than larger curative centres. MP Mr Dzebu argued that in Tsito, a polyclinic offering curative services would be more appropriate.[59] In this case, bias towards 'modern,' curative services persisted.

Economic Crisis and the Ghanaian Health Sector

PHC in Ghana faltered for a lack of resources. As Randall Packard has argued, PHC programmes were most successful on a small scale, where extensive resources were available from foreign donors.[60] Danfa, discussed below, is a good example of this. In 1976, the government stated that only 29% of citizens had access to 'modern' health services.[61] Testimonies of women unable to reach medical care reflected the limitations of rural health services. Health implementation struggled under the burden of economic crisis. In 1981, the *Daily Graphic* warned citizens of the health services' imminent collapse if the government could not provide urgently needed drugs and equipment. It said deaths were occurring due to a lack of basic provisions[62] and excessive bureaucracy.[63] One article reported that members of the public were equipping Komfo Anokye Hospital to give its patients a 'ray of hope.'[64] Numerous articles reported the disastrous state of medical staffing, worsened by doctors striking.[65] Lack of archival evidence makes it difficult to assess exactly what was happening within the health services. However, the sheer number of newspaper articles lamenting the situation suggests severe problems.

According to the World Bank, per capita income in Ghana was in decline from 1971 onwards, and inflation was higher than in any other West African nation. The country was facing a growing budget deficit, with no prospects for economic improvement by the end of the decade.[66] In 1978, Budget Planners reported an urgent need to bring hyper-inflation under control and lay the foundations for economic recovery. Meanwhile, non-essential projects were cancelled and, in theory, 'priority … given to the provision and maintenance of economic and social services.'[67] The crisis affected the availability of medical equipment, staff and drugs. It also had wider implications affecting health: for example, lack of food exacerbated nutritional problems.[68] Lack of transport made it harder to reach hospitals.

Adua Tekyiwa lived in Jukwa and described having to wake at dawn to find transport to visit the midwife in Cape Coast during her first pregnancy in 1975.[69] In some cases, transport problems meant that such medical staff as there were could not reach hospitals themselves.[70] Inequalities widened, and real income fell dramatically by the late 1970s.[71] A 1979 World Bank report noted that Ghana's social development was falling behind other sub-Saharan African countries.[72]

Patients attending government hospitals were required to buy drugs they were prescribed privately, but pharmacies lacked stock. The Minister for Health blamed the situation on thefts of drugs from ships arriving in Ghana's harbours.[73] Arguably the larger problem was how lucrative accumulating and selling drugs had become, exacerbating the problem that they were not reaching the poorest sections of society. Since the beginning of the decade, drug imports and distribution had been compromised by the severe monetary crisis, inadequate staff at stores and a lack of vehicles to transport drugs around the country.[74] MP Dr Ankomah testified that 'a visit to the hospitals reveals that warehouses of hospitals have been turned into museums and archives for broken-down vehicles, machinery and equipment.'[75]

The Ministry of Health seemed unable to deal with these problems. In 1974 Nana Amani V of Asebu pointed out that their clinic was not functioning since they required a nurse. An official replied with a short note telling him to advertise for one himself, since the ministry certainly had none spare.[76] MP Alhaji Abdul Moomin asked the Minister for Health, Dr Ocran, in parliament 'whether he [was] aware of the acute shortage of drugs and medical officers in Wa Hospital,'[77] whilst MP Bafour Osafo Gyewu pointed out that the health clinic in Techiman Constituency was not functioning due to 'the absence of a MO and lack of drugs and other equipment.'[78] Of course, the minister was aware of these issues. Staff shortages had long plagued the health sector. Dr Ocran explained: 'the present deplorable staffing position ... is the result of the exodus of trained medical personnel to other countries. The reasons for the exodus are well known.'[79] The reason, explained Nana Efua Ateifi, who was living in Kumasi, was that all the doctors left for Nigeria seeking adequate wages.[80]

Whilst contraceptives were supplied by donors, the crisis affected their distribution and staffing for their prescription. Economic conditions doubtless affected Ghanaians' health choices. As the cost of orthodox medicines rose, turning to herbalists or TBAs was more likely. Furthermore, Ghanaian families chose to limit their family size in these circumstances.[81] Adua Dua remembered that Rawlings, Ghana's military leader after 1981, introduced birth control, because '[b]y then things were quite difficult in the world ... so if you give birth to fewer children you would be able to take good care of them.'[82] Those working in waged professions in towns were hit hardest by the economic crisis, which saw their living wage decrease and the relative cost of feeding, clothing and – importantly – educating children rise.

PHC as 'Women's Work'

As a development project, PHC's discourses of 'community participation' covered up gendered inequalities. Perceptions of women's roles in community development misread the ways in which they balanced productive and reproductive work inside and outside the home. Women had historically been assumed responsible for the biological and social reproduction of communities. Throughout the colonial and postcolonial period 'women's work' campaigns led by missionaries, humanitarians and the state, focused overwhelmingly on women's domestic roles, child welfare and nutrition. The concept of 'women's work,' introduced by early missionaries, with its dual purpose of providing MCH and domesticating women,[83] survived into the independence era.[84] Women's obligations to family came before their economic autonomy, especially in times of crisis.[85] Healthcare work fell to women both domestically and as TBAs. This labour was devalued as development projects required women partake in 'self-help' or volunteerism. A number of recent studies have found that 'self-help'-style labour in African development projects, has legitimised unpaid labour.[86] But there is a further, gendered, dynamic at play in development projects whereby the unpaid labour required for women's work is naturalised. This is partly due to the caring role expected from women perpetuated through humanitarian discourse.

K. P. Agyekum, government minister talking to GAW in 1971, outlined women's roles in rural reconstruction. He encouraged women's 'voluntary social services,' urging them to motivate 'less-fortunate daughters and sisters in rural areas' to take on this 'selfless service.' Women's voluntary work allowed, he argued, 'social advancement' and 'national development.'[87] The praise of voluntary service and the suggestion that it should be extended devalues women's labour. Indeed, Agyekum argued that it was particularly in their 'individual role as mothers' that women could improve the human resources of the nation.[88] In February 1977, the Minister for Health, Dr Beausoleil, wrote for WHO's magazine, *World Health*, discussing MCH in Ghana. Mother and child units, he explained, had difficulties reaching communities in sparsely populated rural areas. He described how mothers were encouraged to bring their children to health centres for immunisation and receive other treatments and care. Ghana was expanding its programme, Beausoleil said, 'to cover the entire population within the framework of its PHC system.'[89] This programme was dependent on women's cooperation. Images printed alongside this article showed queues of women with children on their backs or at their sides. Attendance at the clinic was clearly gendered – *women* were relied upon to invest in new rural health schemes.

By the 1970s, there was some recognition that the modernisation paradigm wasn't working for women. That is, development practice had so far been more beneficial to men than to women. 'Women in Development' (WID) responded to this and attempted to integrate women into developmental economic systems.[90] However, this approach arguably did not move away from gendered assumptions. One example which highlights this is the Ghana Integrated Rural Development Project, implemented in six villages near Tarkwa, beginning in 1974. It was run through the National Vocational Training Institute in Accra, with the assistance of the ILO and UNDP. Its main purpose was to train women in skills to set up 'small scale industries,' producing and selling soap and clothes, which would 'promote the circulation of money within the villages concerned.'[91] Project leaders reported difficulties because of 'tribal disunity and land disputes,' but also because participants did not have time for activities in between 'farms, petty trading, and house-hold activities.'[92] In other words, this development project underestimated how active women already were in their homes and the local economy. As is common in development projects, 'dimensions of gender or culture' were not allowed to override the assumptions made by project planners.[93] As Eva Rathgeber has pointed out, projects like this one rarely undertook feasibility studies which might have highlighted how 'overburdened' women already were.[94]

Interestingly, this women's project also had an – apparently unrelated – health aspect. This began in 1975 specifically to promote MCH.[95] In April 1978 clinics were opened in five villages in south-western Ghana: Agona, Awudua, Attuabo, Simpa and Abontiakoon.[96] In their first month, 782 people – mainly children – received care. Demonstrations were given to women on supplementary foods to prevent child malnutrition.[97] Mothers were told to visit the clinic regularly to prevent this. Pregnant women were advised on diet and on 'preparation for confinement.' They were told they must go to the hospital for delivery, and visits were made to women's homes.[98] The project was based on the premise that families' prosperity would improve if mothers had health education; furthermore, this would feed into nation-building.[99] In a speech opening the training course for 1979, the Rural Development Officer stated that a mother's training really began from the day her child was born. She said: 'mothers do a lot of service to a nation through teaching children well, by giving the child good food you are contributing in no small manner to the health of the nation.'[100] Evidently, motherhood and healthcare were seen as crucial to women's roles in development. In this and many other contexts, the WID paradigm failed to make a radical change from the 'women's work' that came before it. By the late 1970s, feminist scholars such as Achola Okello Pala recognised this, arguing that WID programmes were a continuity of European colonisation that had sought to 'integrate' women into colonial development, expressed through 'concern' for uneducated women and girls.[101]

One aspect of this was nutrition. In *The Ghanaian Woman*, the 'healthy home' was stated as one of the housewife's responsibilities. Bringing up a healthy family, with proper nutrition, it stated, was a contribution to the establishment of the 'healthy nation.'[102] Despite this, small-scale economic development programmes, like the ILO one near Tarkwa, did not train women in agriculture, but rather industries seen as feminine: handicrafts and dress making. Women's involvement in providing nutrition was treated as strictly domestic. But rural development courses on 'housecraft' and 'mothercraft' were attended sporadically. Women preferred programmes that would augment their income outside the home.[103] Ghana's Chief Education Officer in 1975 rejected the idea that women should learn agriculture. He stated: 'leave that to the men, women teachers should get on with their needlework and cookery.' This seems nonsensical given that Ghanaian women certainly worked in agriculture and were responsible for feeding their families. Scholars have shown that the late 1970s saw more pressure on female-headed households as economic contributions from men dwindled compounded by economic collapse.[104]

Family Planning

Challenges to 'Neo-imperial' Population Control

In their own words, Ford Foundation had been 'intimately associated with the planning and implementation' of NFPP.[105] Its 'impact [was] felt across the entire spectrum of activities of the GNFPP from planning through to implementation at the grassroots level and evaluation.'[106] However, their involvement ended in 1975, with final payments being made in 1978. Ford's Katherine McKee wrote to close the project, 'thereby bringing to an end the chapter of direct Foundation involvement in family planning activities in West Africa.'[107] This was a U-turn for Ford, which a few years previously had been pushing for a stronger line in Ghana's population policy.

McKee explained this, perhaps unsurprisingly, by referencing 'political turmoil' in Ghana. From 1966 onwards Ghana was governed by a series of unstable governments and saw three military coups by 1981. But the main reason was 'the Foundation's evolving philosophy regarding approaches to population and development in the developing world.' Lyle Saunders had been sent to Accra to evaluate NFPP in light of this changing philosophy.[108] Ford no longer saw the push to limit births as appropriate. McKee reported that they would be unlikely to support NFPP again because

> population as a discrete sector of Foundation involvement in this region and other parts of the developing world is diminishing in importance … from about 1975, our program's approach has become … more holistic … focusing on provision of MCH services with a primary health care strategy.

This strategy would safeguard the lives of under-fives to ensure their survival which could, she observed, eventually negate the need for large families.[109]

This tells us that organisations pushing population control had been challenged. As early as 1968, the WHO liaison officer with the ECA wrote that demography was a minefield, moving in the 'realms of national population policy, which is highly emotionally charged, and in which the approach of Western countries to Africa has become suspect.'[110] Of course, this was exactly what Ford was doing in Ghana when this letter was written. Emily Callaci points to a strong counter-narrative at the First African Population Conference in Accra in 1971, to the agenda of international agencies, who saw population control as a way to counter poverty. She exposes a general backlash against population activism in Africa from 'Marxists, feminists and anti-colonial thinkers.'[111] In 1974, the World Population Conference had been due to declare a World Population Plan of Action. Matthew Connelly has described the wide-ranging opposition that manifested against this plan. Ex-colonies stressed the neo-imperial nature of population control: organisations like IPPF and UNFPA were staffed by ex-colonial officials; population activism overwhelmingly targeted poor people and countries. It was not so 'far-fetched to imagine,' suggests Connelly, that the plan to 'reduce the number of poor people was really a form of imperialism by other means.'[112] The World

Population Plan *was* adopted, but it was based on reframing the 'population problem.' It reinforced the idea that population was connected to development, but 'endorsed the principle that parenthood is a fundamental human right and saw its application as a means towards improving health and welfare.' Aims included reducing mortality and morbidity, safeguarding the rights of vulnerable populations, promoting the status of women, and advances in the field of health, food and nutrition.[113] Politically, involvement of IOs and NGOs in population control became problematic.

In the 1972 NFPP Progress Report, the secretariat noted that Ghanaian culture remained strongly pronatalist and

> in the face of growing nationalism after long periods of colonial domination, many view foreign assistance for family planning with suspicion that it has the sinister motive of corrupting the youth, destroying long cherished cultural practices and leading to general moral depravity of the nation.[114]

These tensions over international assistance in family planning suggest that it was seen by many as culturally alien and politically loaded. The idea that family planning would lead to moral decline was linked to foreign interference. In this context, pronatalism was nationalist.

Indeed, two rare references to NFPP in the *Daily Graphic* in 1981 were appeals *against* it. On the front page, Dr D. K. Boateng demanded that the government 'suspend family planning scheme,' since it was wasteful under the economic circumstances.[115] A month later, in May, Nee Azuma Kangidi agreed that family planning was 'not in our interest.' Kangidi vividly described family planning as a 'canker' and 'plague of modern civilization.' He argued that family planning was un-Christian: 'I think it is fair to say that those who succumb to the temptations of genocide only obey the commands of Satan.' Furthermore, he compared the populations of Ghana and Britain, arguing that although Britain's population was much larger, family planning was not enforced in the name of development. Family planning, he said, would 'prevent our future leaders from coming into the world.'[116]

In Ama Ata Aidoo's *Changes: A Love Story*, the author explores how changes to Ghanaian society affected women. Opokuya, the more conservative of two female protagonists, and a midwife, has this to say about family planning:

> Meanwhile, our government are behaving like all professional beggars … Under such circumstances, how does the beggar tell the giver to go and stuff his dangerous and experimental contraceptive pills, capsules and injections? … And they call their murderous programmes beautiful names: 'family planning' and 'mother health'.

She goes on to insinuate that the foreign donors must have an alternative motive: '[i]t seemed to her that any time someone else showed such a keen interest in your not making children … he is not just interested in your good health, your prosperity.'[117] Aidoo chooses a midwife to put forward these views – an educated, female character – suggesting they were widespread.

Family Planning and PHC

There was an international debate over how far family planning should be integrated into MCH. Some saw family planning as a stand-alone service to be supplied regardless of surrounding health infrastructure. Others thought that integrating family planning into MCH was essential. In the late 1950s, Dr R. H. O. Bannerman had provided rare family planning services at Korle Bu. By the 1970s, he was working in the Family Health division of WHO in Geneva. He visited Ghana in this capacity in 1970 and wrote that:

> I personally think that [NFPP] is essentially a health project, and in our present state of development should remain essentially so … [WHO] is making every effort to dissuade national authorities from undertaking family planning programmes as activities isolated from health services which, as experience shows, has impeded the sound development of the countries' general health services or affected detrimentally those already in existence.[118]

WHO's and Bannerman's personal position was against stand-alone family planning provision. This was reflected in aid appeals to WHO from NFPP, which emphasised the need to improve general MCH services, something which NFPP did not prioritise overall.[119] In fact, a lack of development was seen as an argument against NFPP. This directly contradicted advocates who saw family planning and population control as a solution for underdevelopment. WHO had, perhaps unsurprisingly, always insisted that family planning was a health issue and part of MCH.

On the other side of the debate was the idea that stemming population growth was more urgent than the time and resources it would take to build health infrastructure. In 1970 Ford's Gordon Perkin, working as an NFPP adviser, wrote a paper stating that the primary objectives of MCH and family planning differed. As he pointed out, the NFPP secretariat was based in the Ministry for Finance and Economic Planning, and its main goal was to reduce population growth. NFPP acted through a number of government ministries and channels to promote contraception, not just the MH. This enabled it, according to Perkin, to reach the 75% of women that did not go through the healthcare system, because MCH was not available to them.[120]

The premise of the Population Council's postpartum program was that women should be targeted for family planning through MCH services.[121] By the early 1970s, it was advocating an MCH-based approach to family planning, where possible, promoted by its own Bernard Berelson and Howard Taylor. These men argued that the establishment of a 'modern' maternity service was a good way to spread family planning.

> [T]he twin purposes are the improvement of maternal and infant care and the provision of modern contraceptives, to the end that the present gap

between the poorer women of the world and their richer counterparts will be narrowed.[122]

Like PHC, their model specifically addressed rural areas. They foresaw an 'associate' of the programme in each village. Significantly, this associate would ideally be female: an 'indigenous midwife, or other modestly educated village-bred person.' They were in touch with Gordon Perkin and the head of MCH in Ghana, Dr Hammond-Quaye.[123] A representative was sent to Ghana at the end of 1972 to discuss the implementation of this approach.[124] However, the Taylor/Berelson model was not implemented, perhaps unsurprisingly given the economic constraints on Ghana's medical services.[125] Furthermore, the result of integrating MCH and family planning arguably saw the former being compromised. Reflecting on development projects in 1970s Africa, Pala stated: 'I have visited villages where, at a time when the village women are asking for better health facilities and lower infant-mortality rates they are presented with questionnaires on family planning.'[126] Although health officials may have been hoping for long-term benefits to MCH from promoting family planning, the approach evidently appeared disingenuous.

Danfa

The Danfa Comprehensive Rural Health & Family Planning Project was joint between the University of Ghana, the MH and the University of California, Los Angeles (UCLA). It also collaborated with NFPP and IPPF and like NFPP, it was mainly funded through USAID.[127] It was well placed to influence Ghanaian health policy. The project was based in villages 8–10 miles from Accra. NFPP was overwhelmingly urban-based and 'directed at more receptive residents of urban areas where the majority of health facilities ... are located.'[128] In contrast, Danfa aimed to 'focus specifically on stimulating adoption by rural families of health, nutrition and family planning practices.'[129] As well as targeting rural areas, the project also sought to embed family planning into BHS. Danfa quickly became an important part of the family planning landscape in Ghana, attracting one of the highest numbers of 'clients.'[130]

Danfa quickly implemented a family planning programme in one of its project areas of 16,000 people.[131] Before that, the programme area was mapped, staff trained and the population surveyed. Its 'attitudes, beliefs, knowledge and practices' with regard to family planning were recorded. Danfa aimed to reduce maternal mortality, which was 5/1,000 births in the project area in 1972.[132] This was considerably lower than the country's average, and could be explained by the close proximity to Accra's medical services, or it could be recorded incorrectly.[133] A 1964 WHO report estimated a country average of 31.4/1,000 births, and it seems unlikely that vast improvements to maternal mortality would have been made in the intervening eight years.[134] The main threats to pregnant women, according to Danfa experts, were haemorrhage, infection, toxaemia and '*excess fertility*.'[135] Health education involved establishing village development and health committees, and MCH and family planning education.[136] Village committees demonstrated the project's community dynamic. Danfa provided daily family planning, antenatal, postnatal and child welfare services, and community nurses and midwives who made domiciliary visits.[137]

Crucially, Danfa's core purpose was to evaluate whether family planning was a service best provided standing alone, or 'as an integral part of a comprehensive health scheme.'[138] In a 1972 research paper, doctors involved with the project emphasised that 'fertility in this region is one of the highest in the world. This is not surprising given Ghana's highly pronatalist cultural history.'[139] The statement that this is one of the most fertile spots *in the world* is simply a discursive device to legitimise targeting this aspect of people's lives. In its 1974 report, Danfa stated that the health of rural people 'rests largely upon achieving population policy goals.'[140] In other words, fertility limitation remained at the heart of the programme. Indeed, it was funded by USAID, which argued that fertility limitation ought to be a core component of MCH programmes.[141] Motivating men and women to embrace family planning was a core activity carried out by health workers who visited villages in the area on rotation.[142]

Danfa's justification for promoting birth control was to 'reduce the risk of death by reducing the number of pregnancies.'[143] Indeed, family planning was the only aspect of MCH that would have a positive effect on maternal mortality.[144] It was not the only organisation targeting rural areas. Sabina Mensah described how fieldworkers rapidly noted that family planning should be community-based. Therefore, she, along with her team in Western Region, organised community outreach as a core component of PPAG's work. This was part of a wider community-based distribution approach to family planning, which assumed that 'basing family planning on local structures and networks would minimize resistance.'[145] Indeed, Danfa's 1972 report already noted 'increasing acceptance of the idea of family planning' and that initial resistance to the IUD was 'diminishing.'[146]

By 1977, the 'family health' model, integrating family planning into MCH, was a core component of MH training. Health workers were trained to evaluate and report on family planning acceptance, and in government policy on family planning that involved both the 'health benefits' and 'the effects of rapid population growth.'[147] It is unclear though how widespread family planning was in MH services. None of the lists of essential drugs to be provided to health posts included contraception, for example.[148] A training manual noted that the fewer pregnancies women had, the less would be the 'risk of death'; this risk increased if children were not properly spaced; women should have the chance to recover 'physically and emotionally' after births.[149] Women's health appears to have been prioritised here.

To promote family planning, health workers were encouraged to enter homes and communities. Problems in 'motivating' couples to use contraceptives were mainly explained by fear due to 'exaggerated, distorted and untrue information' about contraceptives.[150] Another problem noted in the manual was 'traditional behaviour.' In this case, the problematic behaviour was a failure of couples to discuss in advance how many children they wanted, and lack of communication between couples so that 'husbands make major decisions alone.'[151] As discussed in the previous chapter, this notion of *husbands* making unilateral decisions shows only part of the picture of women's lives which often included multiple sex partners and certainly the influence of the *abusua* or extended family.

Traditional Birth Attendants (TBAs)

Since their initiation in Ghana, women had attended antenatal clinics but given birth attended by a TBA. In the 1970s this was still the case. Reasons for this differed as we have seen and may be explained by women's inability to travel to clinics or hospitals in an emergency, or to the benefits of being attended by family, or to the efficacy of local medicines and methods. Sister Doh attributed it particularly to women's reluctance to lie down to give birth.[152] Midwife Magdalene Ackuah agreed, stating that women preferred to squat.[153] In the colonial period, relying on the help of 'native midwives,' 'handywomen' or 'grandmothers' as they were interchangeably known, was denounced by officials as dangerous. The colonial government institutionalised a western-style medical system. This system sought to exclude indigenous medicine.[154] It constructed legal barriers to indigenous medical practice. Whereas in Nigeria there were training programmes for TBAs, in colonial Ghana, the idea was rejected.[155] Since the Accra midwifery school opened in 1928, the state had encouraged women to give birth assisted by qualified midwives. However, in reality there were nowhere near enough midwives to attend all Ghanaian women. One important feature of the shift towards PHC in the 1970s was the acknowledgement of this and attempts to integrate TBAs into MCH.

A negative attitude towards TBAs, and rural mothers in general, prevailed into the 1970s among policymakers and many healthcare professionals. Dr Mensah worked at Effia Nkwanta Hospital in Sekondi from 1973 to 1975. He said that women who came to the hospital from the town were 'enlightened and educated,' whereas those coming from rural areas attended hospital less and were uneducated regarding diet and reporting health problems. Birth attendants in the villages insisted on giving enemas despite the fact that, according to Dr Mensah, they did not know the exact properties of the herbs they used.[156] Rosina Apraku, who trained as a nurse in Eastern Region in the 1970s, said that TBAs could 'do normal delivery' but 'will not know how to deal with problems.'[157] Medical professionals had little confidence in the abilities of those who had not undergone the same medical training as themselves.

But TBAs were harnessed by PHC programmes that saw them as community-based *par excellence*: 'traditional medical practitioners are central personnel in the delivery of [PHC] for rural populations in developing countries.'[158] In 1973 WHO held a series of consultations with representatives from all over the world to 'define the role traditional birth attendants may play in a programme of maternity and family planning care.'[159] However, although traditional healthcare was increasingly seen as necessary, it was not respected. 'Tradition' was only harboured for as long as it took to change it. Furthermore, there were constant misunderstandings as to what 'tradition' looked like.

In 1973, Ghana reported to WHO that 75% of deliveries were attended by a TBA.[160] Patrick Twumasi and Dennis Warren offer this definition:

> traditional birth attendants focus on life crises. They have a special role to play at birth and at puberty ceremonies. In child birth, they are midwives and they are also recognised as godmothers to young children. Throughout Ghana, especially in the rural areas, they are known as specialists in obstetrics. Their range of activities extends into the field of sex education and contraceptive counselling.[161]

According to this, TBAs had pastoral and cultural as well as medical roles. Implicitly, they were women. The WHO agreed that TBAs had broad roles.[162] In a 1973 glossary of terms, WHO defined the TBA as – 'a person (usually a woman) who assists the mother at childbirth … more commonly found in rural than in urban areas.'[163] However, when Danfa began research into TBAs in the early 1970s, they were surprised to find that around half were male.[164] Historically, only women were trained as midwives by the colonial government, disregarding the fact that both men and women played this role.[165] The idea that 'official' midwives would be women became normalised. However, Danfa's identification that half of TBAs were male seems high; it is possible their categorisation was misleading and included healers more generally.

Certainly, male healers possessed knowledge about women's reproductive health. They also passed this knowledge down along generational lines. For example, in Barabadze in Central Region, Nana Esebu's father was a herbalist. He worked as a birth attendant as well as prescribing medicines. She said, 'he was attending to delivery … he knows the medicine [for] when someone is pregnant … and when he administers the medicine the person [got] healed, especially pregnant women [were] able to deliver safely.' He had a good reputation for protecting pregnant women's health, administering precise herbal remedies for each month of pregnancy. Other women from the village said that he also used to help those who were struggling with infertility or frequent miscarriages.[166] Recounting this village history challenges the gendered roles that were made rigid through training programmes and rural health projects.

WHO was concerned that population policies encouraging family planning would put pressure on limited MCH services in developing countries.[167] In 1973, it therefore held consultations with representatives from all over the world to 'define the role traditional birth attendants may play in a programme of maternity and family planning care.'[168] WHO reported that 'in many developing countries organized health services, including MCH, do not yet provide adequate coverage for the population.'[169] They reported that

> some TBAs have 'training' on the job by their predecessors. Others may be a neighbour or an older member of the family who are called upon, or happen to be on the spot, to render assistance to the women in labour.[170]

WHO, therefore, saw an urgent need to train TBAs, as Stacy Leigh Pigg notes, as a 'pragmatic interim solution on the way to "modern" health services.'[171] WHO proposed that TBAs be trained in developing countries 'to bridge the gulf that exists between the ideal (adequate obstetricians, paediatricians, nurse/midwives, midwives, hospital facilities, etc.) and existing conditions.'[172] The 'ideal' was exclusively biomedical and usually hospital-based.

WHO organised a survey of TBAs in Africa in 1973. They sent questionnaires to 34 African countries, of which only three officially recognised TBAs as part of the health service.[173] In the African Region, WHO planned training to bring TBAs 'under supervision' and to 'help them to do clean and safer deliveries'[174] noting, 'the community should be involved in the motivation of traditional birth attendants to accept further training.'[175] Similarly, Danfa stated that 'TBAs can be an important part of … village based PHC programme[s]' especially in integrating biomedical options with existing health systems. Other members of the community, particularly the chiefs, elders and village representatives, would ideally work with schemes training TBAs.[176] Visions for TBA training adhered to PHC doctrine: it should be community-driven and use available resources. However, whilst acknowledging TBAs' value in delivering babies, and as community opinion leaders, the training ultimately aimed to challenge and change 'traditional' practices.

As a result of development agencies' involvement in one Nepalese village, Pigg showed that categories of birth attendants, which differed according to complex individual contexts, were simplified to create one identity of 'TBA.'[177] Arguably, similar processes occurred in Ghana. TBAs formed part of a complex health landscape, which included government health workers, spiritualists and herbalists. Women had diverse relationships with those who attended their deliveries. Some were family members, some were paid, some were not, most were women but some were men, some were village herbalists, others were spiritualists. Knowledge of basic herbal remedies for pregnancy and childbirth was relatively widespread and passed along generations.[178] The idea that TBAs were people who 'happened to be on the spot,' as WHO suggested, underestimated TBAs' expertise. Although they were not trained by any 'official' source, they did learn from more experienced professionals like themselves. TBAs were 'an influential figure, well versed in folklore relating to maternal and infant care and … likely to be among the highly respected members of the community.'[179] Oral histories confirm that TBAs were well respected. However, the hope expressed by WHO that they would 'have contact with a large number of women when they are highly motivated to adopt family planning'[180] was not reflected in interviews: no interviewee learned about family planning through a TBA, and the majority of TBAs did not engage with 'modern' family planning at this time.[181]

Training TBAs

Ekuah Nkrumah's grandmother was a TBA and attended her when she gave birth in the early 1950s. She attended many women in Ekuah's village in Central

Region, about 20 kilometres from Cape Coast. For training, Ekuah said 'the old people didn't go anywhere ... it was something they understood and did on their own.'[182] Similarly, Adjoa Ewusiwa said 'I didn't even learn it ... it was my gift.'[183] Aunty Moses Ackon's knowledge came to her in a dream, in which her aunt was about to give birth. In the dream, her mother, a TBA, told her she was too old to perform deliveries. So, Aunty Moses helped her aunt to give birth, dreaming what to do and which medicines to administer. In the morning, she woke up and her aunt was indeed in labour. Assisted by Aunty Moses, she gave birth to a baby girl. From then on, Aunty Moses worked as a TBA. She did not receive any other training until much later when 'the government summoned all of the birth attendants to the hospital.'[184] The way that TBAs talk about themselves, decades after they began practice, is illuminating. Through claiming that their knowledge was innate, or the result of spiritual intervention, they appear to disregard or take for granted ways in which knowledge was shared and passed. Arguably, these narratives explaining their knowledge keep it sacred, and in the hands of those it belongs to: there was an important spiritual element to the role.

However, interviews clearly showed older TBAs training younger women. Araba Yedua, who we met in Chapter 3, began practising as a TBA in the 1960s. She began 'following' an older TBA, Maame Ashia, at the age of 12. Maame Ashia 'was very much respected' in the local community in Western Ghana. She knew which herbs to give to women at each stage of pregnancy, to help with vomiting, to help the child move around in utero and to help in childbirth. She was expert, especially in difficult placental deliveries. Araba helped Maame Ashia; she admired her work and pregnancy in general. When Ashia died, Araba took over. Araba learnt a lot from the older woman, but nothing concerning hygiene or nutrition. This she learnt later on a training course at the health centre at Agona Nkwanta, the nearest town.[185]

Aunty Moses was not the only woman to remember being 'summoned' to the hospital, when the government started training programmes. Most formal TBA training often came much later. Many informants who had been working as TBAs since the 1960s testified that there was no obligation or opportunity for training until the 1990s or early 2000s.[186] Earlier training programmes targeted specific geographical areas or constituted less formal interventions. Interest in TBAs' roles extended to their possible influence in family planning uptake. In 1972, NFPP proposed a research project into how far 'traditional healers' influenced peoples' attitudes to family planning,[187] and another in 1973 on the subject of training TBAs in family planning.[188] By 1974, NFPP's annual report stated that TBAs 'should be recruited and trained for the provision of health and family planning services at the villages level.'[189] Importantly, their need was associated particularly with the 'village level,' something NFPP had so far avoided.

Aba Yaa Badiwa lived in Abakrampa and worked as a cocoa farmer as well as a TBA. She remembered that at some point in the late 1970s, the government began to get tough on TBAs. They were called to the hospital for training and issued with papers. By the time Rawlings was in power, Aba remembers that those who were not registered faced arrest if anything went wrong with the deliveries they performed. Despite the implicit threats in these interventionist methods, Aba testified TBAs 'were not reluctant [to go]. Most people use the opportunity to go and learn. There are some people who depended so much on the delivery ... there was no way they could stop, so they went.' For others, 'their husbands forced them to stop, because they did not want any trouble.' During the training, the TBAs were taught to ensure smooth delivery, to cut and tie the umbilical cord hygienically, and postnatal care for women. 'You know women are quite complicated,' she told me, 'we are not like men.'[190]

Esi Dwanwa also worked in a village in close proximity to Cape Coast and attended hospital training in the 1970s.[191] Her grandmother had been a TBA and had assisted her mother in giving birth to all her children. Esi worked first as a seamstress and a farmer, and became a TBA after she 'finished marrying.' She attended training for TBAs delivered by doctors and nurses at Cape Coast hospital in the late 1970s. She went for training 'to learn how to do it well.' She admitted that she did not go willingly; people from the hospital came to her village to seek out TBAs. At the hospital they taught them to feel for the head of the baby to understand when a woman was ready to deliver, not to push her to go through labour too quickly and to begin examining the woman after her water had broken.[192] She was told that if there were any complications, women should be brought directly to the hospital. In fact, she later stopped attending to women who had not attended hospital for antenatal checks, as it was too risky. In the end, she saw the training as beneficial.[193] It is possible that, like the Danfa project, there was a local TBA training scheme at Cape Coast hospital in the 1970s that explains this early training. If there was, it did not reach all of the TBAs in the area. However, by 1981 doctors working in Ghana reported to WHO that 'a large number of traditional healers have been educated in modern midwifery,' especially through the Danfa project.[194]

Interestingly, none of the women called for training in the 1970s or 1980s remembered the course covering family planning. However, the government, WHO and NGOs clearly envisaged family planning as a component of TBA training programmes.[195] WHO hoped TBAs would 'have contact with a large number of women when they are highly motivated to adopt family planning.'[196] TBAs were seen as respected members of the community that could persuade women to take it up.

One of Danfa's aims was to train TBAs in a rural setting, to encourage the availability of basic but effective healthcare. The justification for this was that it was cheap and not dependent on transport. Indeed, these factors probably explain the government's motivation for such programmes, given the economic crisis. In the government's *Summary of Primary Health Care Concept*, published when PHC was officially adopted in 1978, three levels of healthcare workers were identified. The first level were community members, such as TBAs. From this group, workers were to be 'selected and compensated by the community itself, but trained ... with emphasis on pregnancy management, child health promotion, environmental sanitation, and mobilisation for health-related community projects.'[197] The idea that health workers should be 'compensated by the community itself' was surely important for a government struggling to provide medical staff. Furthermore, although this was not supposed to be gendered, the areas of healthcare mentioned here, especially pregnancy management and child health promotion, meant that women's free labour was envisaged above all.

However, there was a further justification for this move, to do with a wider rejection of medicalisation, especially of birth and death.[198] A Danfa training manual for TBAs stated that training them:

> allows childbirth to take place in a more natural setting. Rather than being confined to bed in a hospital separated from her infant and running risk of cross infection, the woman can deliver in her own home, surrounded by her family. Bonding of the mother to the infant may be enhanced ... and most village women prefer to deliver at home.[199]

This language equates women's bodily experiences with what is 'natural.' Accordingly, women's place at the centre of their families is seen as natural. Finally, the idea that 'village women' – a category that connotes ignorance, tradition and illiteracy – would prefer to deliver at home glosses over the fact that health services were often simply unavailable.

More organic 'training' happened as the result of pragmatic relationships in individual villages. CHN Munirata Yahaya explained that it was useless to tell people in the community not to go to TBAs; they would not listen and besides there were no other options. Instead, she talked to TBAs, spiritualists, herbalists, encouraging them to bring pregnant women to clinic so that they could 'all do it together so they can learn something.' 'And it worked!' she said, they began to train TBAs. Moreover, women that had been frightened to come to clinics because of strange facilities, equipment or practices were brought in by TBAs. Importantly, Munirata emphasised that 'TBAs were already there for them, you couldn't discourage them from that.'[200] Working in a small village just outside Accra, Florence Boateng remembered a similar dynamic between CHNs and TBAs. She said that she guided TBAs in how to improve their delivery technique and prevent infection: 'you tell them, you teach them, you don't even shout at her, because she doesn't know.' Like Munirata, she said: 'whether we allow them to deliver or not they will do it because the women are familiar with them so it's better that we train them.'[201] In other words, both women accepted the inevitability of women choosing TBAs whom they lived among. Most TBAs I interviewed testified that payment from clients was irregular. If money was given, it was a small amount and usually for herbal remedies rather than women's services directly.[202] Although this may be a way to grumble that their work was not remunerated adequately, TBAs represented a cheaper option.

Florence Boateng said that these informal training relationships led to the establishment of training programmes in the 1990s and 2000s.[203]

Working with 'Tradition'

Julianna Brown, Regional Director for PPAG, worked as a nurse in the 1970s. She said that 'traditional' beliefs were strong in the 1970s. When women were pregnant they did not eat eggs, and they were delivered by TBAs, paying them through the 'barter system.' Couples performed rituals at shrines to avoid pregnancies. They might also use lemon, enemas, douching or abstinence. According to Brown, these kinds of traditional practices 'caused havoc,' due to their inefficacy. She connects an adherence to tradition with a lack of control over fertility. Indeed, most programmes promoting family planning in Ghana in the 1970s and early 1980s disregarded 'traditional' methods including abstinence and withdrawal. Interviewees testified to these being widely used. For example, Araba Yedua did not have intercourse with her husband for ten months following childbirth to avoid pregnancy, Esi Praah waited six months and then only slept with her husband at times of the month when she could not become pregnant, Meriam Alassa waited for a year.[204] Because these arrangements often involved family structures that differed from the Western-centric nuclear model, they were disregarded.

Danfa, like many international health and development programmes, premised their project on the delivery of modernity. Modernity and PHC had a complicated relationship. As van Der Geest and Krause pointed out, 'traditional' in terms of medicine 'throws together every type of thinking and acting that differs from biomedicine.'[205] In this sense, it is not a useful term as it has a tendency to simplify pluralistic health systems like that described throughout this study. PHC was supposed to incorporate 'traditional' aspects of societies' medical cultures. This was something fought for as freshly decolonised nations added their voices to the World Health Assembly.[206] On the other hand, PHC was supposed to bring 'modern' medicine to communities that it had so far eluded. An ambiguous relationship between tradition and modernity was established. Alfred Neumann, head of Danfa, questioned,

> [s]hould we … seek out those individuals who have already accepted other innovations such as new crop procedures, modern styles of clothing, have transistor radios etc. on the theory that such people are more likely to accept … family planning measures?[207]

That is, should they accept that only 'modern' Ghanaians would embrace family planning? Danfa's answer to this question was, ultimately, no. However, the fact that their family planning efforts were framed in this way suggests that they saw tradition as an obstacle.

Meanwhile, Danfa embraced aspects it saw as traditional to encourage the uptake of birth control: they related birth spacing to the 'traditional belief in the need to space children to prevent kwashiorkor.'[208] It stated that TBA training should not only involve teaching 'modern' practices but also take an 'interest in learning more about applying traditional birth practices to deliveries at the health centre.'[209] It sought to endorse traditional practices where it could, and not to criticise those it categorised as 'neutral.' However, a lot of the research that Danfa did into traditional practices was not with the aim of incorporating them. Surveys of TBAs' practices aided them in 'correct[ing] widely practiced but harmful techniques.'[210]

IOs redefined tradition according to its 'good' and 'bad' aspects. For example, the Centre for Scientific Research into Plant Medicine at Mampong-Akwapim's main function was to work with herbalists for the 'purpose of improvement in the areas of hygiene, dosages stability, palatability, presentability etc.' Doctors at the Centre reported to WHO that traditional healers should also work at village health posts to 'educate' the villagers. For this, '*genuine* traditional healers should be trained in simple hygiene, immunisation, the non-supernatural basis of most diseases and preventative medicine.' In other words, once again, traditional healers' work was judged as valuable but only after certain practices had been abolished. Furthermore, traditional healers were categorised as 'genuine' or otherwise, according to unstated criteria. These healers should work at village health posts from which they were encouraged to send clients to health centres 'manned by *experienced* nurses, traditional healers and midwives.' Again, this suggests that TBAs' experience was not valued.[211]

In 1973, according to WHO reports, TBA training was 'intensifying' in Ghana. However, this was 'bitterly opposed' by the Midwives Board.[212] Apparently, they wanted to protect their official status and not have to compete with TBAs. Nevertheless, Danfa's work with TBAs culminated with the production of a training manual in 1977, jointly with the MH. In the manual, 2 of the 15 sessions outlined were on family planning. It instructed that sessions should be short and avoid technical language. Instead, there should be demonstrations, role plays and participatory methods. TBAs were instructed on multiple benefits of family planning: firstly, women would have the opportunity to work and give their children adequate care if they had fewer pregnancies. Families' and communities' living standards would rise. There would be better amenities, jobs, less crime and overcrowding. In this way, benefits of limiting pregnancies would spread to the national level.[213] TBAs were encouraged to promote visions of progress as part of their work with family planning. The traditional role of the birth attendant was juxtaposed to the reward birth control promised: modernity.

Conclusion

Women's identities as female often intersected with their identities as 'rural.' Women were called upon to provide the healthcare necessary to reproduce families in ways that recalled colonial-style 'women's work.' This was exacerbated as MCH became a core component of BHS and PHC programmes implemented by the Ghanaian state. Women were expected to facilitate community-based heathcare, provide correct nutrition and respond to calls for TBA training. Furthermore, women's fertility continued to be targeted as problematic within this new paradigm. Development programme leaders expected rural women to adhere to timeless 'tradition' and approached health provision with this in mind. TBAs in particular had been characterised as uneducated, unhygienic and unknowledgeable since the colonial period. Evidently, sometimes quite the reverse was true. TBAs shared knowledge, especially with younger women who acted as apprentices. Nonetheless, when IOs and the Ghanaian government engaged with them, it was in the role of regulators and educators.

Notes

1 Daniel Immerwahr, *Thinking Small: The United States and the Lure of Community Development* (Cambridge, MA: Harvard University Press, 2014), 13.
2 Randall Packard, *A History of Global Health: Interventions into the Lives of Other Peoples* (Baltimore, MD: Johns Hopkins University Press, 2016), 227.
3 Nitsan Chorev, *World Health Organization Between North and South* (Ithaca, NY: Cornell University Press, 2012), 49–55.
4 Packard, *A History of Global Health*, 235.
5 For more details on the economic crisis between 1971 and 1983, see Takyiwaa Manuh, 'Ghana: Women in the Public and Informal Sectors Under the Economic Recovery Programme,' in *Mortgaging Women's Lives: Feminist Critiques of Structural Adjustment*, ed. Pamela Sparr and Takyiwaa Manuh (London: Palgrave Macmillan, 1994), 64–66.
6 Robert Darko Osei and Remi Jedwab, 'Structural Change in Ghana, 1960–2010,' conference paper delivered at Country Case Studies Workshop: "Structural Change in Developing Countries", World Bank, 2012, 5.
7 James Ferguson, *The Anti-Politics Machine: Development, Depoliticization and Bureaucratic Power in Lesotho*, New edition (Minneapolis, MN: University of Minnesota Press, 1994), xiv–xv.
8 Packard, *A History of Global Health*, 209.
9 M. Gorsky and C. Sirrs, 'The Rise and Fall of "Universal Health Coverage" as a Goal of International Health Politics, 1925–1952,' *American Journal of Public Health* 108 (2018): 334–42.
10 Deborah Atobrah and Benjamin Kwansa, 'Achieving Universal Health Coverage? A Focus on Constructions of Health and Ill-Health in Ghana' (European Conference of African Studies, University of Edinburgh, 2019).
11 Deborah Atobrah, 'Caring for the Seriously Sick in Ghanaian Society: Glimpses from the Past,' *Ghana Studies* 15/16 (2012/2013).
12 Perhaps most famously in the African context: Ester Boserup, *Woman's Role in Economic Development* (London: George Allen & Unwin Ltd, 1970). Women's roles were also debated at length within international organisations; 1975–1985 was the United Nations Decade for Women.
13 Sharon Fonn and T. K. Sundari Ravindran, 'The Macroeconomic Environment and Sexual and Reproductive Health: A Review of Trends over the Last 30 Years,' *Reproductive Health Matters* 19, no. 38 (January 2011): 11.
14 PRAAD, Accra, PD 232: 'Summary of Primary Health Care Concept,' National Health Planning Unit, Accra, 6 February 1978, 2.
15 Jennifer A. Hart, *Ghana on the Go: African Mobility in the Age of Motor Transportation* (Bloomington and Indianapolis: Indiana University Press, 2016), 123.
16 PRAAD, Accra, PD/232: 'Summary of Primary Health Care Concept,' 1.
17 For details of the reversal of many of the Nkrumah-era large-scale development projects, see Dan-Bright S. Dzorgbo, *Ghana in Search of Development: The Challenge of Governance, Economic Management and Institution Building* (Aldershot: Ashgate, 2001), 196–209.
18 PRAAD, Accra, ADM 5/1/573: *Annual Report of the Medical Services of Ghana, 1967*, E. Akwei, Director of Medical Services, Accra, n.d. 4.
19 PRAAD, Accra, ADM 7/5/101: *National Liberation Council Budget Statement, 1969–1970*, J. H. Mensah, Ministry of Finance, Accra, 1969, 17.
20 PRAAD, Accra, ADM 5/1/573: *Annual Report of the Medical Services*, 30.
21 Ibid., 56.
22 Ibid., 30.
23 PRAAD, Koforidua, ERG 1/1/27: 'Minutes of the 5th General Meeting of the Brong-Ahafo Regional Planning Committee,' 11 July 1969, 3.

24 PRAAD, Cape Coast, RG 1/9/6B: 'Fanti Nyankumasi Health Post – Request for Financial Assistance,' 3 June 1971, 1.
25 PRAAD, Cape Coast, RG 1/9/6B: Letter to Minister of Health, Mr S. D. Dombo from Omanhene Nana Sir Tsibu Darku, 3 June 1971.
26 Packard, *A History of Global Health*, 233.
27 PRAAD, Accra, PD 65 Vol II: 'Development of Basic Health Services. Plan of Operation. Second Edition – 1972,' Accra, April 1972, 2.
28 WHO, P9/445/8 GHA: 'Text of Plan of Operation for a Research Project on Community Involvement in Solving Local Health Problems in Ghana,' 1975, 1.
29 WHO, P9/445/8: Letter to Dr J Stromberg, WHO from Dr Julius M. Prince, USAID, 10 January 1975. See enclosure, 2.
30 See plans for Central Region made under Busia in 1971: PRAAD, Cape Coast, RG 1/9/28: 'Development of Basic Health Services in Central Region,' 30 July 1971.
31 PRAAD, Cape Coast, RG 1/9/28: Letter from Regional Medical Officer of Health to Director of Medical Services Accra, 30 July 1971.
32 Erasmus E. A. Agongo et al., 'Primary Health Care Systems: Comprehensive Case Study from Ghana,' PRIMASYS (Accra: World Health Organization, 2017), 13.
33 PRAAD, Cape Coast, RG 1/9/6B: 'Petition against the Siting of the Proposed Health Centre for Swedru-Nyakrom,' 15 May 1971.
34 PRAAD, Cape Coast, RG 1/9/6B: Letter from M. Caurie, addressee and date missing.
35 PRAAD, Cape Coast, RG 1/9/6B: 'Petition against the Siting of the Proposed Health Centre for Swedru-Nyakrom,' 15 May 1971.
36 PRAAD, Accra, PD/232: 'Health Policies for Ghana, January 1978, 1. PHC at the village level was supposed to be carried out on the principle of 'self-reliance' with villages led by Community Development Committees. These Committees were leaders in the community and responsible for directing health work and coordinate decision-making within the community. See WHO, SHS/Reg.Adv.74/WP.12: 'Community Involvement in Solving Local Health Problems (Ghana),' 29 April–3 May 1974, 5.
37 See file: PRAAD, Accra, PD/232 'Circular,' 1978–1993.
38 PRAAD, Accra, PD 232: 'Summary of Primary Health Care Concept,' National Health Planning Unit, Accra, 6 February, 1.
39 PRAAD, Cape Coast, RG 1/9/6B: Application for a Health Clinic at Assin Jakai, 30 May 1973.
40 Ibid.
41 PRAAD, Cape Coast, RG 1/9/6B: Note in file 15 June 1973. As we saw particularly in Chapter 3, distances between populations and health services were consistently prohibitive.
42 PRAAD, Cape Coast, RG 1/9/6B: 'Twifu Praso Health Centre,' 25 August 1971.
43 RAC, Ford Foundation Collection, Grant #07090496, Reel 4048: 'Ghana National Family Planning Programme Progress Report July 1971–June 1972,' Evaluation and Research Unit, Accra, n.d. but 1972, 1–2.
44 I. K. Acheampong, *Radio and Television Broadcast to the Nation by Colonel I. K. Acheampong, Chairman of the National Redemption Council, on the Devaluation and External Debts, on Saturday, 5th February, 1972*, Accra, 1972.
45 WHO, SHS/Reg.Adv.74/WP.12: 'Community Involvement in Solving Local Health Problems (Ghana),' 29 April–3 May 1974, 2.
46 National Redemption Council, *Towards a Brighter Future*, Information Services Department, Accra, n.d., 63.
47 Cape Coast, RG 1/9/28: Formal Opening of Awutu Bawjiase Health Centre by the Regional Commissioner Col. F. G. Bernasko, Wednesday, 29 November 1972. Address by Awutu Odefrey Nai Wyetey Agyeman Larbie II. In fact, this speech was overtly political, making statements of loyalty to the NRC and asking for their intervention into destoolment cases.

48 Packard, *A History of Global Health*, 232.
49 National Redemption Council, *Guidelines for the Five Year Development Plan, 1975–1980*, Accra, January 1975, 37.
50 PRAAD, Cape Coast, RG 1/9/7: 'Advertisement for "Straight" Midwifery, Community Health Nursing and Enrolled Nursing,' 1972.
51 Interview with Munirata Yahaya, Cape Coast, Central Region, 14 February 2018.
52 Interview with Florence Boateng, Ankaful, Central Region, 22 July 2019.
53 Interview with Mary Boanno and Martha Abena, Abrafo, Central Region, 23 July 2019.
54 Interview with Florence Boateng, Ankaful, Central Region, 22 July 2019.
55 EA, 'Workshop of "Training of Trainers in Programmes Designed to Improve the Quality of Rural Life" 5th–23rd May, 1975.'
56 Republic of Ghana, National Assembly, *Parliamentary Debates*, 4 February 1981, col. 35.
57 Ibid., col. 291.
58 Interview with Dr Joseph Atobrah, Sekondi, Western Region, 26 October 2017.
59 Republic of Ghana, National Assembly, *Parliamentary Debates*, 4 February 1981, col. 35.
60 Packard, *A History of Global Health*, 249.
61 Patrick Twumasi, 'History of Pluralistic Medical Systems: A Sociological Analysis of the Ghanaian Case,' *Issue: A Journal of Opinion* 9, no. 3 (1979): 121.
62 'Health Services Collapse if …,' *Daily Graphic*, 19 February 1981, 1.
63 'Bureaucracy at Health Ministry Condemned,' *Daily Graphic*, 24 February 1981, 1.
64 'Good Health Is Paramount,' *Daily Graphic*, 27 February 1981, 2.
65 See, for example, 'Health Workers Protest Against Fee Imposition,' *Daily Graphic*, 30 April 1981, 1 and 'Limann Tells Doctors … Stop Charging Fees,' *Daily Graphic*, 7 May 1981, 1.
66 *Ghana: Economic Position and Prospects*, World Bank, 29 June 1977, 1.
67 PRAAD, Accra, PD/232: 'Annual Estimates 1979–80,' 30 March 1979, 1.
68 *Ghana: Economic Position and Prospects*, World Bank, 29 June 1977, 7. Insufficient rainfall meant that the availability of crops such as sorghum, rice and maize was affected. The effects of this drought were felt in the years following its conclusion in 1977; see *Ghana Economic Memorandum*, World Bank, 24 April 1979, 1.
69 Interview with Adua Tekyiwa, Jukwa, Central Region, 23 July 2019.
70 Republic of Ghana, National Assembly, *Parliamentary Debates,* 4 February 1981, col. 40.
71 *Ghana: Economic Position and Prospects*, World Bank, 29 June 1977, 5.
72 *Ghana Economic Memorandum*, World Bank, 24 April 1979, 1.
73 Republic of Ghana, National Assembly, *Parliamentary Debates*, 4 February 1981, col. 292–293.
74 PRAAD, Accra, PD/192: 'Memorandum to the Committee on Drugs,' 1973, 1–3.
75 Republic of Ghana, National Assembly, *Parliamentary Debates*, 4 February 1981, col. 46.
76 PRAAD, Cape Coast, RG 1/9/7: Letter from Nana Amani V, President of Asebu Traditional Council to Regional Administrative Officer, Cape Coast, 27 May 1974.
77 Republic of Ghana, National Assembly, *Parliamentary Debates*, 4 February 1981, col. 283.
78 Ibid., col. 290.
79 Ibid., col. 284.
80 Interview with Nana Efua Ateifi I, New Ebu, Central Region, 22 July 2019.
81 The drop in the birth rate between 1971 and 1982 reflects this and almost certainly had more to do with economic decline than the availability of contraception. See World Bank Data, 'Birth Rate, Crude (per 1,000 People)' [Last accessed 28/12/2021] https://data.worldbank.org/indicator/SP.DYN.CBRT.IN?end=2019&locations=GH&start=1960&view=chart.

82 Interview with Adua Dua, Abrafo, Central Region, 23 July 2019.
83 For a more general account on missionaries promoting their domestic ideals in Africa, see Jean Comaroff and John Comaroff, 'Homemade Hegemony: Modernity, Domesticity, and Colonialism in South Africa,' in *African Encounters with Domesticity*, ed. Karen Tranberg Hansen (New Brunswick, NJ: Rutgers University Press, 1992), 31–74.
84 Gloria Ampim, 'An Historical Analysis of Maternal and Infant Welfare in Ghana: 1957–1980' (unpublished MPhil thesis, University of Ghana, 2011); Jessica Cammaert, *Undesirable Practices: Women, Children, and the Politics of the Body in Northern Ghana, 1930–1972* (Lincoln, NE: University of Nebraska Press, 2016).
85 Atobrah, 'Caring for the Seriously Sick,' 84–85.
86 Benedetta Rossi, 'What "Development" Does to Work,' *International Labour and Working Class History* 92 (2017): 7–23.
87 EA, 'Speech Delivered by Hon. K. P. Agyekum, Ministerial Secretary, Ministry of Youth, Rural Development and Social Welfare on the Role of Women in Rural Re-construction … to Ghana Assembly of Women,' 2 December 1971, 1.
88 Ibid., 2.
89 E. G. Beausoleil, 'Protecting Ghana's Children,' *World Health*, no. 2 (1977), 30.
90 Eva M. Rathgeber, 'WID, WAD, GAD: Trends in Research and Practice,' *Journal of Developing Areas* 24 (1990): 490–91.
91 PRAAD, Sekondi, WRG 15/3/266: 'Quarterly Progress Report Covering the Period from 1January–30 April, 1978,' 20 April 1978, 1.
92 Ibid., 2.
93 Jennifer Hyndman and Malathi de Alwis, 'Beyond Gender: Towards a Feminist Analysis of Humanitarianism and Development in Sri Lanka,' *Women's Studies Quarterly* 31, no. 3/4 (2003): 213.
94 Rathgeber, 'WID, WAD, GAD,' 492.
95 PRAAD, Sekondi, WRG 15/3/266: 'Annual Report on Integrated Rural Development Assisted Pilot Project Training Laboratory. Tarkwa District Western Region. January–December, 1978,' 3.
96 PRAAD, Sekondi, WRG 15/3/266: 'Days for the Opening of Clinics,' 19 April 1978.
97 PRAAD, Sekondi, WRG 15/3/266: 'Quarterly Report,' 30 April 1978, 2.
98 Ibid., 3.
99 PRAAD, Sekondi, WRG 15/3/266: 'Modern Skills Training: Closing of Course,' 13 March 1979.
100 Ibid.
101 Achola O. Pala, 'Definitions of Women and Development: An African Perspective,' in *African Gender Studies A Reader*, ed. Oyèrónkẹ́ Oyěwùmí (New York: Palgrave Macmillan US, 2005), 299–300.
102 'The Home and the Homemaker,' *The Ghanaian Woman* 2, no. 1&2 (1976), 21–22.
103 EA, 'The Impact of Home Science Impressions and Observations in Ghana,' May 10 1975.
104 Gwendolyn Mikell, 'Pleas for Domestic Relief: Akan Women and Family Courts,' in *African Feminism*, ed. Gwendolyn Mikell (Philadelphia, PA: University of Pennsylvania Press, 1997), 97–99.
105 RAC, Ford Foundation, Grant #07090496, Reel 4048: 'Foundation-Administrated Project. Request no. ID-1059,' 3.
106 RAC, Ford Foundation, Grant #07090496, Reel 4048: Summary Evaluation and Recommendation for Close-Out, DAP 709-0496A B 'Assistance to Family Planning Activities in Ghana,' by Katherine McKee (with contributions from Oyewole P. Owolabi), 20 May 1982, 3.
107 Ibid., 1.
108 Ibid., 1.
109 Ibid., 3.

110 WHO, P13/372/6: Memorandum from WHO Liaison Officer with ECA to Dr Bellervie Director CE, 25 October 1968.
111 Emily Callaci, '"Injectable Development" Depo-Provera and Creation of the Global South,' *Radical History Review* 131 (2018): 93.
112 Matthew Connelly, *Fatal Misconception* (Cambridge, MA: Harvard University Press, 2009), 312.
113 WHO, P13/372/9: 'UNFPA Priorities in Allocation of Resources.' Report by Executive Director, 3 December 1975, 3.
114 RAC, Ford Foundation Collection, Grant #07090496, Reel 4048: 'Ghana National Family Planning Programme Progress Report July 1971–June 1972,' Evaluation and Research Unit, Accra, n.d. but 1972, 3.
115 'Suspend Family Planning Scheme,' *Daily Graphic*, 27 April 1981, 1.
116 'Family Planning is not in Our Interest,' *Daily Graphic*, 19 May 1981, 5.
117 Ama Ata Aidoo, *Changes: A Love Story* (Oxford: Heinemann Educational Publishers, 1991), 16.
118 WHO, P13/372/9: Letter from R. H. O. Bannerman, Chief Medical Officer for Education and Family Health, WHO, to Dr Boi-Doku, 7 December 1970.
119 WHO, P13/372/9 GHA: Letter from Director of Medical Services to WHO Regional Office, 10 December 1972.
120 RAC, Population Council, Box 234 Folder 2176: 'Family Planning: Within and Beyond Maternal and Child Health,' by G. Perkin, 30 October 1970, 3.
121 See Chapter 5 above.
122 WHO, P13/372/12: Letter to Dr Zahra, Director of Family Health, WHO, from Bernard Berelson, Population Council, 10 December 1970.
123 Ibid.
124 WHO, P13/372/12: Memorandum from Dr Zahra, Director of Family Health, WHO to AFRO Regional Director, 6 October 1972.
125 A. Rosenfield and D. Maine, 'Maternal Mortality—A Neglected Tragedy. Where Is the M in MCH?,' *Lancet* 2, no. 8446 (13 July 1985): 85.
126 Pala, 'Definitions of Women and Development,' 300.
127 WHO, P13/372/9: 'Danfa Comprehensive Rural Health and Family Planning Project: Ghana. Semi-Annual Progress Report July 1972–December 1972,' University of California, Los Angeles and University of Ghana, 1973, 3.
128 Daniel A. Ampofo et al., 'The Danfa Family Planning Program in Rural Ghana,' *Studies in Family Planning* 7 (1976): 266. The authors of this paper either worked for the Danfa project or acted as advisers to it.
129 WHO, P 13/372/9: Letter from A. Neumann, Danfa, to Dr Martikainen, WHO, 8 October 1971.
130 RAC, Ford Foundation, Grant #07090496, Reel 4048: 'Ghana National Family Planning Programme Monthly Report on Family Planning Acceptors July, 1972,' Evaluation and Research Unit, Accra, 1972, 5.
131 Lamptey, Wurapa and Nicholas, 'The Evolution of a Primary Health Care Programme: The Danfa Experience 1970–1977,' 253. Dr P. Lamptey and Dr D. Nicholas worked with the Danfa project as advisers.
132 Ampofo et al., 'The Danfa Family Planning Program,' 267.
133 Rosenfield and Maine, 'Maternal Mortality,' 83. This article found that maternal mortality was drastically underreported throughout Africa.
134 WHO, M2/372/3/GHA: Letter from Dr Strudwick WHO AFRO Representative in Ghana to S. Falkland Public Health Administration. Contains enclosure 'Special Report P.H.A./B.H.S. Ghana-1,' 20 November 1964, 23.
135 Lamptey, Wurapa and Nicholas, 'The Evolution,' 252. My italics.
136 WHO, P13/372/9: 'Danfa Comprehensive Rural Health and Family Planning Project: Ghana. Semi-Annual Progress Report July 1972–December 1972,' University of California, Los Angeles and University of Ghana, 1973, 5.

137 Lamptey, Wurapa and Nicholas, 'The Evolution,' 252.
138 WHO, P13/372/9: 'Danfa Comprehensive Rural Health and Family Planning Project: Ghana. Semi-Annual Progress Report July 1972–December 1972,' University of California, Los Angeles and University of Ghana, 1973, 1.
139 Ampofo et al., 'The Danfa Family Planning Program,' 267.
140 Neumann, Alfred, *Danfa Comprehensive Rural Health and Family Planning Project: Ghana. UCLA Annual Progress Report. January–December, 1974*, 1.
141 WHO, P13/372/6: Letter from R. T. Ravenholt, USAID to Albert Zahra, Director of Family Health, WHO, 13 March 1973.
142 Ampofo et al., 'The Danfa Family Planning Program,' 268.
143 WHO, P13/372/9: 'A Programme Manual for Traditional Birth Attendants. Organization, Training, Evaluation,' Accra, December 1977, 2.
144 Rosenfield and Maine, 'Maternal Mortality,' 83.
145 Beth Maina Ahlberg, *Women, Sexuality, and the Changing Social Order: The Impact of Government Policies on Reproductive Behavior in Kenya* (Philadelphia, PA: Gordon and Breach, 1991), 197.
146 WHO, P13/372/9: 'Danfa Comprehensive Rural Health and Family Planning Project: Ghana: Semi-Annual Progress Report July 1972–December 1972,' 16 October 1972, 5.
147 WHO, P13/372/9: *Manual 'A' and 'B' for Health Workers and Serving Personnel*, Ghana Publishing Corporation, Tema, March 1977, 6–7.
148 See, for example, PD 65: 'Approved Lists of Drugs for Health Centres and Health Posts and Maternal and Child Health Centres,' 16 July 1981.
149 WHO, P13/372/9: *Manual 'A' and 'B' for Health Workers and Serving Personnel*, Ghana Publishing Corporation, Tema, March 1977, 6.
150 Ibid., 9.
151 Ibid., 10.
152 Interview with Patience Doris Doh, Koforidua, Eastern Region, 24 January 2018.
153 Interview with Magdalene Juliet Ackuah, Cape Coast, Central Region, 9 February 2018.
154 Twumasi, 'History of Pluralistic Medical Systems,' 122. See also Chapter 1 above.
155 NA, CO 859/838/12001/10: Advisory Committee on Education in the Colonies, *Report of a Sub-Committee on the Education and Welfare of Women and Girls in Africa*, Colonial Office, London, 12th February 1943, 7. See Chapter 2 above.
156 Interview with Dr Mensah, Takoradi, Western Region, 26 October 2017.
157 Interview with Rosina Apraku, Koforidua, Eastern Region, 25 January 2018.
158 Dennis Michael Warren and Mary Ann Tregoning, 'Indigenous Healers and Primary Health Care in Ghana,' *Medical Anthropology Newsletter* 11, no. 1 (1979): 11.
159 WHO, N 2/180/3: 'Information Bulletin I,' 20 February 1973.
160 WHO, N2/180/3: 'Traditional Birth Attendants, Summary of Analysis,' see summary table, 1.
161 Patrick Twumasi and Dennis Michael Warren, 'The Professionalisation,' 118.
162 WHO, N2/180/3 AFR: 'Training and Supervision of Traditional Birth Attendants: Report of a Study Group, Brazzaville, 9–12 December 1975,' by Dr R. H. Bannerman, 2.
163 N 2/180/3 AFR: 'Study Group on the Training and Supervision of Traditional Birth Attendants: Glossary of Terms,' 9–12 December 1975.
164 N 2/180/3: Letter from Alfred Neumann, Danfa, to Dr Pettros-Barvazian, WHO, 29 November 1972.
165 PRAAD, Accra, CSO 5/1/327: 'The Midwives Ordinance,' 1931.
166 Interview with Ama Fosua, Adua Bensua, Nana Esebu and Esi Mensema at Barabadze, Central Region, 30 November 2017.
167 WHO, N2/180/3: 'Consultation on the Role of the Traditional Birth Attendant, 12–19 March 1973,' Geneva, Enclosed in Memorandum from Chief Nursing Officer to Dr E. Braga, WHO, 24 November 1972, 1.

168 WHO, N 2/180/3: 'Information Bulletin I,' 20 February 1973.
169 WHO, N2/180/3: 'Consultation on the Role of the Traditional Birth Attendant, 12–19 March 1973,' Geneva, Enclosed in Memorandum from Chief Nursing Officer to Dr E. Braga, WHO, 24 November 1972, Enclosure: 'Background Documentation,' 1.
170 Ibid., 2.
171 Stacy Leigh Pigg, 'Authority in Translation. Finding, Knowing, Naming and Training 'Traditional Birth Attendants' in Nepal,' in *Childbirth and Authoritative Knowledge: Cross-Cultural Perspectives*, ed. Robbie E. Davis-Floyd, Carolyn F. Sargent, and Rayna Rapp (Berkeley: University of California Press, 1997), 233–62.
172 WHO, N2/180/3 AFR: 'Proposals for Training Traditional Birth Attendants (Empirical Midwives),' Enclosed in Memorandum from Mrs. R. E. Marshall HNS for Regional Director to all Nursing/Midwifery Personnel, 15 May 1974, 2.
173 WHO, N2/180/3: 'Traditional Birth Attendants, Summary of Analysis,' Enclosed in Memorandum from Dorothy Potts HMD/NUR for Regional Director to Chief Nursing Officer, 30 January 1973, 1.
174 WHO, N2/180/3 AFR: 'Proposals for Training Traditional Birth Attendants (Empirical Midwives),' Enclosed in Memorandum from Mrs. R. E. Marshall HNS for Regional Director to all Nursing/Midwifery Personnel, 15 May 1974, 2.
175 WHO, N2/180/3 AFR: 'Training and Supervision of Traditional Birth Attendants: Report of a Study Group, Brazzaville, 9th–12th December 1975,' by Dr R. H. Bannerman, 3.
176 WHO, P13/372/9: 'A Programme Manual for Traditional Birth Attendants. Organization, Training, Evaluation,' Accra, December 1977, 3.
177 Stacy Leigh Pigg, '"Found in Most Traditional Societies" Traditional Medical Practitioners between Culture and Development,' in *International Development and the Social Science: Essays on the History of Politics of Knowledge,* ed. Frederick Cooper and Randall Packard (Berkeley: University of California Press, 1998), 259–90.
178 Interviews carried out between October 2017 and July 2019 with women who had given birth, mainly in rural areas, evidenced this wide array of experiences.
179 WHO, N2/180/3: 'Consultation on the Role of the Traditional Birth Attendant, 12–19 March 1973,' Geneva, Enclosed in Memorandum from Chief Nursing Officer to Dr E. Braga, WHO, 24 November 1972, 1.
180 Ibid., 2.
181 Interviews carried out between October 2017 and July 2019.
182 Interview with Ekuah Nkrumah, Koforidua, Central Region, 27 November 2017.
183 Interview with Adjoa Ewusiwa, New Ebu, Central Region, 22 July 2019.
184 Interview with Aunty Moses, Adjumako, Western Region, 23 October 2017.
185 Interview with Araba Yedua, Gyabenkrom, Western Region, 27 October 2017.
186 Interviews carried out in July 2019 in Abrafo and New Ebu in Central Region testified to this. Women had certificates showing that they had passed TBA training programmes in 2001 and 2006, and had identity badges with their pictures which made them legal practitioners. Florence Boateng, a retired midwife, who worked as TBA trainer, remembered that training programmes for TBAs formally began in 1990. However, before that as a Community Health Nurse she also taught TBAs certain methods informally. Interview Florence Boateng, Ankaful, Central Region, 22 July 2019.
187 RAC, Ford Foundation Papers, Reel 4048: 'The National Family Planning Programme and Social Science Research,' Dr A. A. Armar, January 1972, 1.
188 RAC, Population Council Papers, Box 564 Folder 5422: Memorandum 'Re: Russell Visit to Ghana National Family Planning Programme,' 18 October 1973, 2.
189 RAC, Ford Foundation Collection, Grant #07090496, Reel 4048: 'Ghana National Family Planning Programme Fourth Annual Report (July 1973–June 1974), n.d. but 1974, 8.
190 Interview with Aba Yaa Badiwa, Abakrampa, Central Region, 29 November 2017.

191 Other interviewees mentioned training at this hospital, for example, Georgina Hermance, Moree, Central Region, 28 November 2017. Georgina's mother had been a healer for decades, attending women in childbirth, preparing herbal remedies and helping women to conceive when she was called for training.
192 It was a common theme when interviewing TBAs and midwives that they had been taught when to tell women to start pushing after the cervix was fully dilated, something they were not doing correctly before.
193 Interview with Esi Dwanwa, Koforidua, Central Region, 27 November 2017.
194 WHO, TRM/MTG/81.9: 'Traditional Medicine Role of Collaborating Centres,' by Professor Adjepon-Yamoah and Dr Ampofo, November 1972, 3.
195 WHO, P13/372/9: 'Danfa Comprehensive Rural Health and Family Planning Project: Ghana. Semi-Annual Progress Report July 1972–December 1972,' University of California, Los Angeles and University of Ghana, 1973, 5.
196 WHO, N2/180/3: 'Consultation on the Role of the Traditional Birth Attendant, 12–19 March 1973,' Geneva, Enclosed in Memorandum from Chief Nursing Officer to Dr E. Braga, WHO, 24 November 1972, 2.
197 PRAAD, Accra, PD 232: 'Summary of Primary Health Care Concept,' National Health Planning Unit, Accra, 6 February 1978, 1.
198 Packard, *A History of Global Health*, 241.
199 WHO, P13/372/9: 'A Programme Manual for Traditional Birth Attendants: Organization, Training, Evaluation,' Accra, December 1977, 1.
200 Interview with Munirata Lardi Yahaya, Cape Coast, Central Region, 14 February 2018.
201 Interview with Florence Boateng, Ankaful, Central Region, 22 July 2019.
202 For example, interview with Georgina Hermance, Moree, Central Region, 28 November 2018; interview with Esi Dwanwa, Koforidua, Central Region, 27 November 2018.
203 Interview with Florence Boateng, Ankaful, Central Region, 22 July 2019.
204 Interviews with Araba Yedua, Gyabenkrom, Western Region, 27 October 2017; Esi Praah, Mpatase, Western Region, 25 October 2017; Mariam Alassa, Abra, Western Region, 25 October 2017.
205 Sjaak van der Geest and Kristine Krause, 'Introduction: Studying Health and Health Care in Ghana,' *Ghana Studies* 15/16 (2012/13): 9.
206 Sung Lee, 'WHO and the Developing World: The Contest for Ideology,' in *Western Medicine as Contested Knowledge*, ed. Andrew Cunningham and Bridie Andrews (Manchester: Manchester University Press, 1997), 24–45.
207 WHO, P13/372/9: 'Letter from A Neumann, Danfa, to Dr Morafi, WHO,' 11 February 1972.
208 WHO, P13/372/9: 'Danfa Comprehensive Rural Health and Family Planning Project: Ghana. Semi-Annual Progress Report July 1972–December 1972,' University of California, Los Angeles and University of Ghana, 1973, 5.
209 WHO, P13/372/9: 'A Programme Manual for Traditional Birth Attendants. Organization, Training, Evaluation,' Accra, December 1977, 5. When Adua Dua did her TBA training in 2001, she was keen to explain that 'even the nurses also learn[ed] from us' so that this was not a matter of a unidirectional learning experience.
210 Ibid., 7.
211 WHO, TRM/MTG/81.9: 'Traditional Medicine Role of Collaborating Centres' by Professor Adjepon-Yamoah and Dr Ampofo. November 1972, 1–2.
212 WHO, N2/180/3: WHO, N2/180/3: 'Consultation on the Role of the Traditional Birth Attendant, 12–19 March 1973,' Geneva, Enclosed in Memorandum from Chief Nursing Officer to Dr E. Braga, WHO, 24 November 1972, Table 1.
213 WHO, P13/372/9: 'A Programme Manual for Traditional Birth Attendants. Organization, Training, Evaluation,' Accra, December 1977, 12.

Afterword

At the beginning of this book, I observed that development, population and women's reproductive health had been intertwined during the twentieth century. In many ways, they remain so. Africa is set to make up a quarter of the world's population by 2050.[1] Today, the population growth we see in Africa is accompanied by one of two discourses: either it is a source of hope for a rising continent or it is a spectre of doom hanging not only over Africans but over humanity as a whole, given inevitable environmental crisis. The conversation on population growth in Africa is too often discursively limited to the age-old question of fertility. Western coverage of African demography is reductive and emphasises 'explosive' growth.[2]

Dr Letitia Appiah, leader of Ghana's National Population Council, made a speech for the launch of World Population Day in 2020. Ghana's National Population Council was first launched to support the Population Policy in the 1970s. It was revived and written into the constitution in the early 1990s. Dr Appiah told her audience in 2020 that 12% of women's deaths in Ghana can be linked to maternal causes and that one in three married Ghanaian women does not have their family planning needs met. She called on Ghana's media to support attempts to 'safeguard the health rights of women and girls now.'[3] Like many, Dr Appiah has linked the sexual and reproductive health of women and girls to the nation's development. Commenting on the radio in 2017, she said: '[p]opulation structure is key to development. We use the population to develop, and we develop for the population.' Crucially, she commented that whilst mortality and migration were somewhat under control, fertility was in desperate need of managing.[4] Indeed, at a Workshop on Recent Trends in sub-Saharan Africa in 2015, attendees highlighted fertility as a key determinant in the continent's development.[5] However, at 3.9 Ghana's total fertility rate is actually the lowest in West Africa, showing us that 'Africa' is not a monolith. This figure may also point us to a continuation of 'anti-politics' in Ghana, with population growth and underdevelopment being linked and used to distract from other development challenges.[6]

Those exploring issues in Ghana's MCH provision at the University's medical school also framed this in development terms in 2014 stating that the health of children 'undisputedly determined the future development of the nation' and that maternal mortality affects those women in their prime and therefore 'deprive[s]

DOI: 10.4324/9781003274162-8

the country of young energetic women who can make a significant contribution to the economy.'[7]

However, a majority of African leaders remain ambivalent towards family planning.[8] Opposition to it was shown clearly when John Magufuli, former president of Tanzania, told citizens in 2018 that it was 'important to reproduce' and, since they can feed their children, why would they use birth control?[9] UNFPA in Tanzania responded, emphasising that family planning is a rights issue, not to do with population control.[10] In Kenya, Jimi Wanjigi, 'Kenya's most feared oligarch,' dismissed the negative effects of population growth as fake news and instead encouraged Kenyans to have more babies.[11] In 2019, Ghana's president, Nana Akufo-Addo, promised to find a 'strategy to reap the demographic dividend' and harness Africa's youthful population for development.[12] It's worth noting though that in order to harness the 'demographic dividend,' that is, the economic benefits of this youthful population, a drop in the birth rate must occur. According to Professor Fred Sai, 'godfather of family planning,' African leaders in the twenty-first century lack the 'courage' to push through family planning programmes.[13] Women's reproductive health remains contentious, particularly through the lens of demographic and development policy. This book has delved into the history of that contention. Nevertheless, it merits further study.

Under colonialism, development meant population increase. In this sense, the aspirations of coloniser and colonised converged. But their approaches differed greatly, as colonial governments ultimately worked for greater exploitation and control over colonial people. Nonetheless, as maternal and infant welfare centres were introduced, colonial archives show that African leaders fought to defend their existence. In so doing, they appropriated the humanitarian language of imperialism, used it to argue for their rights to healthcare and arguably to reinforce their own elite status. Even towards the end of the colonial period in Ghana, when discourses of overpopulation began to pervade, officials in London did not extend them to African colonies. Africa was perceived as somewhere there was room for growth. Whilst women's high fertility was not discouraged, the way they gave birth and raised children was more tightly controlled through late colonial development programmes. From the 1940s onwards, medicalisation of pregnancy was normalised. Given Ghana's low population density, it might make sense that high fertility did not trouble either colonial or African politicians. However, this is to see the equation within the narrow limitations of the population to resource availability. Women's health or freedoms do not come into this equation.

After overthrowing Nkrumah and the CPP through a military coup in 1966 though, it made political sense for Ghanaian politicians to harness discourses of overpopulation and the idea that population growth would threaten economic development. How better to make development the responsibility of individual families? Indeed, I emphasise that development was a malleable, shifting and even contradictory concept in the twentieth century. Development meant an intention, a process and a goal. Its specific meaning therefore only becomes clear in particular contexts. Whilst this book owes a lot to Arturo Escobar's conceptualisation of development as ubiquitous, it qualifies the idea that development is a concept used by the powerful to subjectify and control the powerless. In fact, the concept of development has been widely appropriated.[14] Under independent governments in Ghana, 'development' was constantly used to legitimate processes which restrained women's choices over their reproductive health. Even as successive governments prided themselves on healthcare improvements, this was limited by gendered expectations imposed on particular groups of women. One particularly pertinent example of this is organisations' and governments' relationship with traditional birth attendants explored in Chapter 6. Furthermore, investments into healthcare have often fallen short, so that promises made repeatedly between the 1930s and 1980s to extend health services (especially to rural areas) came up short.

In a way, it seems odd to end a study of reproductive health at a point when the NFPP had yet to make much difference to Ghanaians' lives. Most people – even healthcare workers – did not see it as a significant part of Ghana's health services until at least the 1980s. However, this book does important work to show how family planning, since its systematic introduction in Ghana in 1970, has mirrored historical antecedents which made reproductive health a cornerstone of development policy.

So, what came next? As we saw in Chapter 6, the late 1970s and early 1980s saw economic disaster strike Ghana. The dip in birth rates during the period was a result of this, rather than changing attitudes. It also had a devastating effect on maternity services. J. J. Rawlings described Korle Bu hospital in order to emphasise health inequity: for 'less privileged women,'

> The wards are crowded; certain patients sleep on the bare floor even with babies. Their conditions can only be described as deplorable … The less privileged women … are also human. They suffer the same pain in labour.[15]

By the mid-1980s, the birth rate was actually rising in response to economic recovery. The Rawlings government – which constituted a military dictatorship into the 1990s – began a public response to this. Fred Sai recalled that during this period there were discussions about the 'old family planning programme and what needs to be done to put the thing on a better road.'[16] The National Population Council was reformed in 1992 with Sai as its leader.[17] The Population Policy was written into the constitution of Ghana's Fourth Republic.[18] This response was recalled by many of my interviewees, who noted that Rawlings was the one who brought in strong family planning measures. However, Rawlings also pushed back against the 'drive from developed countries to push population control programmes vigorously.' He noted that this caused suspicion of contraceptives among Ghanaians and that donor aid should not be conditional on population programmes being carried out.[19]

Traditional birth attendants also noted that it was Rawlings who forced them into hospital training. A newspaper article in May 1985 celebrated the graduation of 19 'traditional birth attendants' from a programme near Sekondi, noting the important part they would play in Ghana's Primary Health Care (PHC) provision.

PHC was linked to the World Health Organization's goal of 'Health for All by the year 2000.' Western Regional Director of Health Services Dr Ebenezer Binder was also quoted in the article, stressing PHC's low costs.[20] The emphasis on community-based healthcare and low-cost women birth attendants strengthened in the 1980s and 1990s.

Aside from family planning, the 1990s and 2000s saw another challenge in Ghana's reproductive health landscape: HIV/AIDS had a huge impact on the provision of maternal healthcare.[21] The first case in Ghana was diagnosed in 1986.[22] It inspired a new iteration of international health, christened 'global health,' which emphasised the interconnectedness of the globe through disease. HIV/AIDS stimulated donor aid which poured into Africa from the 1990s. However, until 2000 it was thought that HIV drugs should not be used in Africa because of their cost and logistical issues.[23] In the early twenty-first century, HIV/AIDS had become a priority in the field of sexual and reproductive health globally. The HIV/AIDS crisis legitimised greater intervention than ever before, not only in women's and men's health practices but also their sexuality and reproduction. Again, this was frequently justified by a view of health as a variable in economic development.[24] An important effect this had was that international development aid and non-governmental organisations (NGOs) moved away from maternal healthcare to HIV/AIDS provision.[25] Family planning and population control were also neglected.[26]

Abortion access and its legislation are important issues in Ghana's reproductive health landscape and merit further research, despite largely falling outside of the scope of this book. Apparent rising rates of illegal abortion, especially among schoolgirls and educated young women, were one reason that family planning and sex education came to be of interest in the early 1960s.[27] Women's groups in Ghana published arguments for legalising abortion in 1974 in response to IPPF-funded workshops on the topic held in Accra. Dr Bentsi-Enchill, who had worked on family planning at Korle Bu hospital, called upon the government to permit women abortions upon request.[28] But it took until 1985 for the law to be changed. The law on abortion remains within the criminal code (Act 29; 1960) but was amended in 1985 under the PNDC government so that women could access safe abortions in the case of rape, incest, foetal abnormality or danger to the mother's mental or physical health.[29] Abortion activism in the international sphere was stunted in the 1980s by the US resolution at the Mexico City International Conference on Population, 1984. Delegates arrived with high hopes that abortion could be put on the agenda, but the anti-abortion US delegation put a ban on any USAID population funds going to any programme which so much as mentioned abortion.[30] Although this 'global gag rule' has been rescinded by certain US presidents, it has been reintroduced by others and its effects continue to be felt today in Ghana, given its dependence on USAID funding.[31]

Looking back to the 1920s, when maternal and child health "MCH" interventions began in a systematic way in some areas of Ghana, we saw that priority was given to the 'C,' the healthcare of infants and children. This issue began to be addressed in 1985 when Allen Rosenfield and Deborah Maine asked, 'Where is the "M" in MCH?' The issue highlighted in Chapter 6, that women were predominantly considered in PHC in terms of their contributions to their children's health, began to be talked about internationally. This led to the 'Safe Motherhood' agenda, which was introduced during a conference in Kenya, organised by the World Bank in 1987.[32] This conference drew renewed attention to the problem of clandestine abortions, which were responsible for 25–50% of maternal deaths globally.[33] In 1990 around a quarter of all development aid was designated for maternal healthcare although, as mentioned, this was reduced due to attention on HIV/AIDS in the 2000s.[34]

Despite this, maternal health sat at the centre of the Millennium Development Goals. The target was to reduce maternal mortality to below 70 per 100,000 live births. During this period in Ghana the number of women delivered by skilled health professionals grew significantly to 59% by 2008. However, 84% of urban women had skilled assistance compared to only 43% of rural women.[35] Meanwhile, 95% of women received antenatal care.[36] Furthermore, contraceptive use was much more prevalent among wealthy, educated, urban women.[37] Therefore, despite work to ensure safer motherhood, we continue to see prevailing patterns set out since Chapter 1 in this book: women's access to healthcare is inequitable and based on their social status. We also see that women are more likely to seek antenatal care than attendance at delivery.

The 2015 Sustainable Development Goals continued to emphasise reproductive health as an area for improvement. There are targets for reducing maternal and neonatal mortality and for universal access to family planning. Meanwhile the 2019 International Conference for Population and Development stated a 'promise of universal access to sexual and reproductive health.'[38] Despite this, access to quality maternal health services is lacking for many African women where maternal mortality rates remain high.[39] Maternal mortality is 319/100,000 live births in Ghana.[40] Seventy eight per cent of births are now attended by a skilled birth attendant.[41] These rates are affected by a lack of effective contraception, supervised deliveries and facilities, meaning that deaths are preventable.[42] The COVID-19 pandemic has caused severe interruptions to health systems globally, and in Ghana, health system usage declined among pregnant women as services adapted to reduce close contact. This was estimated to lead to 12,200 excess maternal deaths.[43] The fact that the pandemic has interrupted antenatal care, birth attendance and family planning makes women and girls particularly vulnerable to it across Africa.

Ghana's fertility rate now stands at under 4 births per woman as opposed to 6.4 in 1998.[44] There has been a revolution in many Ghanaians' approaches to reproduction. However, when we look closely at the data, we see that there are considerable disparities between the number of children born to urban and rural women. Furthermore, the total number of children born to women drops dramatically according to the amount of education they have received. Those with primary education had an average of five children whilst those with 'more than secondary' education had 2.4.[45] Nineteen per cent of Ghanaian women have an 'unmet need' for contraception.[46] Edward Paice argues that 'explosion' fever ended in the 1990s as international institutions diverted their attention from the 'population problem.'[47] However, development is still seen as contingent on fertility. The 'demographic dividend' narrative is contingent not only on a people-driven version of development based on 'unleashing' its youth and women.[48] It is also 'critical,' in the words of the African Union, that women have access to 'sexual and reproductive health including family planning.' Low fertility is crucial to the demographic dividend.[49]

This brief account of women's reproductive health in Ghana from the 1980s to the present day evokes a number of issues discussed in this book. First of all, there are ongoing health inequities within the country as well as large disparities in fertility according to the region and socio-economic status. Secondly, international development aid has continued to target women and children unevenly, relying on technical solutions to particular diseases like HIV rather than building strong, equitable health systems. We see the ongoing importance of NGOs in Ghanaian health systems, present since the Red Cross took over MCH in the early 1930s. Finally, population continues to be understood in development terms.

Looking into Ghana's past, as this study has done, we begin to better understand its present, emphasising the importance of looking at healthcare across multiple levels. I have used evidence from international and global organisations, national and colonial governments, healthcare workers, and Ghanaian women to show that none of these groups operated in isolation. This is a crucial history to understand in the context of today's global health structures, in which the state competes with NGOs over health services. Arguably, what we see today is an iteration of a historical process dating from the early twentieth century. By understanding that women's reproductive health has been at the core of a series of development projects and aspirations, we see more clearly that women's own decision-making processes and social networks were often at odds with state or non-state organisations' ideas of development.

Women's experiences of changes to reproductive health services have been at the heart of this study. This has been achieved especially through oral histories, and I hope that I have done justice to the life stories and opinions that women generously shared with me. Charting a history across the colonial/postcolonial divide, of a particular, gendered aspect of healthcare is also unique in studies of Ghana. This book has exposed the important point that women's experiences of health do not necessarily reflect that which is presented in development discourse. Women have frequently been characterised as victims, objects of humanitarian benevolence. We see this particularly through the images of women that emanate from Red Cross or Save the Children imaginaries and from discourses of overpopulation that paint women as overburdened, overworked, sacrificed to their own bodies, which they cannot control. Women are also characterised as 'traditional' in a world in which development is almost synonymous with modernisation. These discourses make women seem powerless and ignore the multiplicity of factors that influence their choices over reproduction and reproductive health. The complexities and nuances of women's histories stand against development discourses which characterise them as two-dimensional.

Even whilst women were characterised as powerless, they were expected to perform aspects of development, especially its social side. The progressive woman under colonial rule was hygienic, fed her family well and attended welfare clinics. When family planning was introduced systematically in Ghana for the first time, women were expected not only to engage with it but to do so as 'modern' women. The modern woman limited her family and adhered to scientific, hospital-based healthcare strategies. Meanwhile, the rural women who, in the minds of development planners, were a separate group, were leaned on to make PHC work. Misconceptions over women's roles in communities meant that projects went awry. Through all these iterations, it was women who were responsible for their families' health. For this reason, a particular focus on women's interaction with health systems is more than justified.

It is also justified by the ongoing focus on women's reproductive health in development policy. Controlling women's reproductive health in Africa has often been thought of as crucial to improving the development prospects of the continent. Today, development agendas seek to empower women and see a reduction in women's fertility as the key to enabling women to take part in the continent's development. Whilst international organisations and agencies call for Africa to take advantage of its demographic dividend, let us hope that we do not see women's choices once again being contingent upon development goals at the expense of reproductive justice.

Notes

1 Edward Paice, *Youthquake: Why African Demography Should Matter to the World* (London: Head of Zeus, 2021), 18.
2 Ibid., 7.
3 Remarks by Dr Letitia Adelaide Appiah on the Press Briefing on the 2020 World Population Day Celebration, 8 July, 2020 [Last accessed 02/03/2022] https://www.npc.gov.gh/news/.
4 'Bedroom Decisions Key to Economic Dev't than Boardroom Choices – MyJoyOnline.Com' [Last accessed 25/08/2017] http://www.myjoyonline.com/news/2017/May-23rd/bedroom-decisions-key-to-economic-devt-than-boardroom-choices.php.
5 Cheikh Mbacké, 'The Persistence of High Fertility in Sub-Saharan Africa: A Comment,' *Population and Development Review* 43, no. 1 (2017): 330.
6 Edward Paice, *Youthquake*, xvi.
7 Lorna A. Renner, Samuel A. Oppong and Bamenla Q. Goka, 'The Way Forward,' in *Topical Issues in Maternal and Child Health in Ghana*, ed. Jennifer E. Welbeck et al., University of Ghana Readers, no. 9 (Tema, Ghana: Digibooks Ghana Ltd, 2014), 185–89.
8 Mbacké, 'The Persistence of High Fertility in Sub-Saharan Africa.'
9 '"No Need for Birth Control": Tanzanian President's Views Cause Outrage,' *The Guardian*, 11 September, 2018 [Last accessed 18/09/2019] https://www.theguardian.com/global-development/2018/sep/11/no-need-for-birth-control-tanzanian-presidents-views-cause-outrage.
10 'Family Planning is a Human Right,' 14 August, 2018 [Last accessed 20/08/2019] https://tanzania.unfpa.org/en/news/family-planning-human-right-17.
11 Paice, *Youthquake*, 1–2.

12 Ralph Ranali, 'Ghana's President Says Young People are Africa's Greatest Asset,' *Harvard Kennedy School*, 8 April, 2019 [Last accessed 23/2/2022] https://www.hks.harvard.edu/faculty-research/policy-topics/public-leadership-management/ghanas-president-says-young-people-are.
13 David Holmes, 'Fred Sai: The Godfather of Family Planning,' *The Lancet* 380, no. 9855 (2012): 1731.
14 Escobar, *Encountering Development.*
15 J. J. Rawlings, *No Turning Back (A Message to the Nation)*, Accra, 29 July 1982.
16 MacFarlane, Deborah, Interview with Dr Fred Sai for *Smith College Population and Reproductive Health Oral History Project*, 11 March, 2004, 58.
17 Ibid., 59.
18 'Statement of Ghana, H. E. Flt-Lt. Jerry John Rawlings,' *United Nations Population Information Network*, Cairo, 5–13 September 1994, 1.
19 Ibid., 5–6.
20 '19 Birth Attendants End Training,' *Daily Graphic,* 8 May, 1985, 5.
21 John Iliffe, *The African AIDS Epidemic: A History* (Oxford: James Currey, 2006).
22 The MEASURE Project and Ghana AIDS Commission, *AIDS in Africa during the Nineties: Ghana. A Review and Analysis of Survey and Research Results* (North Carolina: University of North Carolina, 2003).
23 Vinh-Kim Nguyen, *The Republic of Therapy: Triage and Sovereignty in West Africa's Time of AIDS* (Durham, NC: Duke University Press, 2010), 4.
24 Packard, *A History of Global Health*, 276.
25 Shane Doyle, 'Maternal Health, Epidemiology and Transition Theory in Africa,' in *Epidemiological Change and Chronic Disease in Sub-Saharan Africa*, ed. Megan Vaughan, Kafui Adjaye-Gbewonyo, and Marissa Mika, Social and Historical Perspectives (London: UCL Press, 2021), 106.
26 MacFarlane, Deborah, Interview with Dr Fred Sai for *Smith College Population and Reproductive Health Oral History Project*, 11 March, 2004, 60.
27 Holly Rose Ashford, 'The Christian Council, Moral Citizenship and Sex Education in Ghana, 1951 – 1966,' *History of Education* 51, no. 1 (2022): 1–23; Frederick T. Sai, *With Heart and Voice: Fred Sai Remembers* (Cambridge: Barton, 2010).
28 'Workshop on Abortion,' *The Ghanaian Woman* 1, no. 3 (1974): 16–20.
29 Patience Aniteye and Susannah H. Mayhew, 'Globalisation and Transitions in Abortion Care in Ghana,' *BMC Health Services Research* 19, no. 1 (2019): 3.
30 MacFarlane, Deborah, Interview with Dr Fred Sai for *Smith College Population and Reproductive Health Oral History Project*, 11 March, 2004, 72.
31 Aniteye and Mayhew, 'Globalisation and Transitions in Abortion Care in Ghana,' 2.
32 Ann Starrs, 'Preventing the Tragedy of Maternal Deaths. A Report on the International Safe Motherhood Conference,' Nairobi, Kenya, 1987.
33 Ibid., 6.
34 Doyle, 'Maternal Health, Epidemiology and Transition Theory in Africa,' 106.
35 ICF Macro, *Millennium Development Goals in Ghana: A New Look at Data from the 2008 Ghana Demographic and Health Survey* (Calverton, MD: ICF Macro), 2010, 16.
36 Ibid., 19.
37 Ibid., 18.
38 ICPD25, 'Nairobi Statement on ICPD25: Accelerating the Promise' [Last accessed 30/05/2022] https://www.un.org/en/conferences/population/nairobi2019.
39 Estelle M. Sidze, Martin K. Mutua and Hermann P. Donfouet, 'Towards Achieving Equity in Utilisation of Maternal Health Services in Selected Sub-Saharan African Countries: Progress and Remaining Challenges in Priority Countries,' in *Women and Sustainable Human Development: Empowering Women in Africa*, ed. Maty Konte and Nyasha Tirivayi, Gender, Development and Social Change (Cham: Springer International Publishing, 2020), 111–24.

40 Faith Agbozo and Albrecht Jahn, 'COVID-19 in Ghana: Challenges and Countermeasures for Maternal Health Service Delivery in Public Health Facilities,' *Reproductive Health* 18, no. 1 (2021): 2.
41 'World Population Dashboard Ghana' [Last accessed 23/02/2022] https://www.unfpa.org/data/world-population/GH.
42 Renner, Oppong, and Goka, 'The Way Forward,' 189.
43 Agbozo and Jahn, 'COVID-19 in Ghana,' 2.
44 World Bank, 'Fertility Rate, Total (Births per Woman) | Data,' The World Bank Data [Last accessed 30/07/2019] https://data.worldbank.org/indicator/SP.DYN.TFRT.IN?locations=GH.
45 Ghana Statistical Service (GSS), Ghana Health Service (GHS), and ICF, *Ghana Maternal Health Survey 2017* (Accra, Ghana: GSS, GHS, and ICF), 2018, 44.
46 'World Population Dashboard Ghana' [Last accessed 23/02/2022] https://www.unfpa.org/data/world-population/GH.
47 Paice, *Youthquake*, 9.
48 African Union, *AU Roadmap on Harnessing the Demographic Dividend through Investments in Youth*, 2017, 4.
49 Ibid., 19–20.

Bibliography

Archives

UK

BDL: Bodleian Library Special Collections, Oxford, UK
BRC: British Red Cross Archives, London
CRL: Cadbury Research Library, University of Birmingham, UK
CUL: Cambridge University Library
NA: The National Archives, London, UK
NCL: New College Library, Edinburgh, UK
SOAS: School of Oriental and African Studies Archive, London, UK
Wellcome: The Wellcome Library Archive Collection, London, UK

Ghana

EA: Ghana Historical Society, University of Ghana, Legon, Accra: Private Papers of Evelyn Amarteifio
KBMS: Korle Bu Medical School Archive
PRAAD, Accra: Public Records and Archives Administration Department, Accra, Ghana
PRAAD, Cape Coast: Public Records and Archives Administration Department, Cape Coast, Ghana
PRAAD, Koforidua: Public Records and Archives Administration Department, Koforidua, Ghana
PRAAD, Kumasi: Public Records and Archives Administration Department, Kumasi, Ghana
PRAAD, Sekondi: Public Records and Archives Administration Department, Sekondi, Ghana

Switzerland

LN: League of Nations Archive, Geneva, Switzerland
WHO: World Health Organization Archive, Geneva, Switzerland

USA

RAC: Rockefeller Archive Center, Sleepy Hollow, New York
UN: United Nations Archives, New York

Newspapers, Magazines and Periodicals

Chronicle of the World Health Organization (Geneva)
Daily Graphic (Accra)
Daily Mirror (Accra)
MyJoyOnline (Accra)
The Evening News (Accra)
The Ghanaian Times (Accra)
Ghana Today (Accra)
The Gold Coast Independent (Accra)
The New Ghana (Accra)
The Times of West Africa (Accra)
The Guardian (London)
World Health Magazine (Geneva)

Interviews

All interviews were conducted by the author in October 2017 – February 2018 or in July 2019. Unless they are marked with an asterisk, all interviews were conducted in local languages and translated into English. Those marked with † requested to remain annonymous. Interpretation was carried out with the assistance of a research assistant and with the exception of those carried out in English were also translated and transcribed by a research assistant.

Aunty Moses Ackon, Adjumako, Western Region, 23rd October, 2017
Mary Sampson, Adjumako, Western Region, 23rd October, 2017
Sophia Ampah, Adjumako, Western Region, 23rd October, 2017
Aishatu Manuh, Adjumako, Western Region, 23rd October, 2017
Abena Manuh, Adjumako, Western Region, 23rd October, 2017
Ama Aku, Mpatase, Western Region, 24th October, 2017
Hannah Bowah, Mpatase, Western Region, 24th October, 2017
Mary Bowah, Mpatase, Western Region, 24th October, 2017
Yaa Korenkyewa, Mpatase, Western Region, 24th October, 2017
Akua Nkwiwaa, Abra, Western Region, 25th October, 2017
Mariam Alassa, Abra, Western Region, 25th October, 2017
Esi Praah, Abra, Western Region, 25th October, 2017
Dr. Patrick Mensah*†, Takoradi, Western Region, 26th October, 2017
Dr. Joseph Atobrah*†, Sekondi, Western Region, 26th October, 2017
Esi Atta, Gyabenkrom, Western Region, 27th October, 2017
Esi Kofua, Gyabenkrom, Western Region, 27th October, 2017
Harriet Sekyi-Yorke*, Gyabenkrom, Western Region, 27th October, 2017
Araba Yedua, Gyabenkrom, Western Region, 27th October, 2017
Esi Dwana, Koforidua, Central Region, 27th November, 2017
Esi Yawa, Koforidua, Central Region, 27th November, 2017
Ekua Nkrumah, Koforidua, Central Region, 27th November, 2017
Lucy Amissah, Koforidua, Central Region, 27th November, 2017
Georgina Hermance, Moree, Central Region, 28th November, 2017
Cecilia Essuan, Moree, Central Region, 28th November, 2017
Cecilia Fynn-Essien, Cape Coast, Central Region, 28th November, 2017
Aba Yaa, Abakrampa, Central Region, 29th November, 2017

Efua Ayana, Abakrampa, Central Region, 29th November, 2017
Aunty Angela, Abakrampa, Central Region, 29th November, 2017
Ekua Saba, Barabadze, Central Region, 30th November, 2017
Group 1: Ama Fosua, Adua Bensua, Nana Esebu and Esi Mensema, Barabadze, Central Region, 30th November, 2017
Group 2: Ekuah Esawa, Mary Edu, Aba Donky, Asko Nkrumah and Mary Ahin, Barabadze, Central Region, 30th November, 2017
Group 3: Ekuah Mensah, Ekuah Ama, Efua Kaya, Esi Adjumah and Comfort Kwenu, Barabadze, Central Region, 30th November, 2017
Patience Doris Doh*, Koforidua, Eastern Region, 24th January, 2018
Rosina Apraku*, Koforidua, Eastern Region, 25th January, 2018
Gertrude Engmann*†, Adiembra, Western Region, 30th January, 2018
Dr Daniel Otchere*, Takoradi, Western Region, 31st January, 2018
Sabina Mensah*, Anaji, Western Region, 2nd February, 2018
Jemima Crentsil*, Takoradi, Western Region, 2nd February, 2018
Aba Sekum, Aboadze, Western Region, 6th February, 2018
Comfort Donkoh, Aboadze, Western Region, 6th February, 2018
Efua Akyenoba, Aboadze, Western Region, 6th February, 2018
Aunty Esi, Aboadze, Western Region, 6th February, 2018
Sarah Anderson, Aboadze, Western Region, 6th February, 2018
Juliana Brown*, Abura, Central Region, 9th February, 2018
Magdalene Juliet Ackuah*, Cape Coast, Central Region, 9th February, 2018
Dr Seth Amuah*†, Cape Coast, Central Region, 12th February, 2018
Aba Efrim, Nkanfoa, Central Region, 13th February, 2018
Ama Yemaba, Nkanfoa, Central Region, 13th February, 2018
Esi Sekyua, Nkanfoa, Central Region, 13th February, 2018
Munirata Lardi Yahaya*, Cape Coast, Central Region, 14th February, 2018
Nathaniel Amarteifio*, Accra, Greater Accra, 21st February, 2018
Adjoa Ewusiwa, New Ebu, Central Region, 22nd July, 2019
Nana Efua Ateifi I, New Ebu, Central Region, 22nd July, 2019
Maame Abu, New Ebu, Central Region, 22nd July, 2019
Florence Boateng*, Ankaful, Central Region, 22nd July, 2019
Adua Tekyiwa, Jukwa, Central Region, 23rd July, 2019
Efua Ata, Abrafo, Central Region, 23rd July, 2019
Yadia Eya, Abrafo, Central Region, 23rd July, 2019
Mary Boanno and Martha Abena, Abrafo, Central Region, 23rd July, 2019
Adua Dua, Abrafo, Central Region, 23rd July, 2019

Reports and Documents

'Bedroom Decisions Key to Economic Dev't than Boardroom Choices' [Last accessed 25/08/2017] http://www.myjoyonline.com/news/2017/May-23rd/bedroom-decisions-key-to-economic-devt-than-boardroom-choices.php.
'Family Planning is a Human Right', 14th August, 2018. [Last accessed 20/08/2019] https://tanzania.unfpa.org/en/news/family-planning-human-right-17.
'Remarks by Dr. Letitia Adelaide Appiah on the Press Briefing on the 2020 World Population Day Celebration', 8th July, 2020. [Last Accessed 03/03/2011] https://www.npc.gov.gh/news/.

'Statement of Ghana, H. E. Flt-Lt. Jerry John Rawlings' United Nations Population Information Network, Cairo, 5–13 September 1994, 1.

Acheampong, I. K., *Economic Measures for Financial Year 1973–1974*, Ministry of Finance, 30th August, 1974.

Acheampong, I. K., *Radio and Television Broadcast to the Nation by Colonel I. K. Acheampong, Chairman of the National Redemption Council, on the Devaluation and External Debts, on Saturday, 5th February, 1972*, Accra, 1972.

Annual Colonial Reports. No. 1207. Gold Coast Report for 1922–1923, Government Press, Accra, 1923.

Annual Colonial Reports. No. 1255. Gold Coast Report for 1923–1924, Government Press, Accra, 1925.

Annual Colonial Reports. No. 1386. Gold Coast Report for 1926–1927, Government Press, Accra, 1927.

Annual Colonial Reports. No. 1504. Gold Coast Report for 1929–1930. No. 1504, Gold Coast Colony, 1930.

Annual Report on the Social and Economic Progress of the People of the Gold Coast 1938–39, Government Press, Accra, 1939.

Cardinall, A. W. *The Gold Coast, 1931*. Government Printer, Accra, 1933.

Covenant of the League of Nations. Accessed: http://avalon.law.yale.edu/20th_century/leagcov.asp [Last accessed 18/07/2018].

Dawson-Amoah, Catherine, 'The PPAG Story', unpublished presentation given in Accra.

Ghana Statistical Service (GSS), Ghana Health Service (GHS), and ICF, *Ghana Maternal Health Survey 2017*, GSS, GHS, and ICF, Accra, Ghana, 2018.

Ghana Statistical Service, *Ghana 2021 Population and Housing Census Volume 1: Preliminary Report*, September 2021, 5.

Ghana: Economic Position and Prospects, World Bank, 29th June, 1977.

Gold Coast Government, *Annual Report on the Social and Economic Progress of the people of the Gold Coast, 1935–36*, Accra, 1936.

Gold Coast Government, *Report of the Commission of Enquiry into the Health Needs of the Gold Coast*, Accra, 1952.

Gold Coast Government, *Report of the Commission of Enquiry into the Health Needs of the Gold Coast*, Government Printing Dept., Accra, 1953.

Gold Coast Government, *Report of the Ministry of Health 1952*, Accra, 1953.

Gold Coast Government, *Report of the Ministry of Health 1953*, Government Printing Dept., Accra, 1955.

Gold Coast Government, *Report on the Medical and Sanitary Department for the Financial Year 1927–28*, Government Printing Dept., Accra, 1928.

Gold Coast Government, *Report on the Medical and Sanitary Department for the Financial Year 1928–29*, Government Printing Dept., Accra, 1929.

Gold Coast Government, *Report on the Medical and Sanitary Department for the Financial Year 1929–30*, Government Printing Dept., Accra, 1930.

Gold Coast Government, *Report on the Medical and Sanitary Department for the Year 1930–31*, Government Printing Dept., Accra, 1931.

Gold Coast Government, *Report on the Medical and Sanitary Department for the Financial Year 1932–33*, Government Printing Dept., Accra, 1924.

Gold Coast Government, *Report on the Medical Department for the Year 1933–1934*, Government Printing Dept., Accra, 1934.

Gold Coast Government, *Report on the Medical Department for the Year 1934*, Government Printing Dept., Accra, 1935.

Gold Coast Government, *Report on the Medical Department for the Year 1935*, Government Printing Dept., Accra, 1936.

Gold Coast Government, *Report on the Medical Department for the Year 1936*, Government Printing Dept., Accra, 1937.

Gold Coast Government, *Report on the Medical Department for the Year 1937*, Government Printing Dept., Accra, 1938.

Gold Coast Government, *Report on the Medical Department for the Year 1938*, Government Printing Dept., Accra, 1939.

Gold Coast Government, *Report on the Medical Department for the Year 1939*, Government Printing Dept., Accra, 1940.

Gold Coast Government, *Report on the Medical Department for the Year 1940*, Government Printing Dept., Accra, 1941.

Gold Coast Government, *Report on the Medical Department for the Year 1941*, Government Printing Dept., Accra, 1942.

Gold Coast Government, *Report on the Medical Department for the Year 1942*, Government Printing Dept., Accra, 1943.

Gold Coast Government, *Report on the Medical Department for the Year 1943*, Government Printing Dept., Accra, 1944.

Gold Coast Government, *Report on the Medical Department for the Year 1944*, Government Printing Dept., Accra, 1945.

Gold Coast Government, *Report on the Medical Department for the Year 1945*, Government Printing Dept., Accra, 1946.

Gold Coast Government, *Report on the Medical Department for the Year 1947*, Government Printing Dept., Accra, 1948.

Gold Coast Government, *Report on the Medical Department for the Year 1948*, Government Printing Dept., Accra, 1949.

Gold Coast Government, *Report on the Medical Department for the Year 1949*, Government Printing Dept., Accra, 1950.

Gold Coast Government, *Report on the Medical Department for the Year 1950*, Government Printing Dept., Accra, 1952.

Gold Coast Government, *Report on the Medical Department for the Year 1951*, Government Printing Dept., Accra, 1953.

Gold Coast Government, *Report on the Medical Department for the Year 1952*, Government Printing Dept., Accra, 1954.

Gold Coast Government, *The Development Plan, 1951. Being a Plan for the Economic and Social Development of the Gold Coast as approved by the Legislative Assembly, September, 1951*, Government Printing Dept., Accra, 1951.

Government of the Gold Coast, *Report on the Medical and Sanitary Department for the Financial Year 1926–27*, Government Printing Dept., Accra, 1927.

ICF Macro, *Millennium Development Goals in Ghana: A new look at data from the 2008 Ghana Demographic and Health Survey*, ICF Macro, Calverton, Maryland.

Keeping Baby Healthy, Health Education Unit, Ministry of Health, Accra, 1962.

MacFarlane, Deborah, Interview with Dr Fred Sai for *Smith College Population and Reproductive Health Oral History Project*, 11th March, 2004.

National Redemption Council, *Guidelines for the Five Year Development Plan, 1975–1980*, Accra, January, 1975.

National Redemption Council, *Towards a Brighter Future*, Information Services Department, Accra, n.d.

Neumann, Alfred, *Danfa Comprehensive Rural Health and Family Planning Project: Ghana. UCLA Annual Progress Report. January–December, 1974*, California, 1975.

Poulton, E. Maclean, *A Report on a Visit to Ghana 12 July – 28 August, 1957*, WHO African Regional Office, 1957.

Proceedings of the Imperial Social Hygiene Congress at the British Empire Exhibition, Wembley, London, 1925.

Quarterly Bulletin of the Health Organisation. Vol II, Geneva, 1933, 106.

Ranali, Ralph. 'Ghana's President says Young People are Africa's Greatest Asset', Harvard Kennedy School, 8th April, 2019 [Last accessed 23/2/2022] https://www.hks.harvard.edu/faculty-research/policy-topics/public-leadership-management/ghanas-president-says-young-people-are.

Rawlings, J. J., *No Turning Back (A Message to the Nation)*, Accra, 29th July, 1982.

The Gold Coast Census of the Population 1948. Report and Tables, Government Printing Dept., Accra, 1950.

UN General Assembly (17th sess.: 1962) *Resolutions Adopted by the General Assembly during its 17th session, 18th September – 20 December 1962*, Resolution 1838, 18th December 1962.

World Bank. "Fertility Rate, Total (Births per Woman) | Data." The World Bank Data. [Last accessed 30/7/2019] https://data.worldbank.org/indicator/SP.DYN.TFRT.IN?locations=GH.

World Health Organization. *Ghana: Summary Country Profile for HIV/AIDS Scale-Up*, World Health Organization, Accra, December 2005.

Published Books and Articles

Abu-Lughod, Lila. "Do Muslim Women Really Need Saving? Anthropological Reflections on Cultural Relativism and Its Others." *American Anthropologist* 104, no. 3 (2002): 783–90.

Adamafio, Tawia. *By Nkrumah's Side: The Labour and the Wounds*. Accra: Westcoast, 1982.

Adams, Vivianne, and Stacey Leigh Pigg. "Introduction: The Moral Object of Sex." In *Sex in Development: Science, Sexuality and Morality in Global Perspective*, edited by Vivianne Adams, and Stacy Leigh Pigg, 1–38. Durham: Duke University Press, 2005.

Addae, Stephen. *The History of Western Medicine in Ghana 1880–1960*. Edinburgh: The Pentland Press, 1997.

Agbozo, Faith, and Albrecht Jahn, 'COVID-19 in Ghana: Challenges and Countermeasures for Maternal Health Service Delivery in Public Health Facilities', *Reproductive Health* 18, no. 1 (19 July 2021), 1–5.

Agongo, Erasmus E. A., Patrick Agana-Nsiire, Nana K. A. Enyimayew, Moses Komla Adibo, and Emmanuel Nonaka Mensah. *Primary Health Care Systems: Comprehensive Case Study from Ghana*. PRIMASYS. Accra: World Health Organization, 2017.

Ahlberg, Beth Maina. *Women, Sexuality, and the Changing Social Order: The Impact of Government Policies on Reproductive Behavior in Kenya*. London: Taylor & Francis, 1991.

Ahlberg, Beth Maina, and Asli Kulane. "Sexual and Reproductive Health and Rights." In *African Sexualities: A Reader*, edited by Sylvia Tamale, 313–39. Capetown: Pambazuka Press, 2011.

Ahlman, Jeffrey. “A New Type of Citizen: Youth, Gender, and Generation in the Ghanaian Builders’ Brigade.” *The Journal of African History* 53, no. 1 (2012): 87–105.

Ahlman, Jeffrey. *Living with Nkrumahism: Nation, State, and Pan-Africanism in Ghana*. Athens: Ohio University Press, 2017.

Aidoo, Ama Ata. *Changes a Love Story*. Oxford: Heinemann Educational Publishers, 1991.

Akuffo, Felix Odei. “Teenage Pregnancies and School Drop-Outs. The Relevance of Family Life Education and Vocational Training to Girls’ Employment Opportunities.” In *Sex Roles, Population and Development in West Africa: Policy Related Studies on Work and Demographic Issues*, edited by Christine Oppong, 154–64. Portsmouth: Heinemann, 1987.

Akyeampong, Emmanuel. ‘Sexuality and Prostitution among the Akan of the Gold Coast c. 1650–1950’ *Past & Present* 156, no. 1 (1997): 144–73.

Akyeampong, Emmanuel. “‘Wo Pe Tam Won Pe Ba’ (‘You like Cloth but You Don’t Want Children’) Urbanization, Individualism and Gender Relations in Colonial Ghana.” In *Africa’s Urban Past*, edited by David Anderson, and Richard Rathbone, 222–33. Oxford: James Currey, 2000.

Allman, Jean. “Fathering, Mothering and Making Sense of ‘Ntamoba’: Reflections on the Economy of Child-Rearing in Colonial Asante.” *Africa: Journal of the International African Institute* 67, no. 2 (1997): 296–321.

Allman, Jean. “Making Mothers: Missionaries, Medical Officers and Women’s Work in Colonial Asante, 1924–1945.” *History Workshop*, no. 38 (1994): 23–47.

Allman, Jean. “Rounding up Spinsters: Gender Chaos and Unmarried Women in Colonial Asante.” *The Journal of African History* 37, no. 2 (1996): 195–214.

Allman, Jean. “The Disappearing of Hannah Kudjoe: Nationalism, Feminism, and the Tyrannies of History.” *Journal of Women’s History* 21, no. 3 (2009): 13–35.

Allman, Jean, and John Parker. *Tongnaab: The History of a West African God*. Indianapolis: Indiana University Press, 2005.

Allman, Jean, and Victoria B. Tashjian. *I Will Not Eat Stone: A Women’s History of Colonial Asante*. Portsmouth, NH: Heinemann, 2000.

Ampim, Gloria. “An Historical Analysis of Maternal and Infant Welfare in Ghana: 1957–1980.” MPhil thesis, University of Ghana, 2011.

Ampofo, Akosua Adomako. “‘When Men Speak Women Listen’: Gender Socialisation and Young Adolescents’ Attitudes to Sexual and Reproductive Issues.” *African Journal of Reproductive Health* 5, no. 3 (December 2001), 196–212.

Ampofo, Akosua Adomako. “Whose “Unmet Need”? Dis/Agreement about Childbearing among Ghanaian Couples.” In *Rethinking Sexualities in Africa*, edited by Signe Arnfred, 115–34. Uppsala: Almqvist & Wiksell Tryckeri AB, 2004.

Ampofo, Akosua Adomako, Micheal Perry Kweku Okyerefo, and Micheal Pervarah, “Phallic Competence: Fatherhood and the Making of Men in Ghana.” *Culture, Society & Masculinity* 1, no. 1 (2009): 59–78.

Ampofo, Daniel A., David D. Nicholas, S. Ofosu-Amaah, S. Blumenfeld, and A. K. Neumann. “The Danfa Family Planning Program in Rural Ghana.” *Studies in Family Planning* 7 (November 1, 1976): 266–74.

Amrith, Sunil S. *Decolonizing International Health: India and Southeast Asia, 1930–65*. Cambridge Imperial and Post-Colonial Studies Series. Basingstoke: Palgrave Macmillan, 2006.

Aniteye, Patience, and Susannah H. Mayhew. ‘Globalisation and Transitions in Abortion Care in Ghana’, *BMC Health Services Research* 19, no. 1 (March 21, 2019), 185–97.

Appiah, Anthony. *In My Father's House: Africa in the Philosophy of Culture*. New York: Oxford University Press, 1992.

Appiah-Kubi, Kofi. *Man Cures, God Heals: Religion and Medical Practice among the Akans of Ghana*. Totowa: Allanheld, Osmun & Co. Publishers, 1981.

Apter, David E. *Ghana in Transition*. New York: Atheneum, 1963.

Hippocrene Books. *Asante Twi Dictionary & Phrasebook*. New York: Hippocrene Books, 2015.

Ashford, Holly Rose. "The Christian Council, Moral Citizenship and Sex Education in Ghana, 1951–1966." *History of Education* 51, no. 1 (2022): 91–113.

Ashford, Holly Rose. "The Red Cross and the Establishment of Maternal and Infant Welfare in the 1930s Gold Coast." *The Journal of Imperial and Commonwealth History* 47, no. 3 (2019): 514–41.

Atobrah, Deborah. "Caring for the Seriously Sick in Ghanaian Society: Glimpses from the Past." *Ghana Studies* 15, no. 16 (2013/2012), 69–102.

Atobrah, Deborah, and Akosua Adomako Ampofo. "Expressions of Masculinity and Femininity in Husbands' Care of Wives with Cancer in Accra." *African Studies Review* 59, no. 1 (April 18, 2016): 175–97.

Atobrah, Deborah, and Benjamin Kwansa. "Achieving Universal Health Coverage? A Focus on Constructions of Health and Ill-Health in Ghana." University of Edinburgh, 2019.

Austin, Dennis. *Politics in Ghana, 1946–1960*. Oxford: Oxford University Press, 1964.

Austin, Dennis, and Robin Luckham, eds. *Politicians and Soldiers in Ghana, 1966–1972*. London: Frank Cass and Co. Ltd., 1975.

Austin, Gareth. "Cash Crops and Freedom: Export Agriculture and the Decline of Slavery in Colonial West Africa." *International Review of Social History* 54, no. 1 (2009): 1–37.

Austin, Gareth. *Labour, Land and Capital in Ghana: From Slavery to Free Labour in Asante, 1807–1956*. New York: University of Rochester Press, 2009.

Austin, Gareth. "Quantifying Transitions in Ghanaian Demographic and Labour History 1800–2000: A Contribution to Comparative History." Paris, 2014.

Austin, Gareth. "Resources, Techniques, and Strategies South of the Sahara: Revising the Factor Endowments Perspective on African Economic Development, 1500–2001." *The Economic History Review* 61, no. 3 (2008): 587–624.

Austin, Gareth, Ewout Frankema, and Ewout Morten Jerven. "Patterns of Manufacturing Growth in Sub-Saharan Africa: From Colonization to the Present." In *The Spread of Modern Industry to the Poor Periphery since 1870*, edited by Kevin O'Rouke, and Jeffrey G. Williamson, 345–73. Oxford: Oxford University Press, 2017.

Awusabo-Asare, Kofi. *Population and Housing Census National Analytical Report*. Accra: Ghana Statistical Service, 2013.

Ayala, Turbay, and Lord Caradon. "Declaration on Population: The World Leaders Statement." *Studies in Family Planning* 1, no. 26 (1968): 1–3.

Baeta, C. G. "Aspects of Religion." In *A Study of Contemporary Ghana. Vol. 2 Some Aspects of Social Structure*, edited by W. Birmingham, I. Neustadt, and E. Omaboe, 240–50. London: George Allen & Unwin Ltd, 1967.

Bannister, David. "Public Health and Its Contexts in Northern Ghana, 1900–2000." PhD Thesis, School of Oriental and African Studies, 2017.

Barnett, Michael N. *Empire of Humanity: A History of Humanitarianism*. Ithaca: Cornell University Press, 2011.

Barnor, M. A. *A Socio-Medical Adventure in Ghana: Autobiography of Dr. M.A. Barnor*. Accra: Vieso Universal, 2001.

Barré, Louise. "Compter pour planifier : dénombrement de la population et « capitalisme d'État » en Côte d'Ivoire (1954–1967)." *Politique africaine* 145, no. 1 (July 27, 2017): 109–28.

Barros, Juanita De. *Reproducing the British Caribbean: Sex, Gender, and Population Politics After Slavery*. Chapel Hill: UNC Press Books, 2014.

Bashford, Alison. "Bioscapes: Gendering the Global History of Medicine." *Bulletin of the History of Medicine* 89, no. 4 (December 28, 2015): 690–95.

Bashford, Alison. "Global Biopolitics and the History of World Health." *History of the Human Sciences* 19, no. 1 (2006): 67–88.

Bashford, Alison. *Global Population: History, Geopolitics, and Life on Earth*. New York: Columbia University Press, 2014.

Baughan, Emily. *Saving the Children: Humanitarianism, Internationalism, and Empire*. Berkeley Series in British Studies 19. Oakland: University of California Press, 2022.

Bell, Heather. "Midwifery Training and Female Circumcision in the Inter-War Anglo-Egyptian Sudan." *Journal of African History* 39 (1998): 293–312.

Berger, Iris. *Women in Twentieth Century Africa*. Cambridge: Cambridge University Press, 2016.

Berry, Sara. "Unsettled Accounts: Stool Debts, Chieftaincy Disputes and the Question of Asante Constitutionalism." *Journal of African History* 39, no. 1 (1998): 39–62.

Biney, Ama. *The Political and Social Thought of Kwame Nkrumah*. New York: Palgrave Macmillan, 2011.

Bledsoe, Caroline H., and Fatoumatta Banja. *Contingent Lives: Fertility, Time, and Aging in West Africa*. Chicago: University of Chicago Press, 2002.

Bleek, Wolf. "Family and Family Planning in Southern Ghana." In *Sex Roles, Population and Development in West Africa: Policy-Related Studies on Work and Demographic Issues*, edited by Christine Oppong, 138–53. Portsmouth: Heinemann, 1987.

Boahen, Adu. "Towards a New Catgorization and Periodization of African Reactions of Responses to Colonialism." In *Africa in the Twentieth Century: The Adu Boahen Reader*, edited by A. Adu Boahen, and Toyin Falola, 342–54. Trenton: Africa World Press, 2004.

Boahen, Adu, and Toyin Falola, eds. *Africa in the Twentieth Century: The Adu Boahen Reader*. Trenton: Africa World Press, 2004.

Boddy, Janice. *Civilizing Women: British Crusades in Colonial Sudan*. Princeton: Princeton University Press, 2007.

Borowy, Iris. *Coming to Terms with World Health: The League of Nations Health Organisation 1921–1946*. Frankfurt am Main: Lang, 2009.

Boserup, Ester. *Woman's Role in Economic Development*. London: George Allen & Unwin Ltd, 1970.

Bourbonnais, Nicole C. *Birth Control in the Decolonizing Caribbean: Reproductive Politics and Practice on Four Islands, 1930–1970*. Cambridge: Cambridge University Press, 2016.

Bourbonnais, Nicole C. "Population Control, Family Planning, and Maternal Health Networks in the 1960s/70s: Diary of an International Consultant." *Bulletin of the History of Medicine* 93, no. 3 (2019): 335–64.

Bourmaud, Philippe. "Internationalizing Perspectives: Re-Reading Mandate History through a Health Policy Lens." *Canadian Bulletin of Medical History* 30, no. 2 (2013): 9–21.

Briggs, Laura. *Reproducing Empire: Race, Sex, Science and U.S. Imperialism in Puerto Rico*. Berkeley: University of California Press, 2003.

"British Empire Red Cross Conference." *British Medical Journal* 1, no. 3620 (May 24, 1930a): 968.
"British Empire Red Cross Conference." *The Lancet* 215, no. 5568 (May 17, 1930b): 1083.
Brobbey, S. A. "Report of the Commission of Inquiry into the Creation of New Regions." Accra: Commission of Inquiry into the Creation of New Regions, June 26, 2018.
Caldwell, J. C. "Africa." In *Family Planning and Population Programs: A Review of World Developments*, edited by Bernard Berelson, 163–80. Chicago: University of Chicago Press, 1966.
Caldwell, J. C. "Family Formation and Limitation in Ghana: A Study of the Residents of Economically Superior Urban Areas." In *Family Planning and Population Programs: A Review of World Developments*, edited by Bernard Berelson, 595–613. Chicago: University of Chicago Press, 1966.
Caldwell, J. C. "Population: General Characteristics." In *A Study of Contemporary Ghana. Vol. 2 Some Aspects of Social Structure*, edited by W. Birmingham, I. Neustadt, and E. Omaboe, 17–75. London: George Allen & Unwin Ltd, 1967.
Caldwell, J. C. "Population Change." In *A Study of Contemporary Ghana. Vol. 2 Some Aspects of Social Structure*, edited by W. Birmingham, I. Neustadt, and E. Omaboe, 78–110. London: George Allen & Unwin Ltd., 1967.
Caldwell, J. C. *Population Growth and Family Change in Africa*. London: C. Hurst & Co., 1968.
Caldwell, J. C. "Population Prospects and Policy." In *A Study of Contemporary Ghana. Vol. 2 Some Aspects of Social Structure*, edited by W. Birmingham, I. Neustadt, and E. Omaboe, 147–200. London: George Allen & Unwin Ltd., 1967.
Caldwell, J. C. "The Social Repercussions of Colonial Rule: Demographic Aspects." In *UNESCO General History of Africa, Vol. VII, Abridged Edition: Africa Under Colonial Domination 1880–1935*, edited by Adu Boahen, 200–208. Berkeley: University of California Press, 1990.
Callaci, Emily. "'Injectable Development' Depo-Provera and Creation of the Global South." *Radical History Review* 2018, no. 131 (May 1, 2018): 82–104.
Cammaert, Jessica. *Undesirable Practices: Women, Children, and the Politics of the Body in Northern Ghana, 1930–1972*. Lincoln: University of Nebraska Press, 2016.
Canning, Kathleen. "The Body as Method? Reflections on the Place of the Body in Gender History." *Gender & History* 11, no. 3 (1999): 499–513.
Cardinall, A. W. *The Gold Coast, 1931*. Accra: Government Printer, 1933.
Chorev, Nitsan. *World Health Organization Between North and South*. Ithaca: Cornell University Press, 2012.
Coghe, Samuël. *Population Politics in the Tropics: Demography, Health and Transimperialism in Colonial Angola*. Cambridge: Cambridge University Press, 2022.
Comaroff, Jean, and John Comaroff. "Homemade Hegemony: Modernity, Domesticity, and Colonialism in South Africa." In *African Encounters with Domesticity*, edited by Karen Tranberg Hansen, 31–74. New Brunswick: Rutgers University Press, 1992.
Connelly, Matthew. *Fatal Misconception*. Cambridge: Harvard University Press, 2009.
Cooper, Frederick. *Africa Since 1940: The Past of the Present*. Cambridge: Cambridge University Press, 2002.
Cooper, Frederick. *Decolonization and African Society: The Labor Question in French and British Africa*. Cambridge: Cambridge University Press, 2008.
Cooper, Frederick. "Modernizing Bureaucrats, Backward Africans, and the Development Concept." In *International Development and the Social Sciences: Essays on the History*

and Politics of Knowledge, edited by Frederick Cooper, and Randall Packard, 64–92. Berkeley: University of California Press, 1998.

Cooper, Frederick, and Randall Packard. "Introduction." In *International Development and the Social Sciences: Essays on the History and Politics of Knowledge*, edited by Frederick Cooper, and Randall Packard, 1–44. Berkeley: University of California Press, 1998.

Cordell, Dennis D., Joel W. Gregory, and Victor Piché. "African Historical Demography: The Search for a Theoretical Framework." In *African Population and Capitalism: Historical Perspectives*, edited by Dennis D. Cordell, Joel W. Gregory, and Victor Piché, 14–32. Madison: University of Wisconsin Press, 1994.

Danquah, Francis K. "Sustaining a West African Cocoa Economy: Agricultural Science and the Swollen Shoot Contagion in Ghana, 1936–1965." *African Economic History* 31, no. 1 (2003): 43–74.

Dolphyne, Florence Abena. *The Emancipation of Women: An African Perspective*. Accra: Ghana Universities Press, 1991.

Dornemann, Maria. "Seeing Population as a Problem: Influences on the Construction of Population Knowledge on Kenyan Politics (1940s–1980s)." In *A World of Populations: Transnational Perspectives on Demography in the Twentieth Century*, edited by Heinrich Hartmann, and Corinna R. Unger, 201–51. New York: Berghahn Books, 2014.

Doyle, Shane. *Crisis & Decline in Bunyoro: Population & Environment in Western Uganda 1860–1955*. Oxford: James Currey, 2006.

Doyle, Shane. "Demography and Disease." In *The Oxford Handbook of Modern African History*, edited by John Parker, and Richard Reid, 38–55. Oxford: Oxford University Press, 2013.

Doyle, Shane. "Maternal Health, Epidemiology and Transition Theory in Africa." In *Epidemiological Change and Chronic Disease in Sub-Saharan Africa: Social and Historical Perspectives*, edited by Megan Vaughan, Kafui Adjaye-Gbewonyo, and Marissa Mika, 106–32. London: UCL Press, 2021.

Drenth, Annemieke van, and Francisca de Haan. *The Rise of Caring Power: Elizabeth Fry and Josephine Butler in Britain and the Netherlands*. Amsterdam: Amsterdam University Press, 1999.

Durojaye, Ebenezer, Gladys Mirugi-Mukundi, and C. G. Ngwena, eds. *Advancing Sexual and Reproductive Health and Rights in Africa: Constraints and Opportunities, Routledge Contemporary Africa*. New York: Routledge, 2021.

Dzorgbo, Dan-Bright S. *Ghana in Search of Development: The Challenge of Governance, Economic Management and Institution Building*. The Making of Modern Africa.Aldershot: Ashgate, 2001.

Engmann, E. V. T. *Population of Ghana, 1850–1960*. Accra: Published for the University of Cape Coast by Ghana Universities Press, 1986.

Escobar, Arturo. *Encountering Development: The Making and Unmaking of the Third World*. Princeton: Princeton University Press, 1995.

Esseks, J D. "Economic Policies." In *Politicians and Soldiers in Ghana, 1966–1972*, edited by Dennis Austin, and Robin Luckham, 37–61. London: Frank Cass and Co. Ltd., 1975.

Feierman, Steven, and John M. Janzen. "Introduction." In *The Social Basis of Health and Healing in Africa*, edited by Steven Feierman, and John M. Janzen, 1–23. 30. Berkeley: University of California Press, 2009.

Feierman, Steven, and John M. Janzen, eds. *The Social Basis of Health and Healing in Africa*. Berkeley: University of California Press, 2009.

Ferguson, James. *Expectations of Modernity: Myths and Meanings of Urban Life on the Zambian Copperbelt*. Berkeley: University of California Press, 1999.

Ferguson, James. *The Anti-Politics Machine: Development, Depoliticization and Bureaucratic Power in Lesotho*, New edition. Minneapolis: University of Minnesota Press, 1994.

Field, M. J. *Religion and Medicine of the Ga People*. Oxford: Oxford University Press, 1961.

Field, M. J. *Search for Security: An Ethno-Psychiatric Study of Rural Ghana*. London: Faber and Faber, 1960.

Fonn, Sharon, and Tk Sundari Ravindran. "The Macroeconomic Environment and Sexual and Reproductive Health: A Review of Trends over the Last 30 Years." *Reproductive Health Matters* 19, no. 38 (2011): 11–25.

Frankema, Ewout, and Morten Jerven. "Writing History Backwards or Sideways: Towards a Consensus on African Population, 1850–2010." *The Economic History Review* 67, no. 4 (2014): 907–31.

Frey, Marc. "Neo-Malthusianism and Development: Shifting Interpretations of a Contested Paradigm." *Journal of Global History* 6, no. 1 (2011): 75–97.

Geest, Sjaak van der, and Kristine Krause. "Introduction: Studying Health and Health Care in Ghana." *Ghana Studies* 15, no. 16 (2013/2012): 7–40.

Ginsburg, Faye, and Rayna Rapp. "Introduction: Conceiving the New World Order." In *Conceiving the New World Order: The Global Politics of Reproduction*, edited by Faye D. Ginsburg, and Rayna Rapp, 1–18. Berkeley: University of California Press, 1995.

Gocking, Roger. *The History of Ghana*. Westport: Greenwood Press, 2005.

Gorsky, Martin. 'Public Health in Interwar England and Wales: Did it Fail?', *Dynamis* 28 (2008): 175–98.

Gorsky, M., and C. Sirrs. "The Rise and Fall of 'Universal Health Coverage'; as a Goal of International Health Politics, 1925–1952." *American Journal of Public Health* 108, no. 3 (January 18, 2018): e1–9.

Grischow, Jeff D. "Kwame Nkrumah, Disability, and Rehabilitation in Ghana, 1957–66." *The Journal of African History* 52, no. 2 (2011): 179–99.

Grischow, Jeff D. *Shaping Tradition: Civil Society, Community and Development in Colonial Northern Ghana, 1899–1957*. Leiden: Brill, 2006.

Grischow, Jeff, and Glenn H. McKnight. "Rhyming Development: Practising Post-Development in Colonial Ghana and Uganda." *Journal of Historical Sociology* 16, no. 4 (December 1, 2003): 517–49.

Grischow, Jeff, and Holger Weiss. "Pan-Africanism, Socialism and the Future: Development Planning in Ghana, 1951–66." In *The Struggle for the Long-Term in Transnational Science and Politics: Forging the Future*, edited by Jenny Andersson, and Eglė Rindzevičiūtė. Routledge Approaches to History 11, 218–240. New York: Routledge, Taylor & Francis Group, 2015.

Gros, Jean-Germain. *Healthcare Policy in Africa: Institutions and Politics from Colonialism to the Present*. Lanham: Rowman & Littlefield Publishers, 2015.

Gupta, Monica Das. "Kinship Systems and Demographic Regimes." In *Anthropological Demography: Toward a New Synthesis*, edited by David I. Kertzer, and Thomas E. Fricke, 36–52. Population and Development Conference on Anthropological Demography. Chicago: University of Chicago Press, 1997.

Gyimah, Stephen Obeng, Jones K. Adjei, and Baffour Kwaku Takyi. "Religion, Contraception, and Method Choice of Married Women in Ghana." *Journal of Religion and Health* 51 (2011): 1359–74.

Hart, Jennifer A. *Ghana on the Go: African Mobility in the Age of Motor Transportation*. Indianapolis: Indiana University Press, 2016.

Hilevych, Yuliya, and Chizu Sato. "Popular Medical Discourses on Birth Control in the Soviet Union during the Cold War: Shifting Responsibilities and Relational Values." In *Children by Choice?: Changing Values, Reproduction, and Family Planning in the 20th Century*, edited by Ann-Katrin Gembries, Theresia Theuke, and Isabel Heinemann, 99–122. Boston: Walter de Gruyter, 2018.

Hillbom, E. "African Demographics: How Many People Are Too Many People?" In *The History of African Development: An Online Textbook for a New Generation of African Students and Teachers*, edited by E. Hillbom, E. Frankema, U. Kufakurinani, and F. Selhausen. African Economic History Network E-book, 2018.

Hodge, Joseph M., and Gerald Hodl. "Introduction." In *Developing Africa: Concepts and Practices in Twentieth-Century Colonialism*, edited by Joseph M. Hodge, Gerald Hodl, and Martina Kopf, 1–34. Manchester: Manchester University Press, 2014.

Hodge, Joseph M. *Triumph of the Expert: Agrarian Doctrines of Development and the Legacies of British Colonialism*. Athens: Ohio University Press, 2007.

Holmes, David. "Fred Sai: The Godfather of Family Planning." *The Lancet* 380, no. 9855 (November 17, 2012): 1731.

Huber, Valeska. "Introduction: Global Histories of Social Planning." *Journal of Contemporary History* 52, no. 1 (January 1, 2017): 3–15.

Hugon, Anne. *Être mère en situation coloniale: Gold Coast, 1910–1950*. Paris: Éditions de la Sorbonne, 2020.

Hugon, Anne. "Korle Bu and the Midwives Hostel as a Site of Memory for Ghanaian Pupil Midwives, 1930s–1950s." *Ghana Studies* 7 (2004): 43–58.

Hugon, Anne. "La Redéfinition de La maternité en gold coast, des années 1920 aux années 1950: projet colonial et réalités locales." In *Histoire Des Femmes En Situation Coloniale Afrique et Asie, XXe Siècle*, edited by Anne Hugon, 145–172. Paris: Editions Karthala, 2004.

Hunt, Nancy Rose. *A Colonial Lexicon: Of Birth Ritual, Medicalization, and Mobility in the Congo*. Durham: Duke University Press, 1999.

Hunt, Nancy Rose. *A Nervous State: Violence, Remedies, and Reverie in Colonial Congo*. Durham: Duke University Press, 2016.

Hunt, Nancy Rose. "Health and Healing." In *The Oxford Handbook of Modern African History*, edited by John Parker, and Richard Reid, 378–395. Oxford: Oxford University Press, 2013.

Hunt, Nancy Rose. "'Le Bébé En Brousse': European Women, African Birth Spacing, and Colonial Intervention in Breast Feeding in the Belgian Congo." In *Tensions of Empire: Colonial Cultures in a Bourgeois World*, edited by Frederick Cooper, and Ann Laura Stoler, 287–321. Berkeley: University of California Press, 1997.

Hunt, Nancy Rose. "Placing African Women's History and Locating Gender." *Social History* 14, no. 3 (1989): 359–79.

Hurd, G. E. "Education." In *A Study of Contemporary Ghana. Vol. 2 Some Aspects of Social Structure*, edited by W. Birmingham, I. Neustadt, and E. Omaboe, 217–39. London: George Allen & Unwin Ltd., 1967.

Huston, Perdita. *Motherhood by Choice: Pioneers in Women's Health and Family Planning*. New York: Feminist Press at CUNY, 1992.

Hutchinson, John F. *Champions of Charity: War and the Rise of the Red Cross*. Boulder: Westview Press, 1996.

Hyndman, Jennifer, and Malathi de Alwis. "Beyond Gender: Towards a Feminist Analysis of Humanitarianism and Development in Sri Lanka." *Women's Studies Quarterly* 31, no. 3/4 (2003): 212–26.
Iliffe, John. *Africans: The History of a Continent*, 2nd edition. Cambridge: Cambridge University Press, 2007.
Iliffe, John. *The African AIDS Epidemic: A History*. Athens, OH: James Currey, 2006.
Immerwahr, Daniel. *Thinking Small: The United States and the Lure of Community Development*. Cambridge: Harvard University Press, 2014.
Ittmann, Karl. "Demography as Policy Science in the British Empire, 1918–1969." *Journal of Policy History* 15, no. 4 (2003): 417–48.
Ittmann, Karl. *Problem of Great Importance*. Berkeley: University of California Press, 2013.
Jerven, Morten. "A West African Experiment: Constructing a GDP Series for Colonial Ghana, 1891–1950." *The Economic History Review* 67, no. 4 (November 1, 2014): 964–992.
Johnson, Jennifer. "The Origins of Family Planning in Tunisia: Reform, Public Health, and International Aid." *Bulletin of the History of Medicine* 92, no. 4 (2018): 664–93.
Johnson-Hanks, J. "Éducation, ethnicité et pratiques reproductives au Cameroun." *Population* 58, no. 2 (2003): 171–200.
Jones, Margaret. "Infant and Maternal Health Services in Ceylon, 1900–1948: Imperialism or Welfare?" *Social History of Medicine* 15, no. 2 (2002): 263–89.
Kaler, Amy. "'Who Has Told You to Do This Thing?' Toward a Feminist Interpretation of Contraceptive Diffusion in Rhodesia, 1970–1980." *Signs* 25, no. 3 (2000): 677–708.
Kay, Geoffrey, and Stephen Hymer, eds. *The Political Economy of Colonialism in Ghana: A Collection of Documents and Statistics, 1900–1960*. Cambridge: Cambridge University Press, 1972.
Kendall, Diana Elizabeth. *The Power of Good Deeds: Privileged Women and the Social Reproduction of the Upper Class*. Rowman & Littlefield, 2002.
Khan, Shahrukh Rafi. *A History of Development Economics Thought: Challenges and Counter-Challenges*. New York: Routledge, 2014.
Klancher Merchant, Emily. *Building the Population Bomb*. Oxford: Oxford University Press, 2021.
Klausen, Susanne. *Race, Maternity and the Politics of Birth Control in South Africa, 1910–1939*. New York: Palgrave Macmillan, 2004.
Kobo, Ousman. "'We Are Citizens Too': The Politics of Citizenship in Independent Ghana." *The Journal of Modern African Studies* 48, no. 1 (March 2010): 67–94.
Kuczynski, R. R. *Demographic Survey of the British Colonial Empire. Vol. 1 West Africa*. London: Oxford University Press, 1948.
Kyei, T. E. *Our Days Dwindle: Memories of My Childhood Days in Asante*. Edited by Jean Marie Allman. Portsmouth: Heinemann, 2001.
Kyei, T. E. *Marriage and Divorce among the Asante: A Study Undertaken in the Course of the Ashanti Social Survey (1945)*. Cambridge African Monographs, no. 14. Cambridge: African Studies Centre, 1992.
Lambert, Keri. "'It's All Work and Happiness on The Farms': Agricultural Development between the Blocs in Nkrumah's Ghana." *The Journal of African History* 60, no. 1 (March 2019): 25–44.
Lamptey, Peter, Fred Wurapa, and David Nicholas. "The Evolution of a Primary Health Care Programme: The Danfa Experience 1970–1977." *Journal of Tropical Pediatrics* 30 (1984): 252–56.

Lee, Sung. "WHO and the Developing World: The Contest for Ideology." In *Western Medicine as Contested Knowledge*, edited by Andrew Cunningham, and Bridie Andrews, 24–45. Manchester: Manchester University Press, 1997.

Lewis, Joanna. *Empire State-Building: War & Welfare in Kenya, 1925–52*. Athens, OH: Ohio State University Press, 2000.

Lindner, Ulrike. "The Transfer of European Social Policy Concepts to Tropical Africa, 1900–50: The Example of Maternal and Child Welfare." *Journal of Global History* 9, no. 2 (July 2014): 208–31.

Lindsay, Jennie. "The Politics of Population Control in Namibia." *Review of African Political Economy*, no. 36 (1986): 58–62.

Lugard, Frederick John Dealtry. *The Dual Mandate in British Tropical Africa*. London: W. Blackwood and Sons, 1922.

Malthus, Thomas Robert. *An Essay on the Principle of Population as it Affects the Future Improvement of Society with Remarks on the Speculations of Mr. Godwin, M. Condorcet and Other Writers*. London: J. Johnson, 1798.

Mamdani, Mahmood. *The Myth of Population Control: Family, Caste and Class in and Indian Village*. New York: Monthly Review Press, n.d.

Mann, Gregory. *From Empires to NGOs in the West African Sahel: The Road to Nongovernmentality*. Cambridge: Cambridge University Press, 2014.

Manton, John, and Martin Gorsky. "Health Planning in 1960s Africa: International Health Organisations and the Post-Colonial State." *Medical History* 62, no. 4 (October 2018): 425–48.

Manuh, Takyiwaa. "Building Institutions for the New Africa: The Institute of African Studies at the University of Ghana." In *Modernization as Spectacle in Africa*, edited by Peter J Bloom, Stephan Miescher, and Takyiwaa Manuh, 268–84. Bloomington: Indiana University Press, 2014.

Manuh, Takyiwaa. "Ghana: Women in the Public and Informal Sectors under the Economic Recovery Programme." In *Mortgaging Women's Lives: Feminist Critiques of Structural Adjustment*, edited by Pamela Sparr, 61–76. London: Palgrave Macmillan, 1994.

Manuh, Takyiwaa. "Women and Their Organizations during the Convention People's Party Period." In *The Ghana Reader*, edited by Kwasi Konadu, and Clifford C. Campbell, 285–91. Durham: Duke University Press, 2016.

Marshall, Dominique. "Children's Rights in Imperial Political Cultures: Missionary and Humanitarian Contributions to the Conference on the African Child of 1931." *The International Journal of Children's Rights* 12, no. 3 (2004): 273–318.

Martínez, Samuel, and Kathryn Libal. "Introduction: The Gender of Humanitarian Narrative." *Humanity: An International Journal of Human Rights, Humanitarianism, and Development* 2, no. 2 (September 8, 2011): 161–70.

Mbacké, Cheikh. "The Persistence of High Fertility in Sub-Saharan Africa: A Comment." *Population and Development Review* 43, no. 1 (2017): 330–37.

Mbacke, Cheikh, and National Research Council. "Family Planning Programs and Fertility Transition in Sub-Saharan Africa." *Population and Development Review* 20, no. 1 (March 1994): 188.

McCarthy, Helen. "Service Clubs, Citizenship and Equality: Gender Relations and Middle-Class Associations in Britain between the Wars." *Historical Research* 81, no. 213 (2008): 531–52.

McCaskie, T. C. "Anti-Witchcraft Cults in Asante: An Essay in the Social History of an African People." *History in Africa* 8 (1981): 125–54.

McClintock, Anne. "'No Longer in a Future Heaven': Women and Nationalism in South Africa." *Transition* 51 (1991): 104–23.
Miescher, Stephan. *Making Men in Ghana*. Indianapolis: Indiana University Press, 2005.
Miescher, Stephan. "'Nkrumah's Baby': The Akosombo Dam and the Dream of Development in Ghana, 1952–1966." *Water History* 6, no. 4 (2014): 341–66.
Mikell, Gwendolyn. "Please for Domestic Relief: Akan Women and Family Courts." In *African Feminism*, edited by Gwendolyn Mikell, 96–140. Philadelphia: University of Pennsylvania Press, 1997.
Mohanty, Chandra Talpade. "Introduction." In *Third World Women and the Politics of Feminism*, edited by Chandra Talpade Mohanty, Ann Russo, and Lourdes Torres, 1–49. Bloomington: Indiana University Press, 1991.
Murillo, Bianca. *Market Encounters: Consumer Cultures in Twentieth-Century Ghana, New African Histories*. Athens: Ohio University Press, 2017.
Population Impact Project. *National Conference on Population and National Reconstruction. April 7–10, 1986. Vol. II: Contributed Papers*. Legon: University of Ghana, 1987.
Newell, Stephanie. *Literary Culture in Colonial Ghana: "How to Play the Game of Life"*. Manchester: Manchester University Press, 2002.
Newell, Stephanie, and Audrey Gadzekpo, eds. *Selected Writings of a Pioneer West African Feminist*. Nottingham: Trent Editions, 2004.
Nguyen, Vin-Kim. *The Republic of Therapy: Triage and Sovereignty in West Africa's Time of AIDS*. Durham: Duke University Press, 2010.
Nott, John Daniel. "Between Famine and Malnutrition: Spatial Aspects of Nutritional Health during Ghana's Long Twentieth Century, c. 1896–2000." PhD Thesis, University of Leeds, 2016.
Nott, John Daniel. "'No one may starve in the British Empire': Kwashiorkor, Protein and the Politics of Nutrition between Britain and Africa." *Social History of Medicine* 34, no. 2 (2021): 553–76.
Nkrumah, Kwame. *The Autobiography of Kwame Nkrumah*. London: T. Nelson, 1957.
Nsarkoh, J. K. *Local Government in Ghana*. Accra: Ghana Universities Press, 1964.
Nugent, Paul. *Africa since Independence*. Basingstoke: Palgrave Macmillan, 2012.
Ofori-Atta, Susan B. G. "Nutritional Deficiencies and Maternal and Child Health in Africa." *Journal of the National Medical Association* 52, no. 1 (January 1960): 41–46.
Omaboe, E. "An Introductory Survey." In *A Study of Contemporary Ghana*, edited by W. Birmingham, I. Neustadt, and E. Omaboe, 1 The Economy of Ghana, 17–33. London: George Allen & Unwin Ltd, 1967.
Opong, Adwoa. "Rewriting Women into Ghanaian History 1950–1966." MPhil thesis, University of Ghana 2012.
Oppong, Christine. "Notes on Cultural Aspects of Menstruation in Ghana," World Health Organization Task Force on Acceptability of Fertility Regulating, Geneva, April 1974, 33–38.
Oppong, Christine. "Responsible Fatherhood and Birth Planning." In *Sex Roles, Population and Development in West Africa: Policy-Related Studies on Work and Demographic Issues*, edited by Christine Oppong, and World Employment Programme, 165–78. Portsmouth: Heinemann, 1987.
Oppong, Christine. *Seven Roles of Women: Impact of Education, Migration and Employment on Ghanaian Mothers*. Geneva: International Labour Office, 1987.
Oppong, Christine, Christine Okali, and Beverley Houghton. "Woman Power: Retrograde Steps in Ghana." *African Studies Review* 18, no. 3 (1975): 71–84.

Osei, Robert Darko, and Remi Jedwab. "Structural Change in Ghana, 1960–2010." *Country Case Studies Workshop Structural Change in Developing Countries*. World Bank, 2012.

Osseo-Asare, Abena Dove. "Writing Medical Authority: The Rise of Literate Healers in Ghana, 1930–70." *The Journal of African History* 57, no. 1 (March 2016): 69–91.

Packard, Randall. *A History of Global Health: Interventions into the Lives of Other Peoples*. Baltimore: Johns Hopkins University Press, 2016.

Paice, Edward. *Youthquake Why African Demography Should Matter to the World*. London: Head of Zeus, 2021.

Pala, Achola O. "Definitions of Women and Development: An African Perspective." In *African Gender Studies a Reader*, edited by Oyèrónkẹ́ Oyěwùmí, 299–311. New York: Palgrave Macmillan US, 2005.

Patterson, K. David. *Health in Colonial Ghana: Disease, Medicine, and Socio-Economic Change, 1900–1955*. Waltham: Crossroads Press, 1981.

Patton, Adell. *Physicians, Colonial Racism, and Diaspora in West Africa*. Gainesville: University Press of Florida, 1996.

Pedersen, Susan. *The Guardians: The League of Nations and the Crisis of Empire*. Oxford: Oxford University Press, 2015.

Pedersen, Susan. "The Maternalist Moment in British Colonial Policy: The Controversy over 'Child Slavery' in Hong Kong 1917–1941." *Past & Present* 171, no. 1 (2001): 161–202.

Pigg, Stacy Leigh. "Authority in Translation: Finding, Knowing, Naming and Training 'Traditional Birth Attendants' in Nepal." In *Childbirth and Authoritative Knowledge: Cross-Cultural Perspectives*, edited by Robbie E. Davis-Floyd, Carolyn F. Sargent, and Rayna Rapp, 233–62. Berkeley: University of California Press, 1997.

Pigg, Stacy Leigh. "'Found in Most Traditional Societies' Traditional Medical Practitioners between Culture and Development." In *International Development and the Social Science: Essays on the History of Politics of Knowledge*, edited by Frederick Cooper and Randall Packard, 259–90. Berkeley: University of California Press, 1998.

Plageman, Nate. *Highlife Saturday Night: Popular Music and Social Change in Urban Ghana*. Indianapolis: Indiana University Press, 2013.

Pobee, John S. *The Anglican Story in Ghana: From Mission Beginnings to Province of Ghana*. Accra: Amanza Ltd., 2009.

Prince, Ruth J. "Situating Health and the Public in Africa: Historical and Anthropological Perspectives." In *Making and Unmaking Public Health in Africa: Ethnographic and Historical Perspectives*, edited by Ruth J. Prince, and Rebecca Marsland, 1 edition, 1–51. Athens, OH: Ohio University Press, 2013.

Putnam, Lara. "Global Child-Saving, Transatlantic Maternalism, and the Pathologization of Caribbean Childhood, 1930s–1940s." *Atlantic Studies* 11, no. 4 (2014): 491–514.

Ranchod-Nilsson, Sita. "(Gender) Struggles for the Nation." In *Women, States and Nationalism: At Home in the Nation?* edited by Mary Ann Tetreault, and Sita Ranchod-Nilsson, 168–85. London: Routledge, 2003.

Rathbone, Richard. *Nkrumah and the Chiefs: Politics of Chieftaincy in Ghana 1951–1960*, 1st edition. Oxford: James Currey, 2000.

Rathbone, Richard. "World War I and Africa: Introduction." *The Journal of African History* 19, no. 1 (1978): 1–9.

Rathgeber, Eva M. "WID, WAD, GAD: Trends in Research and Practice." *Journal of Developing Areas* 24 (1990): 489–502.

Ray, Carina. *Crossing the Color Line: Race, Sex, and the Contested Politics of Colonialism in Ghana*. Athens: Ohio University Press, 2015.

Renne, Elisha P. "Interpreting Population Policy in Nigeria." In *Reproductive States: Global Perspectives on the Invention and Implementation of Population Policy*, edited by Mie Nakachi, and Rickie Solinger, 260–289. Oxford: Oxford University Press, 2016.

Renner, Lorna A., Samuel A. Oppong, and Bamenla Q. Goka. "The Way Forward." In *Topical Issues in Maternal and Child Health in Ghana*, edited by Jennifer E. Welbeck et al., University of Ghana Readers, no. 9, 185–91. Tema, Ghana: Digibooks Ghana Ltd, 2014.

Riedi, Eliza. "Options for an Imperialist Woman: The Case of Violet Markham, 1899–1914." *Albion: A Quarterly Journal Concerned with British Studies* 32, no. 1 (2000): 59–84.

Rist, Gilbert. *The History of Development: From Western Origins to Global Faith*. Translated by Patrick Camiller. London: Zed Books Ltd, 2008.

Roberts, Jonathan. "Remembering Korle Bu Hospital: Biomedical Heritage and Colonial Nostalgia in the 'Golden Jubilee Souvenir'." *History in Africa* 38 (2011): 193–226.

Robertson, Claire C. *Sharing the Same Bowl: A Socioeconomic History of Women and Class in Accra, Ghana*. Indianapolis: Indiana University Press, 1984.

Rodney, Walter. *How Europe Underdeveloped Africa*. Pambazuka Press, 1972.

Rooney, David. *Kwame Nkrumah: The Political Kingdom in the Third World*. London: I.B. Tauris, 1988.

Rosenfield, A., and D. Maine. "Maternal Mortality–A Neglected Tragedy. Where is the M in MCH?" *Lancet* 2, no. 8446 (July 13, 1985): 83–85.

Ross, Loretta, and Rickie Solinger. *Reproductive Justice: An Introduction*. Berkeley: University of California Press, 2017.

Rossi, Benedetta. "What 'Development' Does to Work." *International Labour and Working Class History* 92 (2017): 7–23.

Russell, Beatrice A. S. "Malnutrition in Children under Three Years of Age in Ashanti, West Africa." *Archives of Disease in Childhood* 21, no. 106 (1946): 110–12.

Rusterholz, Caroline. *Women's Medicine: Sex, Family Planning and British Female Doctors in Transnational Perspective, 1920–70*. Manchester: Manchester University Press, 2020.

Sabben-Clare, E. E., David J. Bradley, and Kenneth Kirkwood, eds. *Health in Tropical Africa during the Colonial Period*. Oxford: Clarendon Press, 1980.

Sai, Frederick T. *With Heart and Voice: Fred Sai Remembers*. Cambridge: Barton, 2010.

Sarpong, Peter. *Girls Nubility Rites in Ashanti*. Accra: Ghana Publishing Co., 1977.

Scott, James C. *Seeing Like a State: How Certain Schemes to Improve the Human Condition Have Failed*. Yale Agrarian Studies. New Haven: Yale University Press, 1998.

Sen, Amartya. *Development as Freedom*. Oxford: Oxford University Press, 2001.

Senah, Kodjo. "In Sickness and in Health: Globalization and Health Care Delivery in Ghana." *Research Review* 17, no. 1 (2001): 83–89.

Serra, Gerardo. "'Hail the Census Night': Trust and Political Imagination in the 1960 Population Census of Ghana." *Comparative Studies in Society and History* 60, no. 3 (July 2018): 659–87.

Shank, David A. "Le Pentecôtisme Du Prophète William Wadé Harris." *Archives de Sciences Sociales Des Religions* 44, no. 105 (1999): 51–70.

Sharp, Evelyn. *The African Child: An Account of the International Conference on African Children, Geneva*. London: Weardale Press, 1931.

Sharp, Ingrid, and Matthew Stibbe. "Women's International Activism during the Inter-War Period, 1919–1939." *Women's History Review* 26, no. 2 (March 4, 2017): 163–72.

Sharpless, John. "Population Science, Private Foundations, and Development Aid: The Transformation of Demographic Knowledge in the United State, 1945–1965." In *International Development and the Social Sciences: Essays on the History and Politics of Knowledge*, edited by Randall Packard, and Frederick Cooper, 176–202. Berkeley: University of California Press, 1998.

Siddiqi, Javed. *World Health and World Politics: The World Health Organization and the UN System*. London: Hurst, 1995.

Sidze, Estelle M., Martin K. Mutua, and Hermann P. Donfouet. "Towards Achieving Equity in Utilisation of Maternal Health Services in Selected Sub-Saharan African Countries: Progress and Remaining Challenges in Priority Countries." In *Women and Sustainable Human Development: Empowering Women in Africa*, edited by Maty Konte, and Nyasha Tirivayi, 111–24. Gender, Development and Social Change. Cham: Springer International Publishing, 2020.

Skinner, Kate. "Gendering Citizenship and Decolonizing Justice in 1960s Ghana: Revisiting the Struggle for Family Law Reform." *American Journal of Legal History* 60, no. 3 (September 1, 2020): 357–87.

Skinner, Kate. "'It Brought Some Kind of Neatness to Mankind': Mass Literacy, Community Development and Democracy in 1950s Asante." *Africa* 79, no. 4 (2009): 479–99.

Skinner, Kate, and Peter J. Bloom. "Modernity and Danger: *The Boy Kumasenu* and the Work of the Gold Coast Film Unit." *Ghana Studies* 12, no. 13 (2009): 121–54.

Skinner, Rob, and Alan Lester. "Humanitarianism and Empire: New Research Agendas." *The Journal of Imperial and Commonwealth History* 40, no. 5 (December 1, 2012): 729–47.

Spear, Thomas. "Neo-Traditionalism and the Limits of Invention in British Colonial Africa." *The Journal of African History* 44, no. 1 (March 2003): 3–27.

Staples, Amy L. S. *The Birth of Development: How the World Bank, Food and Agriculture Organization, and World Health Organization Have Changed the World 1945–1965*. Kent: Kent State University Press, 2006.

Stoler, Ann Laura. *Along the Archival Grain: Epistemic Anxieties and Colonial Common Sense*. Princeton: Princeton University Press, 2010.

Summers, Carol. "Intimate Colonialism: The Imperial Production of Reproduction in Uganda, 1907–1925." *Signs* 16, no. 4 (1991): 787–807.

Sundby, Johanne. "Infertility and Health Care in Countries with Less Resources." In *Infertility Around the Globe: New Thinking on Childlessness, Gender, and Reproductive Technologies*, edited by Marcia Claire Inhorn, and Frank van Balen, 247–59. Berkeley: University of California Press, 2002.

Szreter, Simon. "The Idea of Demographic Transition and the Study of Fertility Change: A Critical Intellectual History." *Population and Development Review* 19, no. 4 (December 1993): 659–701.

Tamale, Sylvia. "Ob/Gyn Experiences - Life Stories." In *African Sexualities: A Reader*, edited by Sylvia Tamale, 376–86. Capetown: Pambazuka Press, 2011.

Tetteh, P. A. "Marriage, Family and Household." In *A Study of Contemporary Ghana. Vol. 2 Some Aspects of Social Structure*, edited by W. Birmingham, I. Neustadt, and E. Omaboe, 201–16. London: George Allen & Unwin Ltd., 1967.

The Measure Project and Ghana AIDS Commission. *AIDS in Africa during the Nineties: Ghana. A Review and Analysis of Survey and Research Results*. Chapel Hill: University of North Carolina, 2003.

Thomas, Lynn M. *Politics of the Womb: Women, Reproduction, and the State in Kenya*. Berkeley: University of California Press, 2003.

Tignor, Robert L. W. *Arthur Lewis and the Birth of Development Economics*. Princeton: Princeton University Press, 2005.

Tsikata, Edzodzinam. "Women's Political Organisations, 1951–1987." In *State, Development and Politics in Ghana*, edited by Emmanuel Hansen, and Kwame A. Ninsin, 73–93. London: CODESRIA Book Series, 1989.

Twumasi, Patrick, and Dennis Michael Warren. "The Professionalisation of Indigenous Medicine: A Comparative Study of Ghana and Zambia." In *The Professionalisation of African Medicine*, edited by Murray Last, and G. L. Chavunduka, 117–136. African Seminars: Scholarship from the International African Institute. Manchester: Manchester University Press, 1986.

Twumasi, Patrick. "Ashanti Traditional Medicine." *Transition* 41 (1972): 50–63.

Twumasi, Patrick. "History of Pluralistic Medical Systems: A Sociological Analysis of the Ghanaian Case." *Issue: A Journal of Opinion* 9, no. 3 (1979): 29–34.

Twumasi, Patrick. *Medical Systems in Ghana: A Study in Medical Sociology*. Tema: Ghana Publishing Corporation, 1975.

Vaughan, Megan. *Curing Their Ills: Colonial Power and African Illness*, 1st edition. Cambridge: Polity, 1991.

Walters, Sarah. "African Population History: Contributions of Moral Demography." *The Journal of African History* 62, no. 2 (July 2021): 183–200.

Walters, Sarah. "'Child! Now You Are': Identity Registration, Labor, and the Definition of Childhood in Colonial Tanganyika, 1910–1950." *The Journal of the History of Childhood and Youth* 9, no. 1 (March 1, 2016a): 66–86.

Walters, Sarah. "Counting Souls: Towards an Historical Demography of Africa." *Demographic Research* 34 (January 15, 2016b): 63–108.

Warren, Dennis Michael, and Sr. Mary Ann Tregoning. "Indigenous Healers and Primary Health Care in Ghana." *Medical Anthropology Newsletter* 11, no. 1 (November 1979): 11–13.

White, Luise. *Speaking with Vampires: Rumor and History in Colonial Africa*. Berkeley: University of California Press, 2000.

Wiemers, Alice. *Village Work: Development and Rural Statecraft in Twentieth-Century Ghana*. Ohio: Ohio University Press, 2021.

Yuval-Davis, Nira. *Gender & Nation*. London: Sage Publications, 1997.

Index

For Product Safety Concerns and Information please contact our EU representative GPSR@taylorandfrancis.com
Taylor & Francis Verlag GmbH, Kaufingerstraße 24, 80331 München, Germany

www.ingramcontent.com/pod-product-compliance
Ingram Content Group UK Ltd.
Pitfield, Milton Keynes, MK11 3LW, UK
UKHW020142200926
475702UK00005B/877
9781032227849